Oxford Textbook of

Anaesthesia for Oral and Maxillofacial Surgery

Oxford Textbook of

Anaesthesia for Oral and Maxillofacial Surgery

SECOND EDITION

EDITED BY

Patrick A. Ward

Consultant Anaesthetist
St John's Hospital
NHS Lothian, Scotland

and

Michael G. Irwin

Daniel CK Yu Professor
Department of Anaesthesiology
University of Hong Kong, Hong Kong

OXFORD
UNIVERSITY PRESS

OXFORD
UNIVERSITY PRESS

Great Clarendon Street, Oxford, OX2 6DP,
United Kingdom

Oxford University Press is a department of the University of Oxford.
It furthers the University's objective of excellence in research, scholarship,
and education by publishing worldwide. Oxford is a registered trade mark of
Oxford University Press in the UK and in certain other countries

First Edition published in 2010
Second Edition published in 2023

Impression: 1

Published in the United States of America by Oxford University Press
198 Madison Avenue, New York, NY 10016, United States of America

British Library Cataloguing in Publication Data
Data available

Library of Congress Control Number: 2022942555

ISBN 978–0–19–879072–3

DOI: 10.1093/med/9780198790723.001.0001

Printed in the UK by
Bell & Bain Ltd., Glasgow

Melissa, Florence, and Freddy Ward.
May, Ross, Kyle, Alice, Olivia, and Rachel Irwin.

Preface from first edition

Oral and maxillofacial surgery is the surgical specialty concerned with the diagnosis and treatment of diseases affecting the teeth, mouth, jaws, face, and neck and represents one of the commonest indications for anaesthesia worldwide. The anaesthetic care of oral and maxillofacial patients requires specific knowledge and skills on the part of the anaesthetist. An understanding of the subject matter is fundamental to the safe practice of anaesthesia.

This textbook is intended to go some way to address this need. The anaesthetist can be called upon to provide anaesthesia for patients presenting with impacted or carious teeth, infections of the mucosa and adjacent structures, complex facial injuries, head and neck cancers, salivary gland disease, facial disproportion, temporomandibular joint disorders, cysts, and tumours of the jaws.

Anaesthetists may also be involved in managing patients experiencing chronic and intractable facial pain and provide anaesthesia for multiple trauma involving the face.

Although primarily written for anaesthetists, this textbook will also be of interest to maxillofacial surgeons, anaesthetic practitioners, anaesthetic nurses, and Operating Department Practitioners involved in providing anaesthesia for dental, oral, and max-illofacial surgery. We would also expect the work to be of interest to those anaesthetists currently in training and studying for their professional examinations.

Ian Shaw
Chandra Kumar
Chris Dodds

Preface

Anaesthesia for oral and maxillofacial surgery encompasses a wide range of procedures, treatments, and interventions for an array of pathologies affecting the teeth, mouth, and jaw. There is frequently overlap with other related surgical specialties such as otorhinolaryngology, neurosurgery, plastic surgery, and reconstructive surgery. Since the publication of the first edition of the *Oxford Textbook of Anaesthesia for Oral and Maxillofacial Surgery* in 2010, this subspecialty has continued to develop, with procedures and techniques evolving, new guidelines and standards being introduced, and new research evidence becoming available. This second edition has been completely updated by a new group of authors, adding an original, contemporary, and fresh perspective on existing topics, with the addition of new chapters on human factors in anaesthesia and surgical complications, written from the surgeon's perspective.

The safe perioperative care of patients undergoing oral and maxillofacial surgery necessitates a comprehensive knowledge and understanding of the specific challenges posed by this cohort, and their underlying pathologies and comorbidities, including a full appreciation of the implications of a 'shared airway'. This textbook is primarily intended as a reference tool for anaesthetists of all grades, but will also be of interest to maxillofacial surgeons, anaesthetic practitioners, anaesthetic nurses, recovery and intensive care nurses, and operating department practitioners.

Contents

Abbreviations

2D	two-dimensional
3D	three-dimensional
ACC	American College of Cardiology
ACEI	angiotensin-converting enzyme inhibitor
AFOI	awake fibreoptic intubation
AHA	American Heart Association
ANTS	anaesthetic non-technical skills
ARB	angiotensin II receptor blocker
ASA	American Society of Anesthesiologists
ASA-PS	American Society of Anesthesiologists Physical Status
ATLS	Advanced Trauma Life Support
AVL	awake videolaryngoscopy
BMI	body mass index
CABG	coronary artery bypass grafting
CICO	can't intubate, can't oxygenate
CICV	can't intubate, can't ventilate
CPAP	continuous positive airway pressure
CPET	cardiopulmonary exercise testing
CRM	crisis resource management
CSF	cerebrospinal fluid
CT	computed tomography
DAPT	dual antiplatelet therapy
DAS	Difficult Airway Society
DC/TMD	Diagnostic Criteria for Temporomandibular Disorders
DNM	descending necrotizing mediastinitis
DOAC	direct oral anticoagulant
EEG	electroencephalogram
eFONA	emergency front of neck airway
ERAS	Enhanced Recovery After Surgery
ESA	European Society of Anaesthesiology
ESC	European Society of Cardiology
FiO_2	fraction of inspired oxygen
FONA	front of neck airway
GCS	Glasgow Coma Score
HFNO	high-flow humidified nasal oxygen
IASP	International Association for the Study of Pain
ICHD	International Classification of Headache Disorders
ICU	intensive care unit
IMF	intermaxillary fixation
INR	international normalized ratio
LMA	laryngeal mask airway
MAP	mean arterial pressure
MICA	Myocardial Infarction and Cardiac Arrest
MRI	magnetic resonance imaging
N_2O	nitrous oxide
NAP4	Fourth National Audit Project
NICE	National Institute for Health and Care Excellence
NIHSS	National Institutes of Health Stroke Scale
NMDA	N-methyl-D-aspartate
NSAID	non-steroidal anti-inflammatory drug
NSQIP	National Surgical Quality Improvement Project
OMFS	oromaxillofacial surgery/surgical
OSAS	obstructive sleep apnoea syndrome
PACU	post-anaesthesia care unit
PBM	patient blood management
PCC	prothrombin complex concentrate
PCI	percutaneous coronary intervention
PEG	percutaneous endoscopic gastrostomy
PHN	post-herpetic neuralgia
PIFP	persistent idiopathic facial pain
PONV	postoperative nausea and vomiting
RAE	Ring–Adair–Elwyn
RCRI	Revised Cardiac Risk Index
SAD	supraglottic airway device
SMAS	superficial muscular aponeurotic system
SpO_2	oxygen saturation
SSC	Surgical Safety Checklist
TBSA	total body surface area
THRIVE	transnasal humidified rapid-insufflation ventilatory exchange
TIF	tracheo-innominate artery fistula
TIVA	total intravenous anaesthesia
TMJ	temporomandibular joint
TORS	transoral robotic surgery
VKA	vitamin K antagonist
WHO	World Health Organization

Contributors

Joshua H. Atkins, MD, PhD, CPE   Associate Professor of Anesthesiology & Critical Care, Associate Professor of Otorhinolaryngology: Head and Neck Surgery (Secondary), Perelman School of Medicine at the University of Pennsylvania, Philadelphia, PA, USA

Ian Bailes, BMBCh MA (Oxon), FRCA   Consultant Anaesthetist, Imperial College NHS Trust, London, UK

William P. L. Bradley, MBChB, FANZCA, MAICD   Adjunct Clinical Associate Professor, Monash University, TAS & VIC State Airway Lead, Specialist Anaesthetist, Department of Anaesthesia and Perioperative Medicine, The Alfred, Melbourne, Victoria, Australia

Gordon A. Chapman, MBChB, FRCA, FANZCA, MD   Consultant Anaesthetist, Royal Perth Hospital, Perth, Western Australia, Clinical Senior Lecturer, University of Western Australia, Australia

Chi Wai Cheung, MBBS (HK), MD (HKU), FHKCA, FHKAM (Anaesthesiology), FHKCA (Pain Med), Dip Pain Mgt (HKCA)   Clinical Professor, Department of Anaesthesiology, University of Hong Kong; Honorary Consultant, Department of Anaesthesiology, Queen Mary Hospital and Grantham Hospital and Duchess of Kent Children's Hospital, Chair of Specialty for Anaesthesiology and Adult Intensive Care Services Gleneagles Hospital, Chief of Service Department of Anaesthesiology HKU-Shenzhen Hospital, Hong Kong

Justin P. Curtin, FRACDS (OMS), FRCSEd   Associate Professor in Oral and Maxillofacial Surgery, College of Medicine and Dentistry, James Cook University, Australia

Adam R. Duffen, MBBS, BSc, FRCA   Consultant Anaesthetist, University Hospitals Bristol and Weston, UK

Michelle Gerstman, MBBS, FANZCA, MD   Consultant Anaesthetist, Peter MacCallum Cancer Centre, Melbourne, Australia

Jennifer Gosling, MBBS, BSc, MA, FRCA, FFICM   Senior Registrar in Anaesthesia, St. Mary's Hospital Department of Anaesthesia, Imperial College Healthcare NHS Trust, London, UK

Andrew Herlich, DMD, MD, FAAP, FASA, FAAOMS (H)   Professor Emeritus, Department of Anesthesiology and Perioperative Medicine, University of Pittsburgh School of Medicine, Pittsburgh, PA, USA

Roger H. Y. Ho, MBBS, BSc, MRCP, FRCA, FHKCA, FHKAM (Anaesthesiology)   Associate Consultant, Department of Anaesthesiology, Queen Mary Hospital and University of Hong Kong, Hong Kong

Kimberley Hodge, MBChB, FRCA, PGDip Med Ed   Senior Registrar in Anaesthesia, St. Mary's Hospital Department of Anaesthesia, Imperial College Healthcare NHS Trust, London, Squadron Leader, Royal Air Force, UK

Theresa Wan-Chun Hui, MBBS, FANZCA, FHKAM   Consultant Anaesthetist, Department of Anaesthesiology, The Duchess of Kent Children's Hospital, Hong Kong

Michael G. Irwin, MBChB, MD, FRCA, FCAI, FANZCA, FHKAM   Daniel CK Yu Professor, Department of Anaesthesiology, University of Hong Kong, Hong Kong

Cyrus Kerawala, BDS (Hons), FDSRCS (Eng), MBBS (Hons), FRCS, FRCS (OMFS)   Professor, Consultant Maxillofacial/Head & Neck Surgery, Royal Marsden Foundation Trust, London, UK

Orla J. Lacey, MBChB FRCA   Consultant Anaesthetist, The Royal Marsden NHS Foundation Trust, London, UK

David M. H. Lam, MBChB, FHKCA, FHKAM (Anaesthesiology)   Honorary Clinical Assistant Professor, Department of Anaesthesiology, University of Hong Kong, Hong Kong

Corina Lee, MBChB, FRCA, MRCP   Consultant Anaesthetist, Chelsea & Westminster Hospital, London, UK

Gene Lee, MBBS, FRCA, FANZCA   Consultant Anaesthetist, Department of Anaesthesia and Pain Management, Royal North Shore Hospital and St Vincent's Hospital, Sydney, Australia

Shona Love, BSc (Med Sci), MBChB, MRCS, FRCA   Consultant Anaesthetist, Imperial College NHS Trust, London, UK

Frances Lui, MBChB, FHKCA, FHKAM (Anaesthesiology), FANZCA   Consultant Anaesthetist, Department of Anaesthesiology, Queen Mary Hospital, Honorary Clinical Associate Professor, University of Hong Kong, Hong Kong

Craig Lyons, MBBCh, BAO, FCAI   Senior Registrar, Department of Anaesthesia and Intensive Care Medicine, Galway University Hospitals, Galway, Ireland

James W. D. Mann, MBChB, FRCA   Consultant Anaesthetist, Great Western Hospital, Swindon, Wiltshire, UK

Fauzia Mir, MBBS, FRCA, EDICM, PGCert Med Ed   Consultant Anaesthetist, St George's Hospital, London, UK

Indu Mitra, MRCS, FRCR   Consultant Radiologist, Department of Imaging, Chelsea & Westminster Hospital, London, UK

John Myatt, BSc, MBBS, FRCA   Consultant Anaesthetist, Imperial College NHS Trust, London, UK

Caroline A. R. Nicholas, BSc (Hons Lon), MB BS, FRCA   Consultant Anaesthetist, University Hospitals Sussex NHS Foundation Trust, UK

Ellen P. O'Sullivan, MBBCh, BAO, FRCA, FCAI   Professor and Consultant in Anaesthesia, Department of Anaesthesiology and Intensive Care, St James's Hospital, Dublin, Ireland

Christopher H. Rassekh, MD   Professor of Otorhinolaryngology: Head and Neck Surgery, Perelman School of Medicine at the University of Pennsylvania, Philadelphia, PA, USA

Rebecca Thurairatnam, MBBS, BSc, FRCA   Consultant Anaesthetist, Croydon University Hospital, London, UK

David J. A. Vaughan, MBBS, FRCA   Consultant Anaesthetist, Northwick Park Hospital, Harrow, UK

Tim N. Vorster, BSc (Hons Lon), MBBS, FRCA   Consultant Anaesthetist and Clinical Director Anaesthetics, Perioperative and Clinical Support Services, Queen Victoria Hospital, East Grinstead, UK

Patrick A. Ward, MBChB, BSc, FRCA   Consultant Anaesthetist, St John's Hospital, NHS Lothian, Scotland, UK

Silky Wong, MBBS, FHKCA, FHKAM (Anaesthesiology), FANZCA   Associate Consultant in Anaesthesia, The Duchess of Kent Children's Hospital, Hong Kong

Stanley Sau Ching Wong, MBBS (HK), MD (HKU), FHKCA, FHKAM (Anaesthesiology), FANZCA, FHKCA (Pain Med)   Clinical Assistant Professor, University of Hong Kong, Hong Kong

Vivian Yuen, MD, MBBS, FANZCA, FHKCA, FHKAM   Consultant Anaesthetist, Queen Mary Hospital, Honorary Assistant Clinical Professor, Department of Anaesthesiology, University of Hong Kong, Hong Kong

Preoperative assessment

Roger H. Y. Ho and David M. H. Lam

Introduction

Preoperative assessment for oromaxillofacial surgery (OMFS) can be particularly challenging. OMFS encompasses a wide range of procedures, some of which may overlap with ear, nose, and throat surgery; head & neck surgery; neurosurgery; and/or plastic surgery. The anaesthetist must have a good understanding of the extent and complexities of the surgery being undertaken in order to make an appropriate assessment and formulate an effective plan for anaesthesia and postoperative care. The setting in which these procedures are undertaken may be variable, ranging from the hospital operating theatre to the less familiar environment of the outpatient dental clinic, placing emphasis on the preoperative assessment in determining the most appropriate pathway. The indications for OMFS procedures frequently have anaesthetic implications, where concomitant injuries or associated syndromes/diseases must be considered in the anaesthetist's preoperative evaluation—in particular, the potential for difficult airway management. As with all shared-airway surgery, sound preoperative assessment and planning is essential in ensuring patient safety, while optimizing surgical access and operating conditions.

Range of procedures

OMFS encompasses dentoalveolar procedures (such as general dentistry and wisdom teeth extraction), intraoral surgery, orthognathic surgery, facial cosmetic surgery, major reconstructive surgery with implants or local/distant microvascular free flaps, temporomandibular joint (TMJ) surgery, and craniofacial surgery. The goals of surgery can be broadly classified as functional restorative, structural support, and aesthetic reconstruction.

Airway evaluation and planning

Preoperative assessment of the airway for OMFS should include screening patients for the following:

- Predictors of difficulty in tracheal intubation (oral or nasal).
- Predictors of difficulty in ventilation/rescue oxygenation (via face mask or supraglottic airway device).
- Potential requirement for an awake airway management technique (and ability of patient to cooperate/consent for this approach).
- Ease of a front of neck airway.

In the elective setting, a detailed review of previous anaesthetic records, past medical history, and surgical history should be undertaken. In addition to routine examination of the airway, which includes assessment of mouth opening, dentition, thyromental distance, jaw protrusion, and neck mobility, the OMFS airway examination often necessitates assessment for nasotracheal intubation—screening for potential contraindications, such as nasopharyngeal carcinoma or previous cleft palate repair, and risk factors for epistaxis, such as altered coagulation or nasal polyps. The findings of recent imaging, such as computed tomography or magnetic resonance imaging, may provide additional information (including the specific location of any lesion and degree of airway compression, distortion, or obstruction). Other technologies, including virtual airway endoscopy and three-dimensional printed models, have also been described in the assessment and planning of complex airway management, though are less commonly utilized at present. Should the findings of bedside assessments and routine investigations remain inconclusive, awake nasendoscopy can often provide invaluable information. These assessments and investigations assist the anaesthetist in formulating an airway management strategy, which should comprise a primary airway plan, as well as airway rescue plan(s), in accordance with the UK National Audit Project 4 (NAP4).[1] (Assessment and management of the difficult airway is discussed in greater detail in Chapter 2.)

In the emergency setting (e.g. oromaxillofacial trauma or infection), it is crucial to identify any signs or symptoms indicative of impending airway obstruction—stridor, dyspnoea, hoarseness, drooling, and/or lack of tongue protrusion, requiring urgent airway intervention. Management of the airway may be further complicated by limited mouth opening due to trismus, difficult front of neck access due to previous surgery/radiotherapy, infection, obesity, or the presence of a rigid cervical spinal collar, and/or an uncooperative/combative patient.

A crucial aspect in formulating any airway management strategy is the involvement of the multidisciplinary team—prior discussion with the surgical team (in advance of anaesthesia) is essential to ensure the respective requirements/priorities of each team are met. The anaesthetist may wish the surgeon to be present at induction of anaesthesia if there are concerns that a rescue surgical airway may be required. The position of the airway device/breathing circuit should be specifically discussed, so as not to obscure the surgical field or prevent assessment of bite occlusion (if required). Where significant movement of the head and neck is expected (particularly TMJ surgery), this should be emphasized by the surgical team to the anaesthetist, thus ensuring the airway device is secured appropriately to prevent accidental tracheal extubation. In some procedures, patency of the airway may be compromised postoperatively by bleeding or oedema, therefore a plan for tracheal extubation (technique, timing, and setting) must be agreed preoperatively (and modified as necessary). Clearly, if a tracheostomy, intermaxillary fixation device, or other significant intervention is planned, the anaesthetist and surgeon must have discussed them with each other, and with the patient.

Pathology-specific considerations

Trauma

While the appearance of facial injuries can be distracting, it is critical to prioritize management of trauma patients according to clinical importance, following a systematic approach (as per Advanced Trauma Life Support principles). The goal of the airway assessment in the primary survey is to establish any immediate threat to patency, identifying any signs and symptoms of potential airway obstruction (e.g. tracheal deviation, subcutaneous emphysema, and/or marked soft tissue swelling). Traumatic injuries classically associated with airway obstruction include bilateral anterior mandibular fractures and the Le Fort III fracture (**Fig. 1.1**).

Airway management in the trauma setting should always be presumed to be difficult. Cervical spine movements are often restricted due to the application of a rigid cervical spine collar and/or manual in-line stabilization. Mouth opening may be restricted by pain, muscle spasm, or mechanical obstruction (e.g. a tripod fracture of the zygomatic complex may interfere with movement of the coronoid process of the mandible). The patient may be combative/unable to cooperate with an awake tracheal intubation technique,

and there may be the additional risk of aspiration of blood or broken teeth fragments. Having undertaken initial assessment and stabilization of the patient, the secondary survey should include an 'AMPLE' (Allergy, Medication, Past medical history, Last food and drink, Event) history, full body examination, and relevant investigations. In particular, the mechanism of injury and magnitude of energy transfer are important factors in guiding identification and assessment of injuries. Classification of facial fractures as lower, middle, and/or upper third may also be helpful in identifying concomitant injuries commonly associated at each level. (Management of the oromaxillofacial trauma patient is discussed in detail in Chapter 13.)

Infection

The most common cause of oromaxillofacial infection is impacted teeth, and the resulting dental abscess may cause significant facial swelling and trismus, affecting airway management (rarer causes of infection include tuberculosis, syphilis, and fungal or viral infection in immunocompromised states). Infection usually begins with dental decay and pulpitis, leading to perforation of the bone cortex, allowing the infection to spread to the subperiosteal region. In more severe cases, infection may spread along the fascial planes into the infratemporal fossa, subtemporalis, or even the cervical fascial plane (**Fig. 1.2**), forming a parapharyngeal abscess and even mediastinitis. The classic example of this is Ludwig's angina, in which cellulitis extends over the entire floor of mouth, including both the submandibular and sublingual spaces. Preoperative evaluation of the airway reveals difficulty in swallowing secretions and an inability to protrude the tongue. Neck and/or pretracheal fascial involvement complicates the option of tracheostomy formation. In addition to assessing the extent of local spread, the systemic effects of bacteraemia/sepsis via haematogenous spread must be actively sought and promptly managed according to the Surviving Sepsis Campaign.[3] (Management of oromaxillofacial infection is discussed in greater detail in Chapter 12.)

Congenital anomalies

Cleft lip and palate are among the most common congenital defects requiring surgery. In addition to the primary repair, patients often require subsequent procedures for lip aesthetics, closure of residual palatal defects, bone grafts, alignment of alveolar and dental defects,

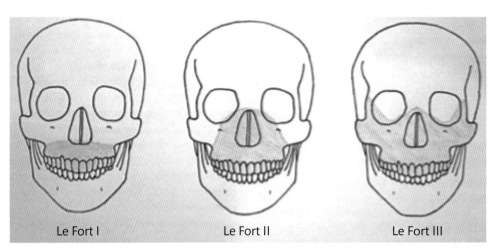

| Le Fort I | Le Fort II | Le Fort III |

Fig. 1.1 The Le Fort classification of facial fractures.[2]

Morosan M, Parbhoo A, Curry N (2012) Anaesthesia and common oral and maxilla-facial emergencies. Continuing Education in Anaesthesia, Critical Care and Pain 12(5), 257–262.

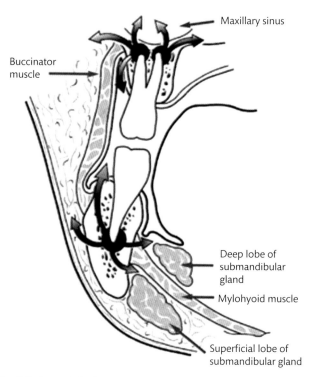

Maxillary sinus

Buccinator muscle

Deep lobe of submandibular gland

Mylohyoid muscle

Superficial lobe of submandibular gland

Fig. 1.2 Spread of odontogenic infection through the fascial planes.

Table 1.1 Congenital syndromes associated with cleft lip and palate

Down syndrome	Microstomia and macroglossia Atlantoaxial subluxation and instability Congenital cardiac disease
Pierre Robin sequence	Micrognathia Glossoptosis Usually easier to intubate with age
Hemifacial microsomia	Hemifacial and mandibular hypoplasia Cervical spine abnormalities Eye and ear malformations Usually more difficult to intubate with age
Treacher Collins syndrome	Micrognathia and maxillary hypoplasia Choanal atresia Eye and ear malformations Usually more difficult to intubate with age

Velocardiofacial syndrome	Microcephaly
	Microstomia, flat nasal bridge,
	  velopharyngeal incompetence, tracheal
	  and laryngeal anomalies
	Congenital cardiac disease
	Small ears, short stature

Stickler syndrome	Micrognathia and flat face Eye, ear, and joint abnormalities Congenital cardiac disease
Klippel–Feil syndrome	Webbed neck and fused cervical vertebrae Congenital cardiac disease Short stature

jaw realignment, and correction of nasal deformity. Although cleft defects per se do not lead to upper airway obstruction and/or difficult airway management, coexisting structural or neuromuscular dysfunction may result in either/both. For example, in Pierre Robin sequence, the combination of micrognathia, glossoptosis, and cleft palate may cause airway obstruction relieved only by prone positioning or insertion of a nasopharyngeal airway, and in some cases necessitating tracheostomy formation. Crucially, beyond the airway examination, the anaesthetist must be aware of the multisystem nature of many of the syndromes associated with cleft anomalies, and make appropriate assessment of cardiac, renal, and skeletal systems as required (Table 1.1).

Malignancy

Airway management may be complicated by distortion, invasion, or compression of tissues by the tumour and/or progressive airway obstruction by the lesion itself. Previous cancer treatments/surgery may also contribute to airway management difficulties (Table 1.2). Consideration should be given to the specific risk factors associated with head and neck cancer, including human papilloma virus, smoking, and alcohol use, and their associated comorbidities—in particular, chronic obstructive lung disease, ischaemic heart disease, alcoholic cardiomyopathy, liver cirrhosis, and alcohol dependence. There is a 10% risk of a synchronous primary cancer elsewhere within the aerodigestive tract, which should be sought through appropriate imaging. Malnutrition is common due to poor appetite, dysphagia, or side effects of chemotherapy and/or radiation mucositis, and dietician input is advocated to optimize nutritional support preoperatively in order to minimize the reduced wound healing, and increased risk of infection/other postoperative complications associated with it. (Management of the oromaxillofacial patient with malignancy is discussed in detail in Chapter 15.)

Free flap transfer

This surgical technique may be employed to provide tissue for reconstruction. Successful flap perfusion (and surgical outcome) relies upon optimization of perioperative haemodynamics (a relative hyperdynamic circulation with high cardiac output and vasodilation is desirable), thus preoperative assessment of cardiorespiratory reserve is crucial in establishing the appropriateness of the planned procedure. Contraindications might include sickle cell disease and untreated polycythaemia rubra vera due to their hypercoagulable states, and flap survival may be compromised in patients with active vasculitis or peripheral vascular disease. Prolonged preoperative fasting should be avoided in order to minimize any fluid deficits.

Table 1.2 Sequelae of oromaxillofacial and head and neck cancer treatments

Maxillectomy and craniofacial resection	Difficult facemask seal Difficult nasotracheal intubation TMJ pseudoankylosis
Tongue, floor of mouth surgery	Trismus Limited mandibular space Fixed tongue
Laryngeal surgery	Laryngeal stenosis Impaired swallowing Aspiration risk
Neck dissection	Damage to cranial nerves IX, X, XII Vocal cord palsy Impaired swallowing Aspiration risk
Radiotherapy	Limited neck extension TMJ ankylosis Osteoradionecrosis of mandible Carotid artery stenosis Poor wound healing

(Management of OMFS patients for free flap reconstruction is discussed in greater detail in Chapter 15.)

Environmental considerations

Minor dental procedures are commonly performed under sedation or general anaesthesia in short-stay ambulatory care centres, and sometimes dental clinics. Accessibility to drugs and equipment, availability of postoperative recovery facilities, staff numbers, and staff training in airway management, resuscitation, and sedation may vary significantly between the settings. Appropriate patient selection through thorough preoperative assessment is crucial in ensuring patient safety in the remote site/day surgical environment. Patient suitability should be based upon assessment of comorbidities and fitness for day surgery, as well as determining the availability of an appropriate escort, geographical proximity, and access to emergency services if required (as described by the Society of Day Surgery[4]). The guidelines for the management of children referred for dental extraction under general anesthesia[5] state that sedation or general anaesthesia is best delivered in the inpatient setting for patients considered to be of high anaesthetic risk, with significant comorbidities or complex dental problems (Table 1.3), where high dependency unit/intensive care is immediately available or may be arranged in advance. (Dental anaesthesia and sedation are covered in greater detail in Chapters 8 and 6, respectively.)

Evaluation of comorbidities

Obesity and obstructive sleep apnoea syndrome

Obesity is defined as a body mass index (BMI) ≥ 30 kg/m²; morbid obesity ≥ 35 kg/m²; and supermorbid obesity ≥ 50 kg/m². There is an increasing number of patients with raised BMI presenting for OMFS, and the pathophysiological consequences of obesity pose significant challenges to the anaesthetist.

Obstructive sleep apnoea syndrome (OSAS) arises from periodic partial or complete collapse of the upper airway during sleep,

Table 1.3 Conditions for dental extraction in the inpatient (hospital) setting

High anaesthetic risk	Anatomically or functionally abnormal airway Significant learning disabilities or behavioural abnormalities Severe anxiety Congenital syndromes associated with increased anaesthetic risk History of adverse reaction to anaesthetic agents History of complications occurring under general anaesthesia Family history of significant problems occurring under general anaesthesia
Significant comorbidities	Severe or poorly controlled asthma Symptomatic cardiac disease, requiring treatment Coagulopathy, anticoagulant therapy, or antiplatelet therapy Impaired renal or hepatic function Unstable metabolic or endocrine disorders Significant neurological or neuromuscular disorders Active systemic infection Haemoglobinopathies Abnormal BMI (<18.5 kg/m² or >30 kg/m²)

Table 1.4 Classification of the severity of OSAS according to the American Academy of Sleeping Medicine Task Force

Apnoea–hypopnoea index	Severity classification
<5	Normal
5–15	Mild
15–30	Moderate
>30	Severe

Sleep-related breathing disorders in adults: recommendations for syndrome definition and measurement techniques in clinical research. The Report of an American Academy of Sleep Medicine Task Force. Sleep. 1999;22(5):667–89.

resulting in decreased (hypopnoea) or complete cessation (apnoea) of airflow. The severity of OSAS is defined by the apnoea–hypopnoea index (the number of apnoea or hypopnoea events per hour) (Table 1.4).[6] These recurrent episodes of hypoxia can lead to significant cardiopulmonary morbidity, such as pulmonary hypertension and cor pulmonale. Patients often have poor sleep quality due to the frequent arousal that occurs during their sleep cycle to restore airway patency,[7] resulting in behavioural disturbances, such as daytime hypersomnolence and sexual dysfunction.

Patients with OSAS presenting for surgery are at increased risk of perioperative airway, respiratory, and cardiovascular complications,[8] and these risks are further increased if the condition remains undiagnosed (and untreated) at the time of surgery.[9] Respiratory complications (e.g. oxygen desaturation, acute respiratory failure, respiratory arrest, and aspiration pneumonia) are the most common, as the underlying pathophysiology of OSAS may be exacerbated by the depressant effects of anaesthetic medications upon respiratory drive, airway protective reflexes, and arousal responses.[8] These problems may be further compounded in patients undergoing major OMFS procedures due to significant alterations in airway anatomy and postoperative oedema.

Obesity per se is not always associated with difficult tracheal intubation; however, many aspects of airway management may be more challenging. Thorough preoperative airway examination should be undertaken, seeking features suggestive of difficult airway management—in particular, a Mallampati score ≥ 3, a high Wilson score, and increased neck circumference. Often, a standard asleep tracheal intubation is both practical and safe (especially following the advent of videolaryngoscopy); however, a robust strategy for airway management must always be in place prior to induction of anaesthesia.

Obese patients are more prone to both restrictive and obstructive respiratory insufficiency—decreased chest wall and lung compliance results in a restrictive defect, while increased adipose tissue within the pharyngeal walls predisposes to airway collapse during normal breathing and contributes to the development of OSAS. Obese patients should therefore be routinely screened for OSAS preoperatively—including identification of any risk factors (Box 1.1),[10] thorough physical examination, use of the STOP-BANG questionnaire (Table 1.5),[8] and appropriate investigations such as electrocardiography, pulse oximetry, pulmonary function tests,[11] and polysomnography.[12] Abnormal spirometry is associated with increased postoperative complications.[13] The STOP-BANG questionnaire is currently the most sensitive, specific, and best-validated screening questionnaire for OSAS. A score of 0–2 indicates 'low risk', 3–4 indicates 'intermediate risk', and a score of ≥ 5 indicates 'high

Box 1.1 Predisposing conditions for obstructive sleep apnoea

- Obesity
- Age 40–70 yr
- Male gender
- Excess alcohol intake
- Smoking
- Pregnancy
- Low Physical activity
- Unemployment
- Neck circumference >40 cm
- Surgical patient
- Tonsillar and adenoidal hypertrophy
- Craniofacial abnormalities (e.g. Pierre Robin, Down's syndrome)
- Neuromuscular disease

Source: Martinez G, Faber P. Obstructive Sleep apnoea. *Continuing Education in Anaesthesia Critical Care & Pain*. 2011; **11**(1): 5–8.

risk' for OSAS. Patients who have an intermediate-to-high risk score are at greater risk of perioperative complications[14] and referral to a sleep specialist for formal evaluation and optimization is recommended. Strategies that may be considered include weight loss, the use of mandibular advancement devices, and non-invasive positive pressure ventilation.[6] Utilization of continuous positive airway pressure/bi-level positive airway pressure devices may reduce the incidence of perioperative hypoxic events in obese patients, regardless of whether OSAS has been formally diagnosed.[11]

Early preoperative identification of OSAS allows initiation of non-invasive ventilation therapy (as indicated) prior to surgery, reducing the overall risk of perioperative complications. Prompt diagnosis also enables the appropriate preoperative planning to occur, influencing the conduct of all aspects of anaesthetic care, including the choice of anaesthetic medications, airway management, and nature of the postoperative care facility. Many patients with OSAS will also suffer from concomitant comorbidities that should be optimized preoperatively.

Obesity is associated with cardiovascular comorbidities such as hypertension, ischaemic heart disease, and arrhythmias. Patients with these conditions should be managed in accordance with the European Society of Cardiology (ESC)/European Society of Anaesthesiology (ESA) guidelines[11] or American College of Cardiology (ACC)/American Heart Association (AHA) guidelines[15] to achieve satisfactory control prior to any elective surgery.

Table 1.5 STOP-BANG questionnaire, utilized as a screening tool for OSAS

Snoring: do you snore loudly (louder than talking or loud enough to be heard through closed doors)?	Yes/No
Tired: do you often feel tired, fatigued, or sleepy during the daytime?	Yes/No
Observed: has anyone observed you stopping breathing during your sleep?	Yes/No
Blood **P**ressure: do you have high blood pressure or are you on treatment for high blood pressure?	Yes/No
BMI: is your body mass index greater than 35 kg/m²?	Yes/No
Age: are you over 50 years old?	Yes/No
Neck circumference: is your neck circumference greater than 40 cm (16 inches)?	Yes/No
Gender: are you male?	Yes/No

Hall A. Sleep physiology and the perioperative care of patients with sleep disorders. BJA Education. 2014;15(4):167–72.

Obesity is an independent risk factor for perioperative renal dysfunction,[16] and although there is no evidence that any particular preoperative optimization strategy is effective in minimizing postoperative renal impairment, general protective strategies such as correcting preoperative anaemia, avoiding nephrotoxic medications, and maintaining adequate volume status should be employed.[17]

Obesity is also commonly associated with metabolic disorders such as diabetes, hyperlipidaemia, and fatty liver disease. Perioperative hyperglycaemia is associated with increased morbidity and mortality in patients undergoing non-cardiac surgery.[18] The 2018 ESA guidelines recommend that laboratory testing to screen for diabetes should be carried out in obese patients prior to elective non-cardiac surgery (if the condition has not already been diagnosed).[11] Glycaemic control should be optimized, with elective surgery delayed in order to achieve this.[19]

Obesity is also associated with anaemia, and deficiencies in various micronutrients such as vitamin D, ascorbic acid, and beta-carotene.[20] These deficits should be identified during preoperative assessment and corrected before elective surgery is undertaken (anaemia is discussed in detail later in this chapter).

Patients with OSAS should have their condition thoroughly reviewed at preassessment, and, if compliant with existing therapy, asymptomatic, and without significant cardiopulmonary sequelae, can be considered appropriate to proceed with surgery as planned without further investigation and/or treatment. The non-invasive ventilation device used by the patient should be brought into hospital on admission and its use continued throughout the perioperative period,[11] unless specifically contraindicated (e.g. if there are surgical concerns following craniofacial surgery). However, patients who have poorly controlled OSAS (or who have developed secondary cardiopulmonary complications) should be referred for further assessment and optimization before elective surgery. In semi-elective/expedited surgery (e.g. cancer surgery), the decision to defer surgery for further investigation and/or treatment for OSAS should take an individualized approach, taking into consideration the urgency and risk of surgery, the severity of OSAS and other comorbidities, and the relative accessibility of proposed investigations/treatments. In urgent or emergency surgery, where preoperative optimization may be precluded, patients considered to be at high risk of OSAS should be presumed to have the condition and managed as such, with measures taken to minimize perioperative complications, including postoperative care in an appropriately staffed and monitored facility.

OSAS is not an absolute contraindication for day surgery, although patient selection is key—taking into consideration the extent of planned surgery, severity of OSAS, comorbidities, anaesthetic technique, postoperative analgesic requirements, and necessity for advanced postoperative monitoring and non-invasive ventilation.

Coronary artery disease and revascularization

Coronary artery disease is a risk factor for perioperative major adverse cardiovascular events.[15] For elective surgery, perioperative cardiac assessment should proceed according to the stepwise approaches described in the 'ESC/ESA guidelines on non-cardiac surgery: cardiovascular assessment and management'[11] or the 'ACC/AHA guideline on perioperative cardiovascular evaluation and management of patients undergoing non-cardiac surgery'.[15] In general, patients presenting with

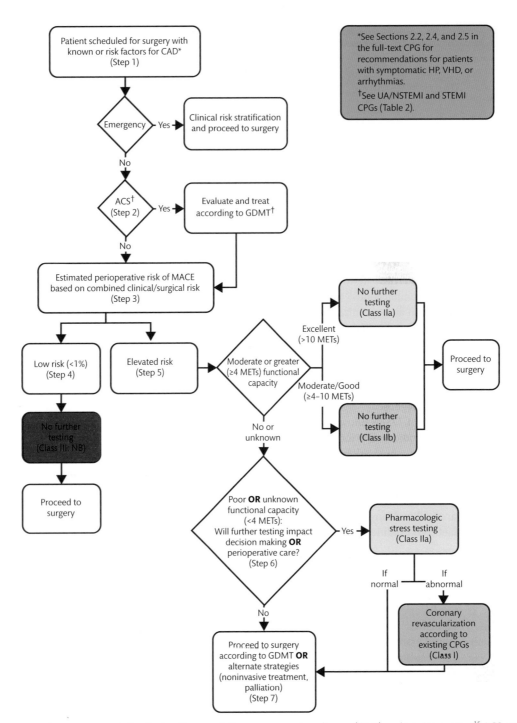

Fig. 1.3 Step-wise approach to assessment of patients with pre-existing coronary artery disease (CAD) undergoing surgery.[15] ACS, acute coronary syndrome; CABG, coronary artery bypass graft; CPG, clinical practice guideline; DASI, Duke Activity Status Index; GDMT, guideline-directed medical therapy; HF, heart failure; MACE, major adverse cardiac event; MET, metabolic equivalent; NB, no benefit; NSQIP, National Surgical Quality Improvement Program; PCI, percutaneous coronary intervention; RCRI, Revised Cardiac Risk Index; STEMI, ST-elevation myocardial infarction; UA/NSTEMI, unstable angina/non-ST-elevation myocardial infarction; VHD, valvular heart disease.

Reproduced with permissions from Fleisher LA, Fleischmann KE, Auerbach AD, Barnason SA, Beckman JA, Bozkurt B, et al. 2014 ACC/AHA guideline on perioperative cardiovascular evaluation and management of patients undergoing noncardiac surgery: a report of the American College of Cardiology/American Heart Association Task Force on Practice Guidelines. Circulation. 2014;130(24):e278–333.

a low combined clinical and surgical risk (<1% risk of a major adverse cardiovascular event) can safely proceed to surgery without additional testing. Many OMFS procedures are considered to be of low surgical risk (e.g. superficial oral and periodontal surgery); however, the presence of ischaemic heart disease alone may elevate the overall risk of major adverse cardiovascular events to ≥1%.[21] In such cases, assessment

of patients' functional capacity is essential, and pharmacological stress testing (and subsequent coronary revascularization) may be indicated (**Figs 1.3 and 1.4**). Routine preoperative coronary angiography or prophylactic revascularization is not recommended to exclusively reduce perioperative cardiac events[22]—an approach supported by the recent Coronary-Artery Revascularisation Prophylaxis (CARP) trial,

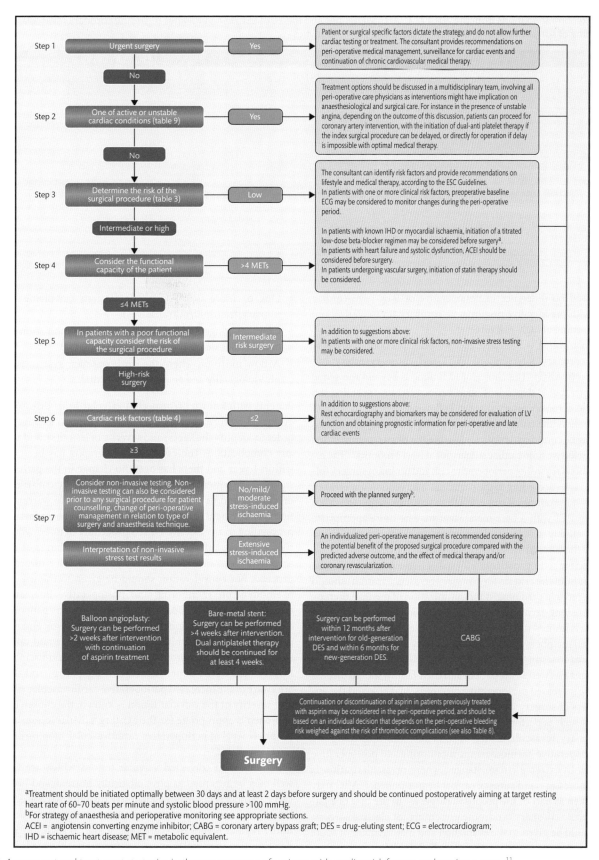

Fig. 1.4 Assessment and treatment strategies in the management of patients with cardiac risk factors undergoing surgery.[11]

Kristensen SD, Knuuti J, Saraste A, Anker S, Botker HE, Hert SD, et al. 2014 ESC/ESA Guidelines on non-cardiac surgery: cardiovascular assessment and management: The Joint Task Force on non-cardiac surgery: cardiovascular assessment and management of the European Society of Cardiology (ESC) and the European Society of Anaesthesiology (ESA). Eur Heart J. 2014;35(35):2383–431. 2014;35(35):2383–431

Table 1.6 Recommendations from the 2014 ACC/AHA guidelines and the 2014 ESC/ESA guidelines regarding coronary revascularization and the timing of surgery following different revascularization modalities

	ACC/AHA guidance[13]	ESC/ESA guidance[9]
Routine preoperative coronary angiography or revascularization prior to elective non-cardiac surgery	Not recommended unless revascularization is otherwise indicated according to existing guidance for stable coronary artery disease	Not recommended unless revascularization is otherwise indicated according to existing guidance for stable coronary artery disease
Recommended duration that elective surgery should be delayed following balloon angioplasty	14 days	14 days
Recommended duration that elective surgery should be delayed following bare-metal stent insertion	30 days	Minimum of 30 days, but ideally 3 months
Recommended duration that elective surgery should be delayed following drug-eluting stent (DES) insertion	6 months for newer-generation DESs 12 months for conventional DESs	6 months for newer-generation DESs 12 months for conventional DESs

Kristensen SD, Knuuti J, Saraste A, Anker S, Botker HE, Hert SD, et al. 2014 ESC/ESA Guidelines on non-cardiac surgery: cardiovascular assessment and management: The Joint Task Force on non-cardiac surgery: cardiovascular assessment and management of the European Society of Cardiology (ESC) and the European Society of Anaesthesiology (ESA). Eur Heart J. 2014;35(35):2383–431

Fleisher LA, Fleischmann KE, Auerbach AD, Barnason SA, Beckman JA, Bozkurt B, et al. 2014 ACC/AHA guideline on perioperative cardiovascular evaluation and management of patients undergoing noncardiac surgery: a report of the American College of Cardiology/American Heart Association Task Force on Practice Guidelines. Circulation. 2014;130(24):e278–333.

which showed no difference in perioperative or long-term cardiac outcomes with preoperative prophylactic coronary revascularization, even in the setting of high-risk surgery.[23]

If revascularization is indicated, the two principal options are percutaneous coronary intervention (PCI) and coronary artery bypass grafting (CABG). The choice of technique is beyond the scope of this chapter, but is dependent upon various factors, including the extent of the coronary artery disease. Following satisfactory CABG revascularization, the risk of subsequent perioperative myocardial ischaemia may be considered relatively low, but it is often recommended to postpone elective non-cardiac surgery for at least 3 months.[24] The recommendations regarding perioperative risk and timing of surgery following PCI varies according to the particular intervention undertaken (**Table 1.6**)—for example, if surgery is time sensitive (required within weeks), then PCI with a bare-metal stent may be more appropriate than a drug-eluting stent to avoid the greater period of anticoagulation required for the latter (discussed in detail later in the chapter).

In the elective setting, patients with stable ischaemic heart disease (who do not fulfil the criteria for coronary revascularization) should still be referred to a cardiologist for optimization of medical therapy and to ensure long-term follow-up. In urgent or emergency surgery, where there is limited time for evaluation and/or optimization prior to surgery, all members of the multidisciplinary team involved in the patient's care (anaesthetist, surgeon, cardiologist, intensivist, and/or haematologist), as well as the patient and their family, should discuss together the increased perioperative cardiovascular risk and the appropriateness of surgery. Specific measures to mitigate risk may be considered, such as performing the surgery at a centre where emergency coronary revascularization is available, and upgrading the level of perioperative haemodynamic monitoring and postoperative care facility. In extreme circumstances, where revascularization is absolutely necessary and surgery cannot be postponed, CABG may be undertaken as part of the proposed surgery.[15] In the case of a patient with acute coronary syndrome presenting for elective surgery, priority should be given to the evaluation and management of acute coronary syndrome according to established guidelines, providing that the condition requiring elective surgery is not life-threatening.

Cardiac murmurs

Patients who present to preoperative assessment with a heart murmur may be classified into three subgroups:

• One or more isolated valvular lesions (involving aortic/pulmonary/tricuspid/mitral valves).
• Complex congenital heart disease with a combination of intra- or extracardiac defects.
• A flow murmur, where the cardiovascular system is otherwise physiologically and anatomically normal.

Patients with known or suspected valvular heart disease should be evaluated by formal echocardiography prior to elective OMFS, in order to identify the site(s) and severity of lesion(s), and to assess for any complications (unless echocardiography has been performed within 1 year and there has been no change in the patient's clinical status).[15] If a patient has a valvular lesion of sufficient severity (based on clinical and/or echocardiographic criteria) to warrant intervention (replacement or repair), then this should be undertaken before proceeding to any elective OMFS procedure of intermediate to high risk.[15] However, if a valvular lesion is present but is of insufficient severity to warrant valvular intervention, elective surgery may still proceed, but consideration should be given to the use of invasive haemodynamic monitoring and postoperative intensive care for ongoing monitoring and/or organ support.[15] For patients with uncorrected valvular lesions who require urgent or emergency surgery, where there is limited time for evaluation and optimization, surgery may proceed providing that there is multidisciplinary team involvement in the patient's care, and the patient and their family are aware of the increased perioperative cardiovascular risk; the type and severity of the valvular lesion is known; the chosen anaesthetic approach is appropriate for the existing valvular lesion; and the appropriate level of perioperative cardiovascular monitoring and support is available.

Patients with corrected valvular lesions which are functioning well may be regarded as physiologically normal, and hence do not carry an increased cardiovascular risk during OMFS procedures unless there are other risk factors present. These patients are normally under regular review by a cardiologist and, as such, any subsequent deterioration in valvular or cardiac function will usually be detected early. Patients with prosthetic metallic valves will require an appropriate perioperative anticoagulation bridging regimen.

Patients with a history of complex congenital heart disease are generally considered to have an increased perioperative cardiovascular risk, but the precise degree of risk is highly variable because it is dependent upon the nature of the pre-existing cardiac condition itself, the extent of previous surgical corrections, the presence of associated complications (e.g. heart failure, pulmonary hypertension, and dysrhythmias), the proposed surgical procedure, and the urgency of surgery. The ESC/ESA guideline[11] and the 2014 ACC/AHA guideline[15] both recommend that preoperative evaluation and any subsequent elective non-cardiac surgery should be carried out by an expert multidisciplinary team at a specialist centre. In the case of urgent or emergency procedures where there is minimal time for evaluation and/or optimization prior to surgery, all clinicians involved in patient care and the patient/family should be made aware of the increased perioperative risk. If it is not practically possible for surgery to be performed at a specialist centre due to the urgency of the condition, expert advice should be sought from an affiliated specialist centre regarding the most appropriate perioperative optimization strategies.

Patients with a physiological flow murmur only are regarded as physiologically normal and do not carry an increased cardiovascular risk during OMFS procedures unless there are other risk factors present. The difficulty lies in determining if the murmur is, in fact, merely a functional flow murmur or if there is a pathological element to it. If other concerns are also identified during the preoperative assessment, then appropriate consideration should be given to further investigation of the murmur.

Arterial hypertension

Uncontrolled arterial hypertension is one of the most common reasons for deferring elective surgery.

Indeed, there is an association between hypertension and adverse perioperative cardiovascular complications, but only when the severity of arterial hypertension is grade 3 or above (Table 1.7).[25,26] As such, the potential benefit of achieving improved blood pressure control in order to minimize cardiovascular complications has to be balanced against the considerable socioeconomic cost, psychological burden upon patients and their families, and the risk of disease progression associated with unnecessary postponement of operations.

The Association of Anaesthetists has published guidelines regarding the management of arterial hypertension in patients scheduled for elective non-cardiac surgery. Firstly, any abnormal blood

Table 1.7 Classification of blood pressure and grade of hypertension

Category	Systolic blood pressure (mmHg)		Diastolic blood pressure (mmHg)
Optimal	<120	and	<80
Normal	120–129	and/or	80–84
High normal	130–139	and/or	85–89
Grade 1 hypertension	140–159	and/or	90–99
Grade 2 hypertension	160–179	and/or	100–109
Grade 3 hypertension	≥180	and/or	≥110
Isolated systolic hypertension	≥140	and	<90

Williams B, Mancia G, Spiering W, Agabiti Rosei E, Azizi M, Burnier M, et al. 2018 ESC/ESH Guidelines for the management of arterial hypertension. Eur Heart J. 2018;39(33):3021–104.

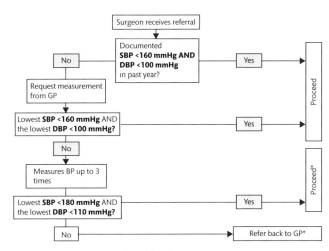

Fig. 1.5 Stepwise approach to blood pressure assessment in patients referred for elective surgery.[28] *The GP should be informed of blood pressure readings in excess of 140 mmHg systolic or 90 mmHg diastolic, so that the diagnosis of hypertension can be refuted or confirmed and investigated and treated as necessary. DBP, diastolic blood pressure; SBP, systolic blood pressure.

Reproduced with permissions from Hartle A, McCormack T, Carlisle J, Anderson S, Pichel A, Beckett N, et al. The measurement of adult blood pressure and management of hypertension before elective surgery: Joint Guidelines from the Association of Anaesthetists of Great Britain and Ireland and the British Hypertension Society. Anaesthesia. 2016;71(3):326-37.

pressure readings should be confirmed by multiple readings, with the use of ambulatory or home blood pressure monitoring if necessary.[27] Grade 2 hypertension or below should be managed according to established guidelines for the treatment of hypertension (e.g. National Institute for Health and Care Excellence guidelines), but surgery may proceed as planned and regular antihypertensive medications continued through the perioperative period. However, if the systolic blood pressure is ≥180 mmHg or diastolic blood pressure ≥110 mmHg (i.e. at least grade 3 hypertension), the patient should be referred for further investigation and treatment prior to surgery (Fig. 1.5).[28] In the case of urgent or emergency operations where there is limited opportunity for preoperative optimization, all those who are involved in the patient's care, as well as the patients and their families, should be made aware of the increased perioperative risk. Specific measures to mitigate the risk should be considered, such as employing invasive haemodynamic monitoring, and providing an enhanced level of postoperative care.

Anaemia

Anaemia is defined by the World Health Organization as a haemoglobin level of <13 g/dL for males and <12 g/dL for females. Preoperative anaemia has been shown to be associated with increased morbidity and mortality in patients undergoing major non-cardiac surgery, as well as an increased risk of allogeneic blood transfusion perioperatively, which itself is associated with significant morbidity.[29] This has led to the development of various perioperative blood conservation strategies and the concept of patient blood management (PBM). PBM involves a patient-centred, multidisciplinary, multimodal, and evidence-based approach to the management of perioperative anaemia. The primary aim of PBM is to avoid unnecessary blood transfusion thereby minimizing the associated morbidity, improving patient outcome, and minimizing resource utilization. This strategy is supported by the World

Table 1.8 The three pillars of PBM: preoperative components

Pillar 1: detection and management of anaemia	Pillar 2: minimization of bleeding and blood loss	Pillar 3: management of anaemia and optimization of tolerance
Aim for assessment of anaemia 4–6 weeks before surgery	Identify and manage bleeding risk (past medical and family history)	Compare estimated blood loss with patient-specific tolerable blood loss
Identify, evaluate, and treat anaemia	Review medications (antiplatelets, anticoagulants)	Assess and optimize patient's physiological reserve, e.g. pulmonary and cardiac function
Treat absolute or functional iron deficiency with oral or intravenous iron	Minimize iatrogenic blood loss	Formulate patient-specific management plan using appropriate blood conservation modalities
Consider erythropoiesis stimulating agents if nutritional anaemia is excluded/treated	Procedure planning and rehearsal	
Refer for further evaluation as necessary		

Au TH, Castillo S, Morrow L, Malesker M. Obstructive sleep apnea and continuous positive airway pressure: A primer for pharmacists2015. 30–3.

Health Organization and many of its principles have been endorsed and adopted internationally, including by the European Society of Anaesthesiology, the National Blood Transfusion Committee in the UK, the National Blood Authority in Australia, and the American Association of Blood Banks in the US. Central to the concept of PBM are the so-called three pillars of PBM (**Table 1.8**):

- Detection and management of anaemia to optimize red cell mass.
- Minimization of blood loss.
- Managing and optimizing patients' tolerance to anaemia.[30]

Each pillar comprises preoperative, intraoperative, and postoperative components. Each pillar should be considered in turn during the preoperative assessment, with appropriate involvement of the multi-disciplinary team (surgeon, anaesthetist, haematologist, and other relevant clinicians).

The first pillar of PBM in the preoperative phase includes all the strategies to detect and manage pre-existing anaemia, such that red cell mass is optimized at the time of surgery. Patients scheduled for major elective surgery (with an estimated blood loss of ≥500 mL)[31] should undergo screening tests for anaemia 4–6 weeks before surgery.[30] Any underlying cause should be identified and treated accordingly. Iron deficiency remains the most common cause of anaemia worldwide and patients with iron deficiency anaemia should be treated with oral iron therapy in the first instance. If the patient has failed oral iron therapy (insufficient response to treatment or intolerance), or if surgery is planned in <6 weeks, intravenous iron therapy is recommended as an alternative (as 3 months are required to replenish body iron stores fully). Other nutritional deficiencies should be treated with haematinics. The use of erythropoietin-stimulating agents may be considered if nutritional deficiencies have been corrected or excluded[30]—the 2018 ESA guidelines suggest that these agents may be used in conjunction with conventional iron therapy to accelerate red cell mass production.[12] Blood tests should be rechecked following a course of appropriate treatment.

The second pillar of PBM includes strategies to minimize bleeding and blood loss. In the preoperative phase, this should include a comprehensive review of the patient's medical background, drug history, laboratory results, and physical examination findings in order to identify conditions which predispose to bleeding and coagulopathy. These conditions (e.g. congenital bleeding disorders) should be corrected and optimized where possible. Patients who are taking anticoagulant medications should undergo an assessment of the thromboembolic risk associated with cessation of anticoagulant therapy versus the risk

of perioperative bleeding associated with continued use. In some cases, a perioperative bridging regimen will be indicated. The proposed surgical procedure and technique should be carefully planned in advance by the surgical team with consideration to the risk of bleeding so that iatrogenic blood loss due to the procedure itself is minimized.

The third pillar of PBM includes strategies to manage and optimize the patient's tolerance to anaemia. This refers to the ability of the patient's cardiopulmonary reserve to compensate for a decrease in oxygen-carrying capacity via an increase in cardiac output. Hence, it is important to assess the functional reserve of the cardiopulmonary system during the preoperative assessment in accordance with the approaches outlined in the 2014 ESC/ESA guideline[11] and 2014 ACC/AHA guideline.[15]

Every attempt should be made to correct anaemia to normal levels by implementing PBM principles prior to proceeding with elective surgery. Some of these principles may still be applicable for patients who require urgent or emergency surgery, though it may still be necessary to proceed despite suboptimal preoperative evaluation and optimization.

Preoperative risk stratification

Although low-risk procedures account for a significant proportion of OMFS caseload, in-hospital mortality has been reported to be around 3% for patients undergoing major head and neck operations within NHS England, while the overall mortality is around 1% for all maxillofacial and head and neck procedures in the UK. It is therefore important to identify patients at increased risk of perioperative morbidity and mortality to allow shared decision-making, informed consent, preoperative optimization, and modification of surgical pathways as required. While various risk stratification tools are available, the accuracy of risk prediction remains uncertain because OMFS accounted for only a small proportion of the surgical procedures included in the databases used during prediction tool development, and consequently there is a paucity of evidence supporting their validity in this particular field.

Prediction of morbidity and mortality

American Society of Anesthesiologists Physical Status (ASA-PS) score

The ASA-PS classification system was first developed in 1941 as a statistical tool for retrospective analysis of hospital records and was updated in 2014 to include BMI, alcohol intake, and smoking. An ASA class is assigned based upon the severity of systemic disease, if any, and the likelihood of survival without an operation being undertaken. The ASA-PS is widely adopted across many specialties, is simple to perform, and is validated for its association with perioperative morbidity and mortality. However, the risk specific to the planned surgical procedure is not taken into account. The ASA-PS is also reported to have poor inter-rater reliability, even among anaesthetists, due to the subjective nature of assessment.

Physiological and Operative Severity Score for the enUmeration of Mortality and Morbidity (POSSUM)

POSSUM was developed by Copeland et al. in 1991 from patients undergoing both elective and emergency gastrointestinal, hepatobiliary, urological, and vascular surgery. It uses 12 physiological and six surgical variables for the calculation of 30-day mortality. Portsmouth-POSSUM (P-POSSUM) is a newer model that requires the same input variables as POSSUM, but uses alternative equations for risk calculation. Both POSSUM and P-POSSUM are well validated in other surgical specialties; however, patients undergoing OMFS procedures were not included in the database. Therefore, the validity of these scores remains uncertain despite one small studying demonstrating reasonable discrimination.[32] In addition to a number of subjective assessments of physiological variables, input of intraoperative findings is also required, which limits the applicability and practicality of these tools in the preoperative setting.

Surgical Outcome Risk Tool (SORT)

In 2014, Protopapa et al. developed SORT from post hoc analysis of data from the 'Knowing the Risk' report of the National Confidential Enquiry into Patient Outcome and Death (NCEPOD), which comprised 16,788 patients undergoing both elective and emergency in-hospital surgical procedures. SORT requires the input of only six preoperative variables: ASA-PS, urgency of surgery, surgical specialty, severity of surgery, presence/absence of cancer, and age. It is simple to use, but it does not calculate morbidity and, to date, has not been validated for OMFS.

American College of Surgeons National Surgical Quality Improvement Project (NSQIP) surgical risk calculator

The NSQIP surgical risk calculator was developed in 2013, based on both inpatients and outpatients undergoing major surgical procedures in the private healthcare setting in the US. It requires input of 21 preoperative variables, such as age, sex, BMI, dyspnoea, previous myocardial infarction, and functional status. NSQIP has the largest data pool, consisting of 1.4 million patients, and predicts procedure-specific morbidity and mortality risks in addition to 14 other postoperative outcomes. However, the tool lacks validation in other populations, and the differing service sector must be taken into account.

Cardiopulmonary exercise testing (CPET)

CPET is the most sensitive and specific exercise capacity test for the purposes of preoperative risk stratification (compared with the shuttle test, 6-minute walk test, and the stair climb test). CPET allows assessment of the cardiopulmonary function by exercising patients on a bike ergometer through four key physiological stages (cardiodynamic, increased cellular respiration, steady state, and incremental work phases), deriving anaerobic threshold, peak oxygen consumption (peak VO_2), and ventilatory equivalents (VE/$VECO_2$)—all of which have been shown to be independent predictors of morbidity, mortality, and length of hospital stay. In addition to risk stratification, CPET can also direct preoperative optimization, identify undiagnosed pathology, and assess effectiveness of neoadjuvant cancer therapies. Its role in risk stratification and decision-making has been explored in a few small studies on patients with head and neck malignancy (with or without tissue reconstruction), and, although the findings are encouraging, further investigation is required.[33,34] It should be noted that CPET carries a reported mortality of 2–4 in 100,000, and is therefore not suitable for all patients, and should be undertaken in an appropriately equipped facility by trained personnel, as recommended by the American Thoracic Society and the Perioperative Exercise Testing and Training Society.[35]

Prediction of cardiac complications

Lee's Revised Cardiac Risk Index (RCRI)

Lee's RCRI was developed in 1999 by Lee et al. from 4315 patients undergoing non-emergency operations, to predict the risk of developing cardiac complications after major non-cardiac operations (including myocardial infarction, pulmonary oedema, ventricular fibrillation, cardiac arrest, and complete heart block). It utilizes six independent factors: high-risk surgery (intraperitoneal, intrathoracic, or suprainguinal vascular procedures); ischaemic heart disease; history of congestive heart failure; cerebrovascular disease (transient ischaemic attack or cerebrovascular accident); diabetes mellitus, on insulin; and preoperative serum creatinine >176 μmol/L). It is simple to use and is highly recommended by consensus guidelines on preoperative evaluation for non-cardiac surgery, including those by the ESC/ESA[11] and ACC/AHA.[15] Only one independent predictor refers to the nature of the planned operation, and its applicability to patients undergoing emergency or minor procedures remains unclear.

NSQIP Myocardial Infarction and Cardiac Arrest (MICA)

NSQIP-MICA was developed in 2011 from a multicentre study of 211,410 patients. It uses five predictors of perioperative myocardial infarction or cardiac arrest: type of surgery, functional status, abnormal serum creatinine, ASA, and age. NSQIP-MICA outperforms the RCRI in discriminative power among patients undergoing vascular surgery and is recommended for cardiac risk stratification by the ESA, whose consensus view is that NSQIP-MICA and Lee's RCRI are complementary in providing prognostic perspective in the decision-making process.

Biomarker assays

Preoperative blood levels of natriuretic peptides (brain natriuretic peptide or N-terminal pro-brain natriuretic peptide) and C-reactive protein have been shown to have incremental predictive value in several observational studies.[36-38] However, there are no data to suggest that targeting these biomarkers for treatment and intervention will reduce the postoperative risk. As such, the ESA does not recommend routine preoperative biomarker sampling in all patients for risk stratification purposes, but suggests brain natriuretic peptide levels may be used to provide independent prognostic information on perioperative and late cardiac events in high-risk patients undergoing major surgery.

Exercise capacity testing

This was described earlier in the 'Cardiopulmonary exercise testing (CPET)' section.

Perioperative management of medications

Many of the patients undergoing OMFS procedures take regular long-term medications for chronic medical conditions. Patients' medication history should be reviewed preoperatively by *all* the clinicians involved in their perioperative care, but in practice, this responsibility often resides with the anaesthetist, in their role as perioperative physician. Many organizations provide guidance on the perioperative management of long-term medications in patients undergoing non-cardiac surgery, including the ESC, ESA, ACC, and AHA. In general, long-term medications which are considered to exert beneficial effects during the perioperative period, or which may result in morbidity with abrupt cessation, should be continued, while those medications which are thought to increase anaesthetic or surgical risk should be discontinued.

Dual antiplatelet therapy

Dual antiplatelet therapy (DAPT) is currently indicated in patients following PCI for coronary artery disease and as an antithrombotic therapy following acute ischaemic stroke.

In the context of PCI, DAPT refers to the combination of aspirin with a $P2Y_{12}$ receptor antagonist, such as clopidogrel, prasugrel, or ticagrelor, to reduce the risk of coronary artery restenosis and stent thrombosis. This is especially important in the perioperative period, as the stress response to surgery has both proinflammatory and prothrombotic effects; however, the protective effects must be balanced with the increased bleeding risk. Thus, decisions regarding the perioperative continuation/cessation of DAPT must involve the multidisciplinary team, comprising a surgeon, anaesthetist, cardiologist, and haematologist. In elective surgery, if the procedure is deemed to have a low surgical bleeding risk (Table 1.9),[39] then the risk of stent thrombosis outweighs the risk of bleeding and hence DAPT should be continued. If, however, the risk of bleeding is moderate to high, then interruption of DAPT for surgery may be considered if the minimum recommended period of DAPT post-stent implantation has been completed. The 2017 ESC focused update

Table 1.9 Assessment of surgical bleeding risk in non-cardiac surgery

Surgical bleeding risk	Blood transfusion requirement	Type of surgery
Low	Usually not required	Peripheral, plastic, and general surgery biopsies Minor otolaryngology, and general surgery Endoscopy Anterior chamber eye surgery Dental extractions
Intermediate	Frequently required	Visceral surgery Otolaryngology Reconstructive surgery
High	Possible bleeding in a closed space	Intracranial neurosurgery Posterior chamber eye surgery

Oprea AD, Popescu WM. Perioperative management of antiplatelet therapy. Br J Anaesth. 2013;111 Suppl 1:i3–17.

on DAPT[40] recommended a minimum of 30 days of uninterrupted DAPT following PCI, regardless of stent type. The 2016 ACC/AHA focused update[41] recommends a minimum of 30 days for bare-metal stents, but a minimum of 3 months and optimally 6 months for drug-eluting stents (the risk of ischaemic events is higher with drug-eluting stents in the immediate months following PCI). A 6-month duration of DAPT may also benefit patients who are at increased ischaemic risk due to acute coronary syndrome at presentation or those who have undergone complex coronary revascularization procedures.

Ticagrelor, clopidogrel, and prasugrel should be stopped for at least 3, 5, or 7 days respectively before surgery to allow for adequate recovery of platelet function. Aspirin, as a sole antiplatelet agent, should be continued where possible unless the risk of bleeding is deemed to be excessively high. If it is necessary to discontinue both antiplatelet agents, a perioperative bridging strategy with short-acting, rapidly reversible intravenous antiplatelet agents such as cangrelor should be considered. The optimal time to restart DAPT following surgery should be a multidisciplinary decision, but ideally within 48 hours. Surgery in this group of patients should be performed at centres where 24-hour emergency PCI facilities are available. In the case of emergency surgery that cannot be delayed beyond the recommended minimum period of DAPT therapy post PCI, the multidisciplinary team must reach a consensus decision—where possible, DAPT should be continued to minimize the risk of catastrophic perioperative thrombosis; aspirin should be continued even if the $P2Y_{12}$ inhibitor is withheld; and if cessation of both agents is deemed necessary, then an intravenous bridging therapy should be considered.

In the context of acute cerebrovascular event prevention, DAPT usually refers to the combination of aspirin with clopidogrel or extended-release dipyridamole. It is beyond the scope of this chapter to discuss the approach to antithrombotic therapy in acute ischaemic stroke. Depending on the underlying aetiology and the stroke severity, a number of antithrombotic therapies are available, including monotherapies (with aspirin or clopidogrel alone), or DAPT.[42] The recommended duration of therapy is also variable, from 3 weeks in the case of a minor ischaemic stroke (National Institutes of Health Stroke Scale (NIHSS) ≤3) in the setting of small vessel disease,[43] to 3 months for higher severity ischaemic stroke (NIHSS >3) due to intracranial large artery atherosclerosis.[44] For patients taking DAPT at the time of surgery, the decision to continue/discontinue antiplatelet agents should be determined by the multidisciplinary team and guided by an individualized risk assessment of bleeding versus thrombosis. In general, aspirin monotherapy should be continued unless the bleeding risk is excessively high, or if bleeding may result in a catastrophic consequence (e.g. closed space surgery). Dipyridamole and clopidogrel should be stopped for at least 2 and 7 days respectively before surgery to allow platelet function to recover.

Aspirin

Aspirin irreversibly inhibits the action of cyclo-oxygenase enzymes COX-1 and COX-2. Its antithrombotic effects are mediated via its action on platelet COX-1. It is a mainstay of treatment in both the primary and secondary prevention of acute coronary syndrome and stroke. Although it may be useful in reducing perioperative thrombotic complications, its antithrombotic effects may also increase the risk of intra- and postoperative bleeding. In addition, the abrupt discontinuation of aspirin may also separately produce a rebound effect, resulting in a temporary prothrombotic state, which increases the risk of major adverse cardiovascular events. The 2014 ESC/ESA guidelines[11] and the 2014 ACC/AHA guidelines[15] both endorse an individualized approach to the perioperative management of patients on aspirin, considering the bleeding risk versus the risk of thrombotic complications. If the bleeding risk outweighs the potential cardiovascular benefits, aspirin should be stopped at least 7 days prior to surgery to allow for sufficient recovery of platelet function. Otherwise, it is reasonable to continue aspirin perioperatively, especially for patients with high-risk coronary artery disease or cerebrovascular disease.

Vitamin K antagonists

Vitamin K antagonists (VKAs) such as warfarin have a wide range of indications, from stroke prophylaxis in atrial fibrillation to the prevention of thromboembolic complications in patients with mechanical heart valves. VKAs exert their anticoagulant effects by inhibiting the action of vitamin K, thereby reducing the production of vitamin K-dependent coagulation factors II, VII, IX, and X. These factors are involved in various parts of the coagulation cascade, leading to the final formation of a stable fibrin clot. VKAs therefore increase the perioperative bleeding risk. The threshold at which surgery is considered safe to proceed with minimal increased risk of bleeding is generally regarded as an international normalized ratio (INR) ≤ 1.5. The interruption of VKAs for surgery can be especially hazardous in patients at particularly high risk of thromboembolic events, including:

- Atrial fibrillation and high CHA_2DS_2-VASc score ≥ 4 (**Table 1.10**)[45] (i.e. high risk of thromboembolic stroke).
- Mechanical prosthetic heart valves.
- Mitral valvular repair within the last 3 months.
- Recent venous thromboembolism or embolic stroke within the last 3 months.
- A history of thromboembolic events during previous discontinuation of anticoagulation.
- Hypercoagulable states (e.g. congenital thrombophilia syndromes or nephrotic syndrome).

Table 1.10 The CHA_2DS_2-VASc score, used to assess the risk of ischaemic stroke in patients with atrial fibrillation

Risk factor	Score
Congestive heart failure/left ventricular dysfunction (ejection fraction $\leq 40\%$)	1
Hypertension	1
Age ≥ 75 years	2
Diabetes mellitus	1
Stroke/transient ischaemic attack/thromboembolism	2
Vascular disease (previous myocardial infarction/peripheral vascular disease/aortic plaque)	1
Age 65–74 years	1
Sex categories (i.e. female sex)	1
Maximum score	9

Lip GY, Nieuwlaat R, Pisters R, Lane DA, Crijns HJ. Refining clinical risk stratification for predicting stroke and thromboembolism in atrial fibrillation using a novel risk factor-based approach: the euro heart survey on atrial fibrillation. Chest. 2010;137(2):263–72.

If the bleeding risk is deemed to be low, then it may not be necessary to interrupt VKA anticoagulation at all throughout the perioperative period. However, if the bleeding risk is high, and VKA anticoagulation has to be stopped perioperatively, then bridging anticoagulation with unfractionated heparin or therapeutic-dose low-molecular-weight heparin may be required, keeping the duration of subtherapeutic anticoagulation to a minimum. For patients taking warfarin for indications other than those listed above, the risk of perioperative bleeding with bridging therapy likely outweighs the risk of perioperative thromboembolic complications, such that routine bridging is probably not indicated even while VKA anticoagulation is interrupted.[46,47] Bridging regimens vary between institutions, but generally warfarin is withheld 3–5 days prior to surgery, and the international normalized ratio (INR) checked daily. Bridging therapy with unfractionated heparin or low-molecular-weight heparin is commenced once the INR is subtherapeutic. If the INR remains high on the day before surgery, vitamin K may be given to hasten normalization of INR, with surgery proceeding once the INR is ≤ 1.5. The timing of the discontinuation of the bridging agent is based upon its biological half-life, allowing sufficient time for clearance—intravenous unfractionated heparin, with a half-life of approximately 45 minutes, is usually discontinued 4–5 hours prior to surgery, while low-molecular-weight heparin, with a half-life of 3–5 hours, is usually discontinued 24 hours before surgery. Following surgery, the bridging agent should be restarted as soon as adequate haemostasis is achieved, typically by postoperative day 1 or 2. VKAs are also usually restarted on the same day, at the usual maintenance dose with or without an additional booster.[11] The INR is monitored daily, and the bridging agent stopped once the INR is within therapeutic range.

For urgent procedures, requiring the anticoagulant effect of VKAs to be rapidly reversed (within hours to days), the VKA should be discontinued and low-dose vitamin K (2.5–5.0 mg) given either orally or intravenously. For emergency procedures, where immediate reversal is required, the recommended reversal agent is now prothrombin complex concentrate (PCC). The dose is dependent on the initial INR and the weight of the patient. If PCC is not available, fresh frozen plasma at a dose of 12–15 mL/kg, can be given. These products produce a significant prothrombotic effect, which can be catastrophic in patients with an already high thromboembolic risk, so their use should be limited to life-threatening haemorrhage associated with a prolonged INR.

Direct oral anticoagulants

Direct oral anticoagulants (DOACs), also known as non-VKA direct oral anticoagulants (NOACs), are a newer class of anticoagulants now in widespread use (e.g. dabigatran, rivaroxaban, and apixaban). They exert their effects by directly inhibiting a specific factor in the coagulation cascade: dabigatran inhibits factor II (thrombin), while rivaroxaban and apixaban inhibit factor Xa. Due to their direct mechanism of action, they have a relatively rapid onset of action. Elimination depends upon adequate renal function, so there is the potential for accumulation in patients with renal impairment. The preoperative cessation period for DOACs is therefore variable, and depends on renal function and assessment of perioperative bleeding risk[48] (**Table 1.11**). In general, DOACs should be withheld for a time period two to three times their biological half-lives for surgery with low bleeding risk, and four to five times for surgery with moderate–high bleeding risk.[49]

Table 1.11 Recommended cessation periods between last dose of a DOAC and surgery

Renal function and related half-life	DOAC and current dose	Timing of last dose before surgery (number of hours)	
		Low bleeding risk surgery (2–3 half-lives between last dose and surgery)	High bleeding risk surgery (4–5 half-lives between last dose and surgery)
Creatinine clearance (CrCl) ≥50 mL/min half-life: 7–8 hours (hr)	Apixaban 5 mg twice daily	24	48–72
CrCl 30–49 mL/min half-life: 17–18 hr		48	72
CrCl ≥50 mL/min half-life: 5–9 hr	Rivaroxaban 20 mg once daily	24	48–72
CrCl 30–49 mL/min half-life: 9–13 hr		48	72
CrCl ≥50 mL/min half-life: 12–17 hr	Dabigatran 150 mg twice daily	24	48–72
CrCl 30–49 mL/min half-life: 13–23 hr		48–72	96

McIlmoyle K, Tran H. Perioperative management of oral anticoagulation. BJA Education. 2018;18(9):259–64.

As they have a quick onset of action, they should only be restarted after surgery when haemostasis has been adequately achieved and postsurgical bleeding risk is low. Bridging therapy is not usually recommended because the duration required for the drug to be withheld prior to surgery is short and its anticoagulant effect is rapidly achieved on re-initiation, *except* in patients where the risk of thromboembolism is unacceptably high. In these cases, the multidisciplinary team must decide upon the optimal perioperative anticoagulation strategy.

For emergency procedures requiring the immediate reversal of dabigatran, the recommended first-line agent is idarucizumab—a humanized monoclonal antibody fragment which binds to dabigatran. Activated PCC or four-factor PCC may be used as second-line alternatives.[50] Haemodialysis remains a further option if neither idarucizumab nor PCC products are available.[51] For patients requiring urgent reversal of factor Xa inhibitors, the current recommended first- and second-line options are four-factor PCC and activated PCC, respectively.[50] A specific reversal agent (andexanet) was approved by the US Food and Drug Administration in 2018 but is not yet in widespread use. Haemodialysis is not useful in the elimination of factor Xa inhibitors. Fresh frozen plasma is no longer recommended for the reversal of DOACs. **Table 1.12** summarizes the available reversal agents.[50]

Statins

Statins (3-hydroxy-3-methylglutaryl coenzyme A reductase inhibitors) are lipid-lowering agents used in the primary and secondary prevention of adverse cardiac events in patients with cardiovascular risk factors. They are also effective in improving perioperative cardiovascular outcomes in these patients. The exact mechanisms by which statins confer cardiovascular protection remain unclear, but may be related to both pleiotropic effects (e.g. coronary plaque stabilization) as well as lipid-lowering effects. Both the 2014 ESC/ESA guidelines[11] and the 2014 ACC/AHA guidelines[15] endorse the perioperative continuation of existing statin therapy in patients undergoing non-cardiac surgery. For patients who are not already on statin treatment, there is probably no benefit in initiating statins preoperatively unless they already meet the existing criteria for statin therapy, especially since potential adverse side effects may be significant (e.g. statin-induced myopathy and rhabdomyolysis).[11] For patients that do meet the criteria, statins should be commenced as soon as possible, and ideally no less than 2 weeks before surgery, to allow maximal plaque-stabilizing benefit.[11] Since these patients have a high baseline cardiovascular risk, it would also be reasonable to continue with statin therapy beyond the perioperative period, at least until further review, in order to minimize long-term cardiovascular risk.

Angiotensin antagonists

There remains considerable debate as to whether angiotensin-converting enzyme inhibitors (ACEIs) and angiotensin II receptor blockers (ARBs) should be continued throughout the perioperative period. ACEIs and ARBs preserve organ function and have prognostic benefits for patients with heart failure and/or left ventricular systolic dysfunction. The main concern with the perioperative continuation of these agents is the increased risk of intraoperative hypotension, especially following induction of anaesthesia, although this has not been shown to be associated with

Table 1.12 VKA and DOAC reversal agents and their suggested use

Reversal agent	VKA (warfarin)	Factor IIa inhibitor (dabigatran)	Factor Xa inhibitor (apixaban, edoxaban and rivaroxaban)
Four-factor prothrombin complex concentrate (4F-PCC)	First line	Second line	First line
Activated prothrombin complex concentrate	Not indicated	Second line	Second line
Idarucizumab	Not indicated	First line	Not indicated
Fresh frozen plasma	If 4F-PCC is unavailable	Not indicated	Not indicated

a difference in major adverse cardiovascular outcomes.[52] There is also no strong evidence of cardiovascular risk reduction with continuation of existing treatment, despite the theoretical benefits.[53] Current guidelines therefore recommend that continuation of existing ACEI or ARB medication in the setting of non-cardiac surgery should at least be considered, especially if the indication for initiation was stable heart failure and/or left ventricular systolic dysfunction. For patients taking these medications for hypertension alone, temporary discontinuation (at least 24 hours prior to surgery) should be considered, due to the risk of intraoperative hypotension. If treatment is continued, blood pressure should be closely monitored intraoperatively and significant hypotension avoided. For patients with stable heart failure and/or left ventricular systolic dysfunction who are not yet taking ACEIs or ARBs, preoperative initiation of these medications at least 1 week before surgery should also be considered.[11] If ACEIs or ARBs are discontinued before surgery, they should be restarted as soon as possible following surgery (if haemodynamically stable), as inappropriate cessation of existing therapy is associated with impaired cardiovascular outcomes.[11,15]

Beta-blockers

Beta-blockers may provide a degree of perioperative cardioprotection by reducing myocardial oxygen consumption through a decrease in both heart rate and contractility. Multiple meta-analyses on perioperative beta-blocker usage have shown a significant reduction in adverse cardiac events (e.g. myocardial infarction, atrial fibrillation), especially in patients at high risk of myocardial ischaemia.[54] For patients already on existing beta-blocker therapy, consensus supports their continuation throughout the perioperative period, as preoperative discontinuation is associated with increased mortality. Conversely, the POISE trial demonstrated that the preoperative introduction of beta-blockers was associated with stroke, hypotension, bradycardia, and an increase in all-cause mortality[55] (though the study received criticism for its design, which led to increased hypotensive episodes and a higher incidence of stroke in the study population). The 2014 ESC/ESA guidelines and the 2014 ACC/AHA guidelines recommend that preoperative beta-blocker initiation (with cardioselective atenolol or bisoprolol first line) should be considered in patients at high risk of perioperative myocardial ischaemia (known ischaemic heart disease, or at least two clinical risk factors according to Lee's RCRI, or ASA status ≥3) if they are undergoing high-risk surgery.[11] However, in patients without these clinical risk factors or in those undergoing low-risk surgery, the potential harm of perioperative initiation of beta-blockers may outweigh the benefits, and is therefore not recommended (even if the patient has been identified as meeting existing criteria for long-term beta-blocker therapy). In such cases, beta-blockers should be commenced as soon as possible after surgery. If the decision is made to initiate beta-blockers prior to surgery for the purposes of perioperative cardiac risk reduction, treatment should not be started on the day of surgery. Instead, at least 2 days (and ideally up to 30 days) should be allowed for dose titration to achieve optimal heart rate and blood pressure targets. If there are long-term indications to support their use, then it would be reasonable to continue them beyond the perioperative period.

Conclusion

Preoperative assessment should target the challenges specific to the underlying oromaxillofacial condition and planned operative procedure. A risk stratification tool should be employed during this process to facilitate optimal planning of the perioperative care. This is particularly important in patients with extensive comorbidities undergoing major OMFS. Long-term medications should be thoroughly reviewed, and appropriately adjusted in order to ensure safe perioperative patient care and the best patient outcome.

REFERENCES

1. Cook TM, Woodall N, Frerk C, Fourth National Audit P. Major complications of airway management in the UK: results of the Fourth National Audit Project of the Royal College of Anaesthetists and the Difficult Airway Society. Part 1: anaesthesia. *Br J Anaesth.* 2011;**106**(5):617–631.

2. Morosan M, Parbhoo A, Curry N. Anaesthesia and common oral and maxillo-facial emergencies. *Cont Educ Anaesth Crit Care Pain.* 2012;**12**(5):257–262.

3. Rhodes A, Evans LE, Alhazzani W, Levy MM, Antonelli M, Ferrer R, et al. Surviving Sepsis Campaign: international guidelines for management of sepsis and septic shock: 2016. *Intensive Care Med.* 2017;**43**(3):304–377.

4. Bailey CR, Ahuja M, Bartholomew K, Bew S, Forbes L, Lipp A, et al. Guidelines for day-case surgery 2019: guidelines from the Association of Anaesthetists and the British Association of Day Surgery. *Anaesthesia.* 2019;**74**(6):778–792.

5. Association of Paediatric Anaesthetists of Great Britain and Ireland. Guidelines for the management of children referred for dental extraction under general anesthesia: guidelines from the Association of Paediatric Anaesthetists of Great Britain & Ireland, the Royal College of Anaesthetists, the Association of Anaesthetists of Great Britain & Ireland, the Association of Dental Anaesthetists, the British Society of Paediatric Dentistry, GDP, and the Royal College of Nursing. 2011. https://www.bspd.co.uk/Portals/0/Public/Files/Guidelines/Main%20Dental%20Guidelines.pdf

6. Sleep-related breathing disorders in adults: recommendations for syndrome definition and measurement techniques in clinical research. The Report of an American Academy of Sleep Medicine Task Force. *Sleep.* 1999;**22**(5):667–689.

7. American Society of Anesthesiologists Task Force on Perioperative Management of Patients with Obstructive Sleep Apnea. Practice guidelines for the perioperative management of patients with obstructive sleep apnea: an updated report by the American Society of Anesthesiologists Task Force on Perioperative Management of patients with obstructive sleep apnea. *Anesthesiology.* 2014;**120**(2):268–286.

8. Hall A. Sleep physiology and the perioperative care of patients with sleep disorders. *BJA Educ.* 2014;**15**(4):167–172.

9. Abdelsattar ZM, Hendren S, Wong SL, Campbell DA, Jr., Ramachandran SK. The impact of untreated obstructive sleep apnea on cardiopulmonary complications in general and vascular surgery: a cohort study. *Sleep.* 2015;**38**(8):1205–1210.

10. Martinez G, Faber P. Obstructive Sleep apnoea. *Continuing Education in Anaesthesia Critical Care & Pain.* 2011;**11**(1):5–8.

11. Kristensen SD, Knuuti J, Saraste A, Anker S, Botker HE, Hert SD, et al. 2014 ESC/ESA guidelines on non-cardiac surgery: cardiovascular assessment and management: the Joint Task Force on non-cardiac surgery: cardiovascular assessment and management of the European Society of Cardiology (ESC) and the European Society of Anaesthesiology (ESA). *Eur Heart J.* 2014;**35**(35):2383–2431.

12. De Hert S, Staender S, Fritsch G, Hinkelbein J, Afshari A, Bettelli G, et al. Pre-operative evaluation of adults undergoing elective noncardiac surgery: updated guideline from the European Society of Anaesthesiology. *Eur J Anaesthesiol.* 2018;**35**(6):407–465.

13. Clavellina-Gaytan D, Velazquez-Fernandez D, Del-Villar E, Dominguez-Cherit G, Sanchez H, Mosti M, et al. Evaluation of spirometric testing as a routine preoperative assessment in patients undergoing bariatric surgery. *Obes Surg.* 2015;**25**(3):530–536.

14. Fernandez-Bustamante A, Bartels K, Clavijo C, Scott BK, Kacmar R, Bullard K, et al. Preoperatively screened obstructive sleep apnea is associated with worse postoperative outcomes than previously diagnosed obstructive sleep apnea. *Anesth Analg.* 2017;**125**(2):593–602.

15. Fleisher LA, Fleischmann KE, Auerbach AD, Barnason SA, Beckman JA, Bozkurt B, et al. 2014 ACC/AHA guideline on perioperative cardiovascular evaluation and management of patients undergoing noncardiac surgery: a report of the American College of Cardiology/American Heart Association Task Force on Practice Guidelines. *Circulation.* 2014;**130**(24):e278–e333.

16. Calder CL, Ortega G, Vij A, Chawla K, Nnamdi-Emetarom C, Stephanie S, et al. Morbid obesity is an independent risk factor for postoperative renal dysfunction in young adults: a review of the American College of Surgeons National Surgical Quality Improvement Program database. *Am J Surg.* 2016;**211**(4):772–777.

17. Goren O, Matot I. Perioperative acute kidney injury. *Br J Anaesth.* 2015;**115** Suppl 2:ii3–ii14.

18. Frisch A, Chandra P, Smiley D, Peng L, Rizzo M, Gatcliffe C, et al. Prevalence and clinical outcome of hyperglycemia in the perioperative period in noncardiac surgery. *Diabetes Care.* 2010;**33**(8):1783–1788.

19. Membership of the Working Party, Barker P, Creasey PE, Dhatariya K, Levy N, Lipp A, et al. Peri-operative management of the surgical patient with diabetes 2015: Association of Anaesthetists of Great Britain and Ireland. *Anaesthesia.* 2015;**70**(12):1427–1440.

20. Wolf E, Utech M, Stehle P, Busing M, Stoffel-Wagner B, Ellinger S. Preoperative micronutrient status in morbidly obese patients before undergoing bariatric surgery: results of a cross-sectional study. *Surg Obes Relat Dis.* 2015;**11**(5):1157–1163.

21. Lee TH, Marcantonio ER, Mangione CM, Thomas EJ, Polanczyk CA, Cook EF, et al. Derivation and prospective validation of a simple index for prediction of cardiac risk of major noncardiac surgery. *Circulation.* 1999;**100**(10):1043–1049.

22. Neumann FJ, Sousa-Uva M, Ahlsson A, Alfonso F, Banning AP, Benedetto U, et al. 2018 ESC/EACTS guidelines on myocardial revascularization. *Eur Heart J.* 2019;**40**(2):87–165.

23. McFalls EO, Ward HB, Moritz TE, Goldman S, Krupski WC, Littooy F, et al. Coronary-artery revascularization before elective major vascular surgery. *N Engl J Med.* 2004;**351**(27):2795–2804.

24. Mookadam F, Carpenter SD, Thota VR, Cha S, Jiamsripong P, Alharthi MS, et al. Risk of adverse events after coronary artery bypass graft and subsequent noncardiac surgery. *Future Cardiol.* 2011;7(1):69–75.

25. Howell SJ, Sear JW, Foex P. Hypertension, hypertensive heart disease and perioperative cardiac risk. *Br J Anaesth.* 2004;**92**(4):570–583.

26. Williams B, Mancia G, Spiering W, Agabiti Rosei E, Azizi M, Burnier M, et al. 2018 ESC/ESH guidelines for the management of arterial hypertension. *Eur Heart J.* 2018;**39**(33):3021–3104.

27. Mancia G, Fagard R, Narkiewicz K, Redon J, Zanchetti A, Bohm M, et al. 2013 ESH/ESC guidelines for the management of arterial hypertension: the Task Force for the Management of Arterial Hypertension of the European Society of Hypertension (ESH) and of the European Society of Cardiology (ESC). *Eur Heart J.* 2013;**34**(28):2159–2219.

28. Hartle A, McCormack T, Carlisle J, Anderson S, Pichel A, Beckett N, et al. The measurement of adult blood pressure and management of hypertension before elective surgery: joint guidelines from the Association of Anaesthetists of Great Britain and Ireland and the British Hypertension Society. *Anaesthesia.* 2016;**71**(3):326–337.

29. Shander A, Knight K, Thurer R, Adamson J, Spence R. Prevalence and outcomes of anemia in surgery: a systematic review of the literature. *Am J Med.* 2004;**116** Suppl 7A:58S–69S.

30. Thakrar SV, Clevenger B, Mallett S. Patient blood management and perioperative anaemia. *BJA Educ.* 2016;**17**(1):28–34.

31. Munoz M, Acheson AG, Auerbach M, Besser M, Habler O, Kehlet H, et al. International consensus statement on the peri-operative management of anaemia and iron deficiency. *Anaesthesia.* 2017;**72**(2):233–247.

32. Scott N, Jones J, Hulbert J, Kittur MA, Parkin R, Silvester KC, et al. Possum scoring and risk prediction in head and neck surgery. *Br J Oral Maxillofac Surg.* 2014;**52**(8):e53.

33. Lalabekyan BB, Tetlow N, Moonesinghe R, Martin D, Burdett E, Otto J, et al. Cardiopulmonary exercise testing and cardiopulmonary morbidity in patients undergoing major head and neck surgery. *Br J Oral Maxillofac Surg.* 2021;**59**(3):297–302.

34. Fernandes N, Hussain M, Ho M, Kanatas A, Fabbroni G, Ong TK, et al. The value of cardiopulmonary exercise testing as a prognostic indicator for head and neck cancer patients considered for primary surgery. *Br J Oral Maxillofac Surg.* 2018;**56**(10):e62.

35. Levett DZH, Jack S, Swart M, Carlisle J, Wilson J, Snowden C, et al. Perioperative cardiopulmonary exercise testing (CPET): consensus clinical guidelines on indications, organization, conduct, and physiological interpretation. *Br J Anaesth.* 2018;**120**(3):484–500.

36. Dernellis J, Panaretou M. Assessment of cardiac risk before non-cardiac surgery: brain natriuretic peptide in 1590 patients. *Heart.* 2006;**92**(11):1645–1650.

37. Rodseth RN, Padayachee L, Biccard BM. A meta-analysis of the utility of pre-operative brain natriuretic peptide in predicting early and intermediate-term mortality and major adverse cardiac events in vascular surgical patients. *Anaesthesia.* 2008;**63**(11):1226–1233.

38. Karthikeyan G, Moncur RA, Levine O, Heels-Ansdell D, Chan MT, Alonso-Coello P, et al. Is a pre-operative brain natriuretic peptide or N-terminal pro-B-type natriuretic peptide measurement an independent predictor of adverse cardiovascular outcomes within 30 days of noncardiac surgery? A systematic review and meta-analysis of observational studies. *J Am Coll Cardiol.* 2009;**54**(17):1599–1606.

39. Oprea AD, Popescu WM. Perioperative management of antiplatelet therapy. *Br J Anaesth.* 2013;**111** Suppl 1:i3–i17.

40. Valgimigli M, Bueno H, Byrne RA, Collet JP, Costa F, Jeppsson A, et al. 2017 ESC focused update on dual antiplatelet therapy in coronary artery disease developed in collaboration with EACTS: the Task Force for dual antiplatelet therapy in coronary artery disease of the European Society of Cardiology (ESC) and of the European Association for Cardio-Thoracic Surgery (EACTS). *Eur Heart J.* 2018;**39**(3):213–260.

41. Levine GN, Bates ER, Bittl JA, Brindis RG, Fihn SD, Fleisher LA, et al. 2016 ACC/AHA guideline focused update on duration of dual antiplatelet therapy in patients with coronary artery disease: a report of the American College of Cardiology/American Heart Association Task Force on Clinical Practice Guidelines. *J Am Coll Cardiol.* 2016;**68**(10):1082–1115.

42. Hackam DG, Spence JD. Antiplatelet therapy in ischemic stroke and transient ischemic attack. *Stroke.* 2019;**50**(3):773–778.

43. Prasad K, Siemieniuk R, Hao Q, Guyatt G, O'Donnell M, Lytvyn L, et al. Dual antiplatelet therapy with aspirin and clopidogrel for acute high risk transient ischaemic attack and minor ischaemic stroke: a clinical practice guideline. *BMJ.* 2018;**363**:k5130.

44. Chimowitz MI, Lynn MJ, Derdeyn CP, Turan TN, Fiorella D, Lane BF, et al. Stenting versus aggressive medical therapy for intracranial arterial stenosis. *N Engl J Med.* 2011;**365**(11):993–1003.

45. Lip GY, Nieuwlaat R, Pisters R, Lane DA, Crijns HJ. Refining clinical risk stratification for predicting stroke and thromboembolism in atrial fibrillation using a novel risk factor-based approach: the Euro Heart Survey on atrial fibrillation. *Chest.* 2010;**137**(2):263–272.

46. Douketis JD, Spyropoulos AC, Kaatz S, Becker RC, Caprini JA, Dunn AS, et al. Perioperative bridging anticoagulation in patients with atrial fibrillation. *N Engl J Med.* 2015;**373**(9):823–833.

47. January CT, Wann LS, Calkins H, Chen LY, Cigarroa JE, Cleveland JC Jr, et al. 2019 AHA/ACC/HRS Focused Update of the 2014 AHA/ACC/HRS guideline for the management of patients with atrial fibrillation: a report of the American College of Cardiology/American Heart Association Task Force on Clinical Practice Guidelines and the Heart Rhythm Society. *J Am Coll Cardiol.* 2019;**140**(2):e125–e151.

48. McIlmoyle K, Tran H. Perioperative management of oral anticoagulation. *BJA Educ.* 2018;**18**(9):259–264.

49. De Caterina R, Husted S, Wallentin L, Andreotti F, Arnesen H, Bachmann F, et al. New oral anticoagulants in atrial fibrillation and acute coronary syndromes: ESC Working Group on Thrombosis-Task Force on Anticoagulants in Heart Disease position paper. *J Am Coll Cardiol.* 2012;**59**(16):1413–1425.

50. Tomaselli GF, Mahaffey KW, Cuker A, Dobesh PP, Doherty JU, Eikelboom JW, et al. 2017 ACC expert consensus decision pathway on management of bleeding in patients on oral anticoagulants: a report of the American College of Cardiology Task Force on Expert Consensus Decision Pathways. *J Am Coll Cardiol.* 2017;**70**(24):3042–3067.

51. Camm AJ, Lip GY, De Caterina R, Savelieva I, Atar D, Hohnloser SH, et al. 2012 focused update of the ESC Guidelines for the management of atrial fibrillation: an update of the 2010 ESC Guidelines for the management of atrial fibrillation. Developed with the special contribution of the European Heart Rhythm Association. *Eur Heart J.* 2012;**33**(21):2719–2747.

52. Hollmann C, Fernandes NL, Biccard BM. A systematic review of outcomes associated with withholding or continuing angiotensin-converting enzyme inhibitors and angiotensin receptor blockers before noncardiac surgery. *Anesth Analg.* 2018;**127**(3):678–687.

53. Bertrand M, Godet G, Meersschaert K, Brun L, Salcedo E, Coriat P. Should the angiotensin II antagonists be discontinued before surgery? *Anesth Analg.* 2001;**92**(1):26–30.

54. McGory ML, Maggard MA, Ko CY. A meta-analysis of perioperative beta blockade: what is the actual risk reduction? *Surgery.* 2005;**138**(2):171–179.

55. Group PS, Devereaux PJ, Yang H, Yusuf S, Guyatt G, Leslie K, et al. Effects of extended-release metoprolol succinate in patients undergoing non-cardiac surgery (POISE trial): a randomised controlled trial. *Lancet.* 2008;**371**(9627):1839–1847.

2

Difficult airway

Craig Lyons and Ellen P. O'Sullivan

Introduction

The fundamental goal of airway management is to ensure the reliable delivery of oxygen to the lungs. Thirty-nine per cent of airway complications reported to the fourth National Audit Project of the Royal College of Anaesthetists involved patients with acute or chronic head and neck disease.[1] The majority of incidents related to anaesthesia for diagnostic or resection surgery, half of which occurred at induction of anaesthesia, with the remainder arising during maintenance, emergence, or in recovery. Airway management for oral and maxillofacial surgery, therefore, presents unique challenges, requiring an adaptable, diverse skill set that is tailored to the patient's pathology and facilitates the surgical procedure.

Airway assessment

The aim of preoperative airway assessment is to formulate a personalized airway management plan that minimizes the risk of complications. This is particularly important for patients with oromaxillofacial or head and neck pathology, as they commonly have abnormal airways. First of all, it is important to determine the methods by which oxygenation of the patient is likely to be successful, as both primary and rescue strategies. These are primarily face mask ventilation, supraglottic airway device (SAD) insertion, tracheal intubation, and front-of-neck access.

Assessment includes history taking and examination, a review of previous investigations (such as a recent intubation, nasendoscopy, and imaging studies of the airway), and a discussion with the surgeon regarding an appropriate airway plan. However, difficult airway management may be unanticipated, and so several alternative airway strategies must be in reserve for all patients, with adequate equipment and skills for their immediate implementation. Stridor, hoarseness, and intolerance of lying flat are concerning features in the history. Prior radiotherapy of the neck tissues can impair all facets of airway management from face mask ventilation to landmark identification for front-of-neck access. Patient comorbidities should be carefully assessed as they may directly impact airway assessment, such as restricted neck movement in the patient with rheumatoid arthritis and possible obstructive sleep apnoea.

Individual elements of clinical examination have a low positive predictive value for difficult airway management. When combined, their predictive value modestly increases, but not to the degree that they can be relied upon to confirm or exclude a difficult airway for any given patient.[2,3] 'Easy' airway management is ultimately a retrospective diagnosis. Clinical examination includes assessment of obvious facial deformities, facial hair, dentition, and range of neck motion. Mouth opening is assessed by inter-incisor distance. If reduced (<3 cm), it makes direct laryngoscopy challenging and can preclude the insertion of a videolaryngoscope. The modified Mallampati score (1–4) is based on the anatomical structures seen with maximal protrusion of the tongue from an open mouth in the sitting position. A higher score is associated with greater difficulty in airway management. Jaw protrusion is assessed by asking the patient to place their lower incisors as far forward as possible. Failure to advance the lower teeth as far as the upper teeth is predictive of difficult intubation, as is the inability of the lower incisors to bite the vermilion border of the upper lip.[4] Difficult laryngoscopy is associated with a thyromental distance of <6 cm and a sternomental distance of <13.5 cm, which are measured with the head extended from the mental prominence to the thyroid and sternal notches, respectively.[5,6] Patients presenting for major oromaxillofacial or head and neck surgery have typically undergone computed tomographic or magnetic resonance imaging. This should form part of airway assessment, which may be enhanced by discussion with a radiologist. It can be particularly informative in relation to glottic and subglottic pathologies which are not amenable to assessment by clinical examination.

Airway anatomy can be assessed via flexible nasendoscopy, either preoperatively or prior to induction of anaesthesia. An outpatient nasendoscopy may have been undertaken by the surgeon, though findings can become outdated with a rapidly growing tumour. Since it is performed awake, it does not necessarily reflect circumstances under anaesthesia, where loss of pharyngeal tone promotes upper airway obstruction. This caveat also applies to any virtual endoscopic examination undertaken on airway models that have been reconstructed from imaging studies. Nonetheless, nasendoscopy can significantly influence airway management, tipping the balance in favour of awake intubation, or indeed allaying concerns sufficient to proceed with induction of anaesthesia. Ultrasound can also be used to pre-emptively identify the cricothyroid membrane and to guide advancement towards the membrane during the procedure itself.[7]

All documentation of previous airway management should be reviewed. This alone can highlight difficulties which would have otherwise been unanticipated. Likewise, detailed documentation of airway management on this occasion is important for informing clinicians involved in future patient care. All documentation represents a snapshot in time that may not continue to reflect the patient's airway status. Airway assessment does not cease after induction of anaesthesia. The anaesthetist must continually appraise the security of oxygenation, which can be jeopardized by surgical manipulation of the airway and at emergence of anaesthesia.

The airway plan

There is no one-size-fits-all approach to airway management. At all stages, the anaesthetist should assess whether the airway plan, personnel, equipment, or location could be further optimized. A fundamental decision is whether to intubate the trachea with the patient awake (with or without sedation) or under general anaesthesia. No approach to the airway, awake or under anaesthesia, is devoid of complications or guaranteed to bring success.

Traditionally, inhalational induction has been performed in an effort to maintain spontaneous respiration. However, this approach can transition to a scenario where spontaneous respiration becomes inadequate, such as with the loss of airway patency, but the patient is not adequately anaesthetized to allow for satisfactory airway instrumentation. A rescue plan in this scenario would commonly necessitate the administration of neuromuscular blocking drugs. As these agents improve the likelihood of successful oxygenation, their administration from the outset arguably represents a more logical approach. Thus, most anaesthetists would typically select either an awake approach or an intravenous induction with neuromuscular blocking drug when difficulty is anticipated. Awake intubation is chosen when there are heightened concerns that intubation under general anaesthesia could prove problematic. When it is felt that airway management could deteriorate to the point of requiring emergency tracheostomy, it should take place in the operating theatre rather than the induction room. Indeed, such circumstances may require the performance of a tracheostomy under local anaesthesia from the outset.

Repeated airway instrumentation can create a spiral of worsening airway conditions and convert challenging airway management into impossible airway management.[8] Bleeding, soiling, worsening airway oedema, and fragmentation of diseased tissues can all arise. The first attempt at airway management for all patients should, therefore, reflect the anaesthetist's assessment of what constitutes the best attempt. Key elements to consider in this regard include positioning, preoxygenation, apnoeic oxygenation, and neuromuscular blockade. When difficulty is encountered, subsequent attempts are informed in real time by the anaesthetist's perception of the barriers to oxygenation. A key tenet is that repeating the same approach to airway management, and hoping for a different outcome, typically results in continued failure.

During an airway crisis, the specific conduit for oxygen delivery is of secondary importance, as is the degree of ventilation attained. This is reflected in the increasingly used 'can't intubate, can't oxygenate' (CICO) terminology in lieu of 'can't intubate, can't ventilate' (CICV), emphasizing oxygenation as the main priority. If a route of oxygenation is established with difficulty, such as with a SAD, the clinician must appraise whether efforts at tracheal intubation are now appropriate. For example, they may make a further attempt at intubation with laryngoscopy, intubate via a SAD, or allow the patient to wake up (and subsequently perform an awake intubation or postpone surgery). Any intervention risks progression to a CICO scenario.

Monitoring of heart rate, blood pressure, and oxygen saturation is essential during all airway management, as is the use of capnography for confirmation of correct tube placement.

Positioning

Optimal positioning for direct laryngoscopy involves neck flexion and head extension, termed the 'sniffing' position. Obese patients are 'ramped', often with dedicated pillows, such that the external auditory meatus is aligned with the suprasternal notch. This position improves respiratory mechanics and assists with laryngoscopy.[9]

Preoxygenation

Preoxygenation refers to the administration of 100% oxygen to replace the nitrogen present in the lungs and to increase body oxygen stores. It is undertaken prior to an airway intervention, where there is a risk that the supply of oxygen to the lungs may be interrupted. This is not isolated to induction of anaesthesia, also relating to an intraoperative change in airway management and emergence. Preoxygenation delays the onset of hypoxaemia should oxygen delivery become compromised, allowing more time for rescue interventions. Given that difficult airway management is often unpredictable, universal use of preoxygenation is advocated.

Maximal benefit from preoxygenation is derived at induction when performed in an upright position for at least 3 minutes, with confirmation of an adequate face mask seal with capnography and the attainment of an end-tidal oxygen concentration of >0.85.[10] Every effort should be undertaken to overcome an incomplete seal, such as two-handed face mask application, placement of transparent film over facial hair, or the use of a mouthpiece. Preoxygenation is further enhanced by the application of continuous or bilevel positive airway pressure. Despite a limited evidence base, high-flow nasal cannulae are increasingly used for preoxygenation to allow for a smooth transition to apnoeic oxygenation during airway instrumentation.

Neuromuscular blockade

The administration of a neuromuscular blocking drug enhances the likelihood of tracheal intubation, and also of successful rescue attempts at oxygenation via face mask and SAD.[11,12] Maximal neuromuscular blockade should, therefore, be ensured before laryngoscopy, and is frequently achieved by the administration of 1 mg/kg rocuronium. The placement of a quantitative nerve stimulator at induction of anaesthesia offers an objective assessment of the adequacy of neuromuscular blockade, helping to curtail early suboptimal efforts, and is advocated in monitoring guidelines from the Association of Anaesthetists.[13]

Apnoeic oxygenation

Apnoeic oxygenation refers to oxygenation in the absence of spontaneous respiration or positive pressure ventilation.[14] This technique allows for continued oxygenation following onset of apnoea at induction of anaesthesia. By prolonging the time to oxygen desaturation, a stop–start approach to engage in efforts at re-saturation is made less likely, thereby extending the 'safe apnoea time' to allow for definitive airway management.

Oxygen insufflation is most commonly achieved via nasal cannulae, allowing for largely unimpeded airway instrumentation, while other options include face mask, nasopharyngeal catheter, and front-of-neck catheter. Apnoeic oxygenation with low-flow nasal cannulae has been termed NODESAT (nasal oxygen during efforts securing a tube),[15] while a similar approach using high-flow nasal cannulae is commonly known as THRIVE (transnasal humidified rapid insufflation ventilatory exchange).[16] The latter allows for more prolonged oxygenation and can also assist with clearance of carbon dioxide. Optimal settings remain unknown; flow rates of 60–80 L/min at a fraction of inspired oxygen (FiO_2) of 1.0 are the most widely reported.

In an airway crisis, failure of more common oxygenation methods (bag mask ventilation, SAD insertion, and tracheal intubation) is often secondary to loss of upper airway patency, which is also necessary for successful apnoeic oxygenation via nasal or oral routes. Therefore, apnoeic oxygenation is most likely to fail in those circumstances where its success is most desired. It should be regarded as a supplemental effort at oxygenation rather than a primary oxygenation technique. High-flow nasal oxygen can also be used as an intraoperative oxygenation technique for the apnoeic patient in scenarios where the presence of a tracheal tube is impeding short-duration surgery.[17] However, diathermy and laser should be used with caution, given the increased risk of airway fire with an open oxygenation system.

Bag mask ventilation

Bag mask ventilation with 100% oxygen during the apnoeic period enables administration of oxygen between intubation attempts and is a core rescue technique. Difficult face mask ventilation is assisted with a two- or four-handed technique and the use of airway adjuncts such as an oropharyngeal airway. Placement of airway adjuncts must be undertaken with care as they can lead to airway trauma and bleeding, particularly in patients with intraoral pathologies.

Supraglottic airway devices

A SAD is occasionally used in lieu of a tracheal tube for airway management during oral and maxillofacial surgery, particularly for minor procedures. This device does not prevent aspiration. Rotation of the cuff can lead to an inadequate seal that impairs gas exchange or stimulates airway reflexes leading to laryngospasm. Furthermore, efforts at troubleshooting and rectifying problems with this airway device may require a pause in surgery and encroachment upon the surgical field.

SADs can occupy a life-saving role during rescue of the difficult airway by re-establishing oxygenation. They can subsequently offer a conduit for the passage of a tracheal tube.

Second-generation SADs are those with design elements that aim to reduce the risk of aspiration, such as an oesophageal conduit for the diversion of any regurgitant gastric contents away from the respiratory tract and to enable the placement of a gastric tube. Common second-generation SADs include the i-gel (Intersurgical, Wokingham, UK), laryngeal mask airway (LMA) Supreme (Teleflex Medical, Athlone, Ireland), ProSeal LMA (Teleflex Medical, Athlone, Ireland), and Laryngeal Tube Suction (VBM Medizintechnik GmbH, Sulz am Neckar, Germany). These devices exhibit improved safety and efficacy when compared with first-generation SADs.[18]

The reinforced LMA has a flexible wire-reinforced shaft which enables its position to be adjusted to reduce impingement on the surgical site. This flexibility can make insertion more difficult. It is commonly used during dental surgery and tonsillectomy.

In the scenario of difficult airway management, attempts at SAD insertion should be limited, much like attempts at tracheal intubation, as they are associated with trauma and diminishing success. Causes of a malpositioned SAD include folding of the tip of the cuff, lodgement of the cuff tip between the vocal cords, and presence of the epiglottis in the bowl of the SAD.[19] Each attempt at SAD insertion should differ in approach, such as the selection of an alternative type or size. Jaw thrust, laryngoscopy, or the railroading of a SAD over a bougie or orogastric tube can assist with successful siting of the device.[20,21]

Once oxygenation through a SAD is achieved, the anaesthetist must balance the risks and benefits in deciding whether to proceed with this device *in situ*, to attempt intubation via the SAD, or to wake the patient up. Key considerations include aspiration risk, tolerance for spontaneous respiration, available equipment (such as a fibreoptic scope), and urgency of surgery. Intubation via a SAD can be performed blindly or under fibreoptic guidance. The former risks trauma to an already compromised airway and should not be undertaken unless there is no alternative. Fibreoptic placement of a tracheal tube via the SAD can be assisted with an Aintree Intubation Catheter (Cook Medical, Bloomington, IN, USA) which is placed into the trachea over the scope under visualization, followed by removal of the SAD and railroading of the tracheal tube over the Aintree Intubation Catheter.[22]

Direct laryngoscopy

Irrespective of other advancements in airway management, direct laryngoscopy remains the commonest approach to tracheal intubation. Direct laryngoscopy is most commonly performed with a Macintosh blade, but other variations can prove beneficial, such as the hinged tip McCoy blade.[23] Gentle, gradual advancement of the laryngoscope should be undertaken, identifying anatomical landmarks en route to the glottis, in an effort to avoid airway trauma. Elevation of the tongue with the laryngoscope tensions the hyoepiglottic ligament and lifts the epiglottis from the posterior pharyngeal wall. The tip of the laryngoscope blade is placed in the vallecula to maximize epiglottis elevation. An inadequate view may be improved by external laryngeal manipulation. Classically, this is achieved with 'BURP' (backward, upward, rightward pressure) of the larynx.[24] An assistant's thumb and index finger can be manipulated by the laryngoscopist with one hand, while the other hand maintains laryngoscopy, to ensure the manoeuvre provides optimal benefit.

Dynamic head elevation can also enhance the glottic view, and is performed by placing the right hand at the occiput and elevating or lowering the head during laryngoscopy.[25] A bougie or styletted tube can prove invaluable when a poor view persists, while maintaining a low threshold for intubation by other means, such as videolaryngoscopy.

Videolaryngoscopy

Videolaryngoscopy utilizes a laryngoscope containing a video camera or other optical arrangement to indirectly visualize the laryngeal inlet. Benefit is greatest in patients for whom visualization of the glottis by direct laryngoscopy is challenging or even impossible, as the videolaryngoscope can 'look around the corner'.

Videolaryngoscopes can be classified based on whether or not they contain an integrated channel for the passage of a tracheal tube. Unchannelled devices include the McGrath (Aircraft Medical, Edinburgh, UK), C-Mac (Karl Storz, Tuttlingen, Germany), and GlideScope (Verathon Medical, Bothell, Washington, USA). Channelled devices include the Airtraq (Prodol Meditec, Vizcaya, Spain) and the Pentax Airway Scope (Ambu, Copenhagen, Denmark). The King Vision (King Systems, Noblesville, IN, USA) can accommodate both channelled and unchannelled laryngoscope blades. The Airtraq uses mirrors and prisms rather than a video camera to obtain a view of the laryngeal inlet. Some videolaryngoscopes have modifications to aid intubation success, such as a steeper angulated D-blade for the C-Mac laryngoscope, and an Airtraq designed for nasal intubation. User familiarity with both channelled and unchannelled laryngoscopes is essential if they are to be relied upon in a time-critical airway crisis.

Videolaryngoscopy avoids the need to obtain a view of the laryngeal inlet that is in the direct line of vision of the anaesthetist. This is particularly beneficial where attempted intubation with direct laryngoscopy has proven unsuccessful. Videolaryngoscopy also enables less use of force and multiple individuals can observe the attained view on a monitor, offering advice to the laryngoscopist or collectively deciding upon a change of plan for managing the airway.

The videolaryngoscope and tracheal tube must be cautiously inserted into the airway to avoid damage to pharyngeal structures, the likelihood of which may be enhanced in maxillofacial surgery patients, where the airway may contain disease or have been injured during airway management.

An improved view of the laryngeal inlet does not necessarily equate to an easier intubation. The tracheal tube must navigate the natural upper airway curvature and any pharyngeal pathology. Common pitfalls include advancing the laryngoscope too close to the glottis in an effort to obtain a 'perfect' view. Advancement of the tracheal tube tends to collide with the right arytenoid cartilage or pass towards the oesophagus. To reduce this likelihood, the clinician should retract the videolaryngoscope to obtain a more 'panoramic' view of the laryngeal inlet, which may reduce the percentage of glottic opening visualized but be of greater overall benefit. Channelled devices help to guide the tracheal tube through the glottic opening. Selection of a smaller diameter tracheal tube and lubrication allows for easier advancement through the channel. For unchannelled videolaryngoscopes, successful intubation is most likely when the curvature of the tracheal tube mirrors that of the curvature of the laryngoscope blade. The use of a bougie or a malleable stylet can assist with this anterior redirection of the tracheal tube. Further obstruction to tracheal tube advancement may arise when the angulated tube contacts the anterior tracheal rings after passing through the glottis. This can be ameliorated with 180° rotation of the tracheal tube. 'Reverse loading' of the tracheal tube on a stylet, such that the tube has a tendency to bend posteriorly down the trachea when it is offloaded off the anterior facing stylet, can also prevent collision with the anterior tracheal wall.[26]

Awake tracheal intubation

All patients are capable of progressing to a CICO scenario on induction of anaesthesia. However, it would be excessive to obviate this risk by subjecting all patients to an awake intubation. Awake intubation is indicated when the anaesthetist appraises that the risk of airway compromise on induction of anaesthesia is unacceptably high, or would be regarded as unacceptable by a group of practitioners making a reasonable appraisal of the circumstances. The opinion, and indeed assistance, of an experienced colleague can be invaluable in this scenario. We advocate a low threshold for awake intubation, a threshold frequently reached by patients undergoing major oromaxillofacial or head and neck surgery. Awake intubation is most commonly performed with a flexible fibreoptic scope. The use of awake videolaryngoscopy (AVL) is increasing, while an awake tracheostomy may be most appropriate for managing airways in greatest jeopardy.

Fibreoptic intubation

Fibreoptic intubation can be performed awake (AFOI), with or without sedation, or under general anaesthesia.

An antisialagogue, such as glycopyrrolate 4 mcg/kg IV, administered 30 minutes before the procedure, can reduce the burden of secretions, increase the efficacy of topical anaesthesia, and offset the bradycardia associated with use of remifentanil or dexmedetomidine.[27] However, tachycardia may be undesirable in patients with significant cardiac disease and can worsen patient anxiety.

Sedation can improve tolerance of awake intubation but is not an essential component of the procedure with optimal topical anaesthesia and a cooperative patient. In all cases, careful titration is essential in order to minimize the risk of airway obstruction. The degree of sedation must be continually appraised during the procedure, and ideally controlled by a second practitioner whose primary focus is not intubation. Vital signs should be monitored and supplementary oxygen administered, such as via high-flow nasal cannulae. The patient should remain capable of responding to a verbal stimulus. Traditional sedative regimens have typically included midazolam and fentanyl. Use of remifentanil, propofol, ketamine, and dexmedetomidine has increased in recent years.[27] No sedative regimen has demonstrated clear superiority. Local drug availability and clinician experience are key determining factors. In many institutions, a remifentanil-based regimen (target-controlled infusion 1–3 ng/mL) is often preferred as this drug effectively blunts airway reflexes, is easily titratable due to its short context-sensitive half-time, and is reversible with naloxone. Dexmedetomidine, though less universally available, produces sedation with excellent patient compliance, antisialagogue effects, and no respiratory depression.

Topical anaesthesia is most commonly achieved with lidocaine, which is available in varying concentrations (1–10%), and combined with other agents, such as phenylephrine (co-phenylcaine). The addition of a vasoconstrictor is useful for topical anaesthesia of the nasal passages to reduce the risk of epistaxis. Cocaine is an alternative agent, though is a controlled drug and less readily available. The safe dose of lidocaine for airway topical anaesthesia is uncertain, with thresholds of 7–9 mg/kg commonly quoted.[28] There is poor correlation between administered dose and serum concentration. Excessive administration of lidocaine can cause local anaesthetic systemic toxicity, most likely to arise during a prolonged effort at intubation and with concomitant local anaesthetic administration for other reasons. Sedation and progression to general anaesthesia precludes assessment of symptoms, such that cardiovascular instability may be the first sign. Clinicians should familiarize themselves with a treatment protocol for this rare event, including the location of lipid emulsion in their department.

Techniques for topical anaesthesia include nebulization, gargling of viscous lidocaine, application of soaked pledgets, and translaryngeal injection. A 'spray-as-you-go' technique enables progressive anaesthesia of the airway with advancement of the fibreoptic scope. Dispersal of local anaesthetic in the airway is achieved through the working channel of the scope by one of two means. The first method involves the filling of syringes with local anaesthetic and air (e.g. a 10 mL syringe with 3 mL of 2% lidocaine and 7 mL of air), such that rapid compression of the plunger pressurizes the syringe and propels the local anaesthetic through the working channel in a jet-like spray. Alternatively, the injection of local anaesthetic through an epidural catheter that has been passed through the working channel can achieve a similar effect.

Dedicated nerve blocks most commonly involve the glossopharyngeal and superior laryngeal nerves (discussed in Chapter 4). Translaryngeal anaesthesia involves puncture of the cricothyroid membrane with a peripheral cannula, while aspirating air in a caudad direction. A 5 mL syringe containing 2 mL of 4% lidocaine is then attached, and the local anaesthetic is injected after the patient is asked to exhale forcefully. This causes the patient to inhale before coughing and aids lidocaine spread to the distal trachea. However, it can cause laryngeal injury and bleeding.

For nasal intubations, the nare that is selected for intubation may be influenced by the site of pathology and by the patient's subjective assessment of nasal patency. Some clinicians commence with serial dilatation of the nares with nasopharyngeal airways of increasing size, coated in lidocaine gel, to increase the likelihood of unobstructed tube passage into the pharynx. The passage of any airway risks trauma, particularly when tissues are friable, and should cease if significant resistance is met.

Scope (and later tube) advancement are assisted by tongue and jaw protrusion, and neck extension. In the unconscious patient, the tongue can be grasped gently with gauze and protruded by an assistant, or a jaw thrust. Airway conduits, such as the Ovassapian and Berman airways, may prove useful for oral tracheal intubation.

Airway deformity can make identification of the glottis challenging, but is aided by slow advancement of the scope. Loss of landmarks should prompt slow withdrawal until the anatomy is discernible. This process may be aided by patient vocalization. If the image becomes blurred, gently touching the mucosa with the tip of the scope can clear the lens. The infrared red intubation system (IRRIS) is a promising device that emits infrared light through the cricothyroid membrane, transilluminating the glottis in a retrograde fashion, such that it is visible through a scope as a blinking beacon to guide advancement.[29]

Once the scope enters the trachea, it is advanced to the carina. This does not guarantee successful tracheal intubation, as advancement of the tube over the scope can prove challenging. Tube advancement is blind as it occurs proximal to the viewpoint of the scope, which uncommonly causes airway trauma. The tube can be warmed in hot water prior to use to soften it and should never be forced—gentle rotation can help facilitate insertion to the glottis.

Tracheal tube selection is important as difficulty with advancement is proportionate to the gap between the scope and tracheal tube.[30] This gap enables the course of the tube to deviate from that of the scope, most commonly towards the right arytenoid cartilage, but also towards the pyriform fossa, epiglottis, or oesophageal inlet. A snug fit makes tracheal tube advancement easier, favouring a narrower diameter tube, a thicker fibreoptic scope, or the placement of an airway adjunct between the scope and the tube, such as an Aintree Intubation Catheter. A conventional polyvinyl chloride tube is more difficult to advance than a flexible tube, such as that used with the intubating LMA, or the Parker flex-tip tube, which has an inward-facing bevel that closely apposes the scope. Contact of the bevel of the tracheal tube with the right arytenoid cartilage can be overcome by 90° anticlockwise rotation of the tube, such that the tip is brought anterior to the arytenoids.

The distance between the tracheal tube and carina is measured as the scope is withdrawn. Final confirmation of tracheal placement is confirmed with detection of carbon dioxide. Cuff inflation is stimulating if the subglottic space is not adequately anaesthetized and is often undertaken after induction of anaesthesia. Rarely, the cuff can rupture on advancement of the tube, and remain undetected until it fails to adequately inflate in the trachea, requiring exchange over a catheter.

Multiple attempts at fibreoptic intubation can lead to mucosal trauma, bleeding, and airway oedema. Rarely, the procedure will need to be abandoned and other methods of airway management selected, which may include AVL or awake tracheostomy. Despite failed AFOI, the anaesthetist may have gained sufficient insight into the patient's airway anatomy to make a judgement that proceeding with induction of anaesthesia is safe. Fibreoptic intubation may retain a role in intubation of that patient, occasionally in tandem with videolaryngoscopy, or via a SAD.

Awake videolaryngoscopy

Awake direct laryngoscopy is not adequately tolerated by patients as the forces necessary to obtain a view of the glottis stimulate airway reflexes and cause adverse autonomic effects. However, AVL is an emerging area.[31] Airway instrumentation is less forceful and stimulating when an indirect view of the laryngeal inlet can be obtained. Stimulation can be further reduced by tolerating a suboptimal view of the glottis and selecting a slender videolaryngoscope, such as the McGrath.[32] Adequate airway topical anaesthesia and sedation are key contributors to success, particularly with blockade of afferent branches of the glossopharyngeal and vagus nerves. A 'spray-as-you-go' local anaesthetic technique is commonly performed as the laryngoscope is progressively advanced.

AVL may be a suitable alternative to AFOI.[33] This approach can succeed when AFOI has failed, such as with severe airway oedema, bleeding, or a large volume of secretions. AVL can more easily displace tissues and create a path for tracheal tube passage. With AVL, tracheal tube placement occurs under vision, allowing for any obstruction to advancement to be diagnosed and corrected. In contrast, the tracheal tube is advanced blindly over the scope during AFOI, risking tissue trauma. An airway which is greatly narrowed is also susceptible to complete occlusion by a fibreoptic scope, while a videolaryngoscope does not pass through the narrowing and could allow for the passage of a smaller diameter tracheal tube.

Limitations of AVL include difficult or impossible insertion due to poor mouth opening or inadequate space between the mouth and chest wall, such as a fixed flexion deformity. Insertion of a videolaryngoscope can also cause tissue trauma, particularly if airway anatomy is abnormal, which may further compromise an already threatened airway.

AVL is most likely to fail when pharyngeal reflexes are not adequately suppressed. However, the videolaryngoscope may still be temporarily tolerated to attain a view of the laryngeal inlet, offering some (but not complete) reassurance to the clinician that intubation would be possible following abandonment of awake intubation and induction of anaesthesia. There is no guarantee that a good view will translate to an easy intubation or even remain under anaesthesia.

Awake tracheostomy

Awake tracheostomies are performed for acute upper airway obstruction, in scenarios where oxygenation by other means has failed, is not secure, or is inappropriate to attempt.[34,35] Rescue tracheostomy may be required after a cricothyroidotomy has failed to obtain airway access. Awake tracheostomy should be strongly considered for an anticipated difficult airway, where other awake intubation techniques such as fibreoptic or videolaryngoscopic intubation proved unsuccessful, and where the anaesthetist judges the risks associated with induction of anaesthesia to be greater than a pre-emptive surgical airway.

Local anaesthesia alone may suffice in enabling this procedure to be performed. However, hypoxaemia, fear, and procedural demands for neck extension can all impair essential patient cooperation. Sedative drugs must be carefully titrated.

While tracheostomy is performed with the aim of avoiding serious morbidity and mortality, it also carries the risk of the same, including life-threatening haemorrhage and loss of the airway. Greatest risk is associated with emergency tracheostomies, which have been classically surgical in nature, but can also be undertaken by a percutaneous dilational technique.[36]

Retrograde intubation

Retrograde intubation involves advancement of a tracheal tube over a guide that has been percutaneously introduced into the trachea and passed in a retrograde manner through the vocal cords and out through the mouth or nose.[37] The emerging guide offers a route for anterograde tube passage, assisting with navigation around upper airway abnormalities and avoiding the need to visualize the laryngeal inlet. The technique is, therefore, most beneficial with upper airway deformities, or where more common techniques prove challenging, such as airway bleeding that is preventing adequate visualization with a fibreoptic scope.

Following topical anaesthesia and optional sedation, the cricothyroid or cricotracheal membrane is punctured with an appropriate needle. The Tuohy epidural needle is commonly used, as its bevel assists with cephalad direction of the guide. Peripheral vascular access catheters or introducer needles from central venous access kits are alternatives. The lumen of the larynx is located with needle advancement by aspiration of air, followed by advancement of the catheter in a cephalad direction into the larynx.

A guide is then advanced, most commonly a 'J'-tipped guidewire from a central venous access kit, or an epidural catheter. The former is more visible and stiff, allowing for easier guide retrieval and subsequent tube advancement. Its 'J'-tip can assist with passage through upper airway obstacles and can be grasped by forceps to lift the wire from the pharyngeal mucosa and retrieve it by mouth, if the wire has not emerged with simple advancement. Should nasal intubation be necessary, but the guide has appeared by mouth, a catheter can be placed through the nose and retrieved by mouth. This can act as a conduit for the retrograde advancement of the guide through the nose, or the guide can be tied to the end of the catheter and pulled out through the nose.

Advancement of the tracheal tube over the guide can be difficult. It is important to keep the guide taut, so that it does not loop in the pharynx or allow for tube advancement into the oesophagus. However, excessive tension can depress the guide into the tissues, impede the passage of the tube, and increase the risk of tissue trauma. Difficulty with advancement also arises secondary to the large gap between the guide and the tube, allowing the tube to impinge upon adjacent structures, such as the arytenoid cartilages. Looping of the retrograde guide through the Murphy's eye can offer a remedy. A hollow anterograde guide can also be placed over the retrograde guide to reduce this problematic gap, such as a suction catheter or airway exchange catheter.[38] With fibreoptic-aided retrograde intubation, the retrograde guidewire can be placed through the distal end of the working channel. The scope is loaded with a tracheal tube and is then railroaded into the trachea, allowing for tube placement under visualization.[38]

Contraindications to retrograde intubation include subglottic pathologies and coagulopathy. Complications include bleeding, infection, surgical emphysema, vocal cord injury, and oesophageal puncture.

Blind nasal intubation

This technique of airway management involves the gradual advancement of a tracheal tube from the nostril to the trachea, guided by breath sounds or tactile sensation, rather than visualization. Key to success is optimal patient positioning, which involves lateral rotation of the head towards the side of intubation, along with hyperextension of the neck.[39] Intubation is also aided by the preformed curve of the tracheal tube. In the breathing patient, the tube is advanced during inhalation and the anaesthetist assesses for airflow via the tube during exhalation. In the apnoeic patient, there is greater obstruction to tube advancement with loss of upper airway tone and the respiratory cycle is no longer present to assist the anaesthetist. Greater reliance is placed on tactile sensation, whereby the anaesthetist may sense obstruction to tube advancement at the vallecula or glottis, or appreciate forward motion of the tube into the trachea by palpation of the front of the neck.

The value of this technique is increasingly limited, as a blind technique has greater likelihood of causing trauma to the airway, creating a time-critical scenario where management options become limited and airway patency is compromised. Its role may be greatest in a resource-poor setting.

Cricothyroidotomy

Cricothyroidotomy is universally recommended in all major airway management guidelines as a rescue oxygenation technique, following failure of face mask ventilation, conventional tracheal intubation, and SAD insertion.[40]

The laryngeal handshake can aid cricothyroid membrane identification. The thumb and middle finger pass down over the thyroid laminae to reach the cricoid cartilage, allowing the index finger to land upon the cricothyroid membrane.[41] Difficulty in identifying the membrane by inspection and palpation greatly increases the failure rate of cricothyroidotomy. The membrane should, therefore, be identified as a component of preoperative assessment, assisted by ultrasound if necessary.

Successful cricothyroidotomy is reliant on timely performance and both technical and non-technical skills. A scalpel or cannula cricothyroidotomy is possible. Dedicated equipment sets are available. Scalpel cricothyroidotomy with familiar equipment is increasingly favoured—a number 10 blade, a bougie, and a 6.0 mm internal diameter cuffed tracheal tube. A 'stab, twist, bougie, tube' technique has been described.[41] A vertical rather than horizontal incision is made when the membrane is impalpable, followed by blunt dissection with the hands to locate the larynx.

The presence of a nearby surgeon may prove invaluable in assisting with rescue efforts should an airway crisis progress to this scenario.

Intubation for maxillomandibular fixation

Nasotracheal intubation is typically used in lieu of orotracheal intubation in order to enable maxillomandibular fixation during reduction of facial fractures. Occasionally, complex facial fractures may contraindicate or obstruct passage of a nasal tube. Tracheostomy can be performed if injuries are extensive. Retromolar and submental intubation techniques are alternatives for patients who are likely to require only short-term ventilatory support and for whom the clinician wishes to avoid tracheostomy-associated complications. A submental technique can also be suitable for a number of elective surgeries, for example, Le Fort III osteotomies, skull base surgeries, repair of cancrum oris defects, and complex cleft lift and palate surgeries.[42]

Retromolar intubation

Retromolar intubation was first described by Bonfils in 1983, using an eponymous rigid fibrescope.[43] The retromolar space is bounded by the last molar, the maxillary tuberosity, and the anterior aspect of the ascending ramus of the mandible. The tracheal tube can rest in this space, allowing for complete dental occlusion. The space can also act as a conduit for the use of a flexible fibrescope or rigid intubating fibrescope, and to enable passage of a suction catheter into the oropharynx.

To discern whether the retromolar space is large enough to accommodate the tracheal tube, the patient's index finger can be placed in the space and they are asked to slowly occlude the teeth. The extraction of a third molar, to expand an otherwise inadequate retromolar space, has been reported. A small diameter, reinforced tracheal tube is also helpful. Effort must be made to avoid deforming the tube when it is fixed with wire ligature.

A gap created by loss of teeth can fulfil a similar purpose to the retromolar space, accommodating tube passage for dental occlusion. Risks of retromolar intubation include mucosal trauma, inadequate dental occlusion, and accidental extubation.

Submental intubation

A submental intubation is one that externalizes the proximal end of the tracheal tube through the floor of the mouth and submental region. To perform submental intubation, the trachea is first intubated by mouth using a reinforced tracheal tube.[42] The universal connector of the selected tube must be easy to detach. An orocutaneous tunnel is created in order to divert the proximal end of the tracheal tube through the floor of the mouth. Under aseptic technique, a 15 mm incision is made in the submental region, paralleling the inferior border of the mandible, on the contralateral side to the fracture. The optimal site for incision has been contested and is based largely on clinician desire to avoid certain anatomical structures.

Blunt dissection is performed with forceps adjacent to the mandible, passing through fat, platysma, deep cervical fascia, the mylohyoid muscle, and between the two heads of digastric muscles, before the forceps is observed to indent the oral mucosa. The mucosa is then incised to enable passage of the forceps into the cavity. The forceps blades are separated to enlarge the orifice sufficient to enable tube passage. Following a period of 100% oxygen delivery, the pilot balloon is deflated and pulled through the submental incision by the forceps. This is followed by removal of the tracheal tube connector and pull through of the tube, before reconnection and confirmation of tube placement with capnography. The tube is sutured and taped in place. Following surgery, the tube can be returned to the orotracheal position or left submentally for subsequent extubation. In order to reduce the likelihood of hypoxaemia which can arise with challenging tube retrieval and reconnection, some clinicians utilize a second tracheal tube.[44] Following orotracheal intubation, a reinforced tracheal tube is advanced from the exterior through the submental incision into the oropharynx. At this point, the orotracheal tube is removed, and the submental tube is advanced into the trachea (approaches to submental intubation are also discussed in Chapters 3 and 10).

Complications of submental intubation include bleeding, damage to adjacent structures (such as the lingual nerve, sublingual gland, and submandibular duct), desaturation due to tube positioning, displacement of the tube (leading to extubation or endobronchial intubation), superficial skin infection, and scar formation.

Tracheal extubation

During tracheal extubation, the anaesthetist aims to maintain an uninterrupted delivery of oxygen to the lungs, as the patient transitions to an independent state of airway protection and gas exchange that no longer relies on the presence of a tracheal tube. There is often an underappreciation of the risks associated with extubation. In the fourth National Audit Project, one-third of major anaesthesia-related airway complications occurred on emergence or in recovery, and commonly involved patients who underwent head and neck surgery.[1] Guidance on extubation has been issued by the Difficult Airway Society.[45]

Like intubation, challenges at extubation can be anatomical or physiological, and are exacerbated by human factors.[46] Airway reflexes may be exaggerated or obtunded. Exaggerated reflexes can lead to laryngospasm, which is most likely to arise in a light plane of anaesthesia, with the presence of blood and secretions acting as stimuli. Obtunded airway reflexes can lead to airway obstruction or aspiration, secondary to the residual effects of anaesthetic agents, opioids, and neuromuscular blocking drugs. Initial airway instrumentation and surgical interventions can adversely affect the airway, including oedema, bleeding, haematoma formation, and nerve injury.

During intubation, the anaesthetist assumes full control of the patient by pharmacological means. In contrast, extubation is somewhat associated with a loss of control, as responsibility is progressively transferred back to the patient to manage their own airway. Like intubation, extubation must be tailored to the needs of the patient. Ultimately, the anaesthetist must be prepared for reintubation and demonstrate awareness of the resources available to assist them in this regard, such as personnel and equipment. They must ask whether airway management at induction was predictive of a difficult extubation, or if the status of the airway has changed in the interim. Consequently, the airway being managed by the anaesthetist at extubation may represent an airway not previously encountered. A classical scenario is the airway following intermaxillary fixation, where wire cutters should be available to enable oral access for emergency reintubation.

Decisions regarding suitability for extubation must be individualized. Multisystem assessment of the patient is crucial. Consciousness, haemodynamics, respiratory effort, acid–base status, thermoregulation, and analgesia are examples of areas that should be optimized before extubation. Extubation should never be hurried. Indeed, extubation may be postponed for hours or days, in order to create more favourable airway circumstances, such as the resolution of oedema. The risk of airway compromise may be such that elective

tracheostomy is performed, during the initial surgery or in the post-operative period.

The upper airway must be thoroughly suctioned before extubation, ideally under direct vision to reduce the risk of trauma. Endoscopic or laryngoscopic assessment may be necessary to ensure the absence of clots in the upper airway. The presence of a throat pack in the airway must be clearly signposted at insertion in order to ensure retrieval before extubation. A gastric tube, if present, should be aspirated. If neuromuscular blocking drugs have been used, a train of four ratio >0.9 should be confirmed by quantitative nerve stimulator monitoring before extubation, as residual neuromuscular blockade demonstrates a clear association with postoperative complications. Rapid return of neuromuscular function can be attained with the administration of sugammadex where rocuronium and vecuronium have been administered.

Preoxygenation at a FiO_2 of 1.0 should precede extubation. Head-up tilt is the increasingly favoured position for extubation, as it improves respiratory mechanics and is a familiar position for airway intervention. Airway oedema may benefit from steroid administration and adrenaline nebulization.[47] Corticosteroids can reduce laryngeal oedema and the likelihood of failed extubation, but require administration at least 4 hours prior to extubation for benefit. The presence of a cuff leak is a positive sign, but is not sufficiently sensitive or specific to exclude a problem on extubation.

Deep extubation reduces the likelihood of coughing and associated adverse haemodynamic effects but can lead to upper airway obstruction and is not recommended. Alternatively, the Bailey manoeuvre involves the exchange of a tracheal tube for a SAD in a deep plane of anaesthesia before emergence. This can also enable fibre-optic assessment of laryngeal and tracheal motion following the resumption of spontaneous respiration but prior to emergence.

Airway exchange catheters are thin, blunt-ended hollow tubes that are passed through the tracheal tube and remain in the airway on extubation.[48] They offer a conduit for the administration of oxygen via standard anaesthesia circuitry or jet ventilation, and can act as a guide for the passage of a tracheal tube in the event of reintubation. The distal end of the catheter should remain above the carina. There is a risk of barotrauma with both jet ventilation or continued oxygen insufflation when the path for gas egress is compromised. If reintubation is necessary, both laryngoscopy and the selection of a small tracheal tube can assist with railroading of the tracheal tube over the catheter. Gum elastic bougies and suction catheters are inferior substitutes for airway exchange catheters, as they typically do not allow for oxygen administration and can cause trauma, but they may be the only catheters available for use in resource-poor countries.

Opioids suppress airway reflexes. Remifentanil, administered by infusion, can allow for a patient to emerge from anaesthesia to the point of being fully awake while remaining tube tolerant. The volatile agent or propofol is discontinued in advance of extubation, allowing adequate time for drug washout, while the remifentanil infusion is continued. Patients can be encouraged to breathe while the remifentanil infusion is titrated down until normal respiration resumes and the tracheal tube can be safely removed with the patient fully conscious. Efforts to hasten extubation by vigorous stimulation are inappropriate. Adequate spontaneous respiration should be ensured. Venous catheters should be aspirated or flushed of remifentanil and other agents no longer required, in order to avoid their adverse effects in the recovery room or ward. Respiratory status must be closely monitored with this approach, as patients remain at risk of apnoeic periods after extubation.

Particular caution must be applied to patients with intermaxillary fixation, such as ensuring tracheal extubation is undertaken when the patient is fully conscious and that wire cutters are immediately available (discussed in detail in Chapter 17).

Any complaint of difficult breathing by the patient following extubation, or observation of the same by nursing staff, demands urgent clinician assessment. History and examination should be undertaken to identify stridor or evidence of haematoma formation, which may indicate impending airway compromise, before abnormalities of vital signs or blood gas parameters are detected.

For patients being admitted to the intensive care unit, monitoring during transfer should replicate that seen prior to transfer, including capnography. The on-call anaesthesia service should be informed about the patient and an airway management plan agreed upon in the event of deterioration, with all necessary equipment located near the patient.

Human factors

Difficult airway management can be caused or complicated by human factors. During an airway crisis, several issues may unfold simultaneously, each demanding of attention during this time-critical scenario. The inability to rapidly prioritize this information to the point where it can impair decision-making is known as cognitive overload. An overwhelmed anaesthetist may become fixated on one aspect of care to the overall detriment of the patient. For example, repeated attempts at intubation can lead to airway trauma and jeopardize the delivery of oxygen to a patient who is easy to oxygenate by other means, such as bag mask ventilation.

Cognitive aids, such as the Vortex model of airway management or the airway algorithms of the Difficult Airway Society, aim to focus on the challenge at hand, suggesting methods of optimizing their current approach or alternative interventions, some of which may not have occurred to them. Verbalizing one's thought process enables those in attendance to be aware of the problem and positions them to offer optimal assistance. This may include questioning that thought process and recognizing that any individual, irrespective of traditional hierarchy, may be instrumental in solving the problem at hand.

Conclusion

All patients require an airway management plan that is tailored to their needs. This plan must consider the patient's airway anatomy and broader clinical state, the skill set of the anaesthetist, the requirements for surgery, and the resources available. The shared airway has its own unique challenges and the surgery itself may create particular difficulties with extubation, such as anatomical changes and intermaxillary fixation. Surgical instruments and throat packs must be carefully documented for removal. During difficult airway management, the anaesthetist must remember that the immediate and principal goal is to secure oxygenation, which does not necessarily equate to tracheal intubation.

REFERENCES

1. Cook TM, Woodall N, Frerk C; Fourth National Audit Project. Major complications of airway management in the UK: results of the Fourth National Audit Project of the Royal College of Anaesthetists and the Difficult Airway Society. Part 1: anaesthesia. *Br J Anaesth.* 2011;**106**(5):617–631.

2. Shiga T, Wajima Z, Inoue T, Sakamoto A. Predicting difficult intubation in apparently normal patients: a meta-analysis of bedside screening test performance. *Anesthesiology.* 2005;**103**(2):429–437.

3. Kheterpal S, Martin L, Shanks AM, Tremper KK. Prediction and outcomes of impossible mask ventilation: a review of 50,000 anesthetics. *Anesthesiology.* 2009;**110**(4):891–897.

4. Khan ZH, Mohammadi M, Rasouli MR, Farrokhnia F, Khan RH. The diagnostic value of the upper lip bite test combined with sternomental distance, thyromental distance, and interincisor distance for prediction of easy laryngoscopy and intubation: a prospective study. *Anesth Analg.* 2009;**109**(3):822–824.

5. Randell T. Prediction of difficult intubation. *Acta Anaesthesiol Scand.* 1996;**40**(8):1016–1023.

6. Al Ramadhani S, Mohamed LA, Rocke DA, Gouws E. Sternomental distance as the sole predictor of difficult laryngoscopy in obstetric anaesthesia. *Br J Anaesth.* 1996;**77**(3):312–316.

7. Kristensen MS, Teoh WH, Rudolph SS. Ultrasonographic identification of the cricothyroid membrane: best evidence, techniques, and clinical impact. *Br J Anaesth.* 2016;**117**(1): i139–i148.

8. Mort TC. Emergency tracheal intubation: complications associated with repeated laryngoscopic attempts. *Anesth Analg.* 2004;**99**(2):607–613.

9. El-Orbany M, Woehlck H, Salem MR. Head and neck position for direct laryngoscopy. *Anesth Analg.* 2011;**113**(1):103–109.

10. Nimmagadda U, Salem MR, Crystal GJ. Preoxygenation: physiologic basis, benefits, and potential risks. *Anesth Analg.* 2017;**124**(2):507–517.

11. Warters RD, Szabo TA, Spinale FG, DeSantis SM, Reves JG. The effect of neuromuscular blockade on mask ventilation. *Anaesthesia.* 2011;**66**(3):163–167.

12. Lundstrøm LH, Duez CH, Nørskov AK, Rosenstock CV, Thomsen JL, Møller AM, et al. Avoidance versus use of neuromuscular blocking agents for improving conditions during tracheal intubation or direct laryngoscopy in adults and adolescents. *Cochrane Database Syst Rev.* 2017;**5**:CD009237.

13. Dalton AJ, Millar F. Neuromuscular monitoring and the AAGBI 2016 monitoring guidelines. *Anaesthesia.* 2016;**71**(8):981–982.

14. Lyons C, Callaghan M. Uses and mechanisms of apnoeic oxygenation: a narrative review. *Anaesthesia.* 2019;**74**(4):497–507.

15. Levitan RM. (2010, 9 December). NO DESAT! Nasal oxygen during efforts securing a tube. *Emergency Physicians Monthly.* https://www.epmonthly.com/article/no-desat/

16. Patel A, Nouraei SA. Transnasal humidified rapid-insufflation ventilatory exchange (THRIVE): a physiological method of increasing apnoea time in patients with difficult airways. *Anaesthesia.* 2015;**70**(3):323–329.

17. Lyons C, Callaghan M. Apnoeic oxygenation with high-flow nasal oxygen for laryngeal surgery: a case series. *Anaesthesia.* 2017;**72**(11):1379–1387.

18. Cook TM, Kelly FE. Time to abandon the 'vintage' laryngeal mask airway and adopt second-generation supraglottic airway devices as first choice. *Br J Anaesth.* 2015;**115**(4):497–499.

19. Van Zundert AA, Kumar CM, Van Zundert TC. Malpositioning of supraglottic airway devices: preventive and corrective strategies. *Br J Anaesth*. 2016;**116**(5):579–582.

20. Howath A, Brimacombe J, Keller C. Gum-elastic bougie-guided insertion of the ProSeal laryngeal mask airway: a new technique. *Anaesth Intensive Care*. 2002;**30**(5):624–627.

21. Wong DT, Yang JJ, Mak HY, Jagannathan N. Use of intubation introducers through a supraglottic airway to facilitate tracheal intubation: a brief review. *Can J Anaesth*. 2012;**59**(7):704–715.

22. Berkow LC, Schwartz JM, Kan K, Corridore M, Heitmiller ES. Use of the Laryngeal Mask Airway-Aintree Intubating Catheter-fiberoptic bronchoscope technique for difficult intubation. *J Clin Anesth*. 2011;**23**(7):534–539.

23. Cook TM, Tuckey JP. A comparison between the Macintosh and the McCoy laryngoscope blades. *Anaesthesia*. 1996;**51**(10):977–980.

24. Knill RL. Difficult laryngoscopy made easy with a 'BURP'. *Can J Anaesth*. 1993;**40**(3):279–282.

25. El-Orbany M, Woehlck H, Salem MR. Head and neck position for direct laryngoscopy. *Anesth Analg*. 2011;**113**(1):103–109.

26. Dupanović M, Isaacson S, Borovcanin Z, Jain S, Korten S, Karan S, et al. Clinical comparison of two stylet angles for orotracheal intubation with the GlideScope video laryngoscope. *J Clin Anesth*. 2010;**22**(5):352–359.

27. Johnston KD, Rai MR. Conscious sedation for awake fibreoptic intubation: a review of the literature. *Can J Anaesth*. 2013;**60**(6):584–599.

28. Du Rand IA, Blaikley J, Booton R, Chaudhuri N, Gupta V, Khalid S, et al. British Thoracic Society guideline for diagnostic flexible bronchoscopy in adults. *Thorax*. 2013;**68**:i1–i44.

29. Kristensen MS, Fried E, Biro P. Infrared red intubation system (IRRIS) guided flexile videoscope assisted difficult airway management. *Acta Anaesthesiol Scand*. 2018;**62**(1):19–25.

30. Asai T, Shingu K. Difficulty in advancing a tracheal tube over a fibreoptic bronchoscope: incidence, causes and solutions. *Br J Anaesth*. 2004;**92**(6):870–881.

31. Rosenstock CV, Thøgersen B, Afshari A, Christensen AL, Eriksen C, Gätke MR. Awake fiberoptic or awake video laryngoscopic tracheal intubation in patients with anticipated difficult airway management: a randomized clinical trial. *Anesthesiology*. 2012;**116**(6):1210–1216.

32. McGuire BE. Use of the McGrath video laryngoscope in awake patients. *Anaesthesia*. 2009;**64**(8):912–914.

33. Paolini JB, Donati F, Drolet P. Review article: video-laryngoscopy: another tool for difficult intubation or a new paradigm in airway management? *Can J Anaesth*. 2013;**60**(2):184–191.

34. Fang CH, Friedman R, White PE, Mady LJ, Kalyoussef E. Emergent awake tracheostomy—the five-year experience at an urban tertiary care center. *Laryngoscope*. 2015;**125**(11):2476–2479.

35. Yuen HW, Loy AH, Johari S. Urgent awake tracheostomy for impending airway obstruction. *Otolaryngol Head Neck Surg*. 2007;**136**(5):838–842.

36. Davidson SB, Blostein PA, Walsh J, Maltz SB, VandenBerg SL. Percutaneous tracheostomy: a new approach to the emergency airway. *J Trauma Acute Care Surg*. 2012;**73**(2):S83–S88.

37. Dhara SS. Retrograde intubation—a facilitated approach. *Br J Anaesth*. 1992;**69**(6):631–633.

38. Vieira D, Lages N, Dias J, Maria L, Correia C. Retrograde intubation: an old new technique. *OA Anaesthetics*. 2013;**1**(2):18.

39. Chauhan V, Acharya G. Nasal intubation: a comprehensive review. *Indian J Crit Care Med*. 2016;**20**(11):662–667.

40. Frerk C, Mitchell VS, McNarry AF, Mendonca C, Bhagrath R, Patel A, et al. Difficult Airway Society 2015 guidelines for management of unanticipated difficult intubation in adults. *Br J Anaesth*. 2015;**115**(6):827–848.

41. Levitan RM. (2014, 6 February). Tips and tricks for performing cricothyrotomy. *ACEP Now*. https://www.acepnow.com/article/tips-tricks-performing-cricothyrotomy/

42. Das S, Das TP, Ghosh PS. Submental intubation: a journey over the last 25 years. *J Anaesthesiol Clin Pharmacol*. 2012;**28**(3):291–303.

43. Bonfils P. [Difficult intubation in Pierre-Robin children, a new method: the retromolar route]. *Anaesthesist*. 1983;**32**(7):363–367.

44. Amin M, Dill-Russell P, Manisali M, Lee R, Sinton I. Facial fractures and submental tracheal intubation. *Anaesthesia*. 2002;**57**(12):1195–1199.

45. Difficult Airway Society Extubation Guidelines Group, Popat M, Mitchell V, Dravid R, Patel A, Swampillai C, et al. Difficult Airway Society Guidelines for the management of tracheal extubation. *Anaesthesia*. 2012;**67**(3):318–340.

46. Cavallone LF, Vannucci A. Review article: extubation of the difficult airway and extubation failure. *Anesth Analg*. 2013;**116**(2):368–383.

47. McCaffrey J, Farrell C, Whiting P, Dan A, Bagshaw SM, Delaney AP. Corticosteroids to prevent extubation failure: a systematic review and meta-analysis. *Intensive Care Med*. 2009;**35**(6):977–986.

48. Mort TC. Continuous airway access for the difficult extubation: the efficacy of the airway exchange catheter. *Anesth Analg*. 2007;**105**(5):1357–1362.

3

Surgical airway

William P. L. Bradley and Gordon A. Chapman

Introduction

Oxygenation is the cornerstone of anaesthesia and airway management. This is usually achieved by a supraglottic approach. However, there are times when infraglottic access may be required. Surgical airways in oral and maxillofacial surgery may be performed as elective or emergency procedures.

Elective procedures include the temporary or permanent tracheostomy performed as part of a surgical procedure, submental intubation, the laryngostomy following total laryngectomy, as well as transtracheal jet ventilation. Usually, obstruction of the upper airway due to perioperative or infective swelling is temporary and a tracheostomy may only be required until these resolve. Urgent and planned procedures would include the percutaneous or surgical tracheostomy in the intensive care unit (ICU) patient to expedite weaning and facilitate tracheobronchial toilet.

Emergency surgical airway procedures include the awake tracheostomy where an oral or nasal intubation may be deemed impossible or contraindicated. Emergency surgical airways in anaesthesia are most commonly associated with the 'can't intubate, can't oxygenate' (CICO) scenario. The CICO scenario is a relatively rare event with an estimated incidence of approximately 1 in 5000 to 1 in 10,000 general anaesthetics.[1,2]

It is essential that a thorough airway assessment is performed to ensure the appropriate airway plans are put in place to minimize the risk of hypoxia to the patient. Non-technical and human factors are also important, and the anaesthetist should be cognisant of their role in managing the surgical airway. In addition to the relevant chapters in this textbook (see Chapters 1, 2, and 18), the Australian and New Zealand College of Anaesthetists has produced downloadable online airway resources available to compliment these areas (https://libguides.anzca.edu.au/airway).

Several conditions (including previous surgery, radiotherapy, fixed cervical spine deformities, acute or chronic infective or inflammatory conditions, neoplastic disease of the neck, larynx, or trachea, obesity, trauma, and neck deformities such as torticollis) may distort the anatomy or make surface landmarks difficult to palpate. Infection, oedema related to an allergic reaction, and haemorrhage may make surgical access to the airway more difficult due to loss of normal surgical tissue planes.

Anatomy

Knowledge of the anatomy of the larynx, trachea, and surrounding structures is critical for successful infraglottic airway access and avoiding the potential risk of trauma to surrounding structures especially when the anatomy is distorted.

The larynx is comprised of six cartilages:

- Thyroid cartilage.
- Cricoid cartilage.
- Epiglottis cartilage.
- Arytenoid (paired) cartilage.
- Corniculate (paired) cartilage.
- Cuneiform (paired) cartilage.

The cricothyroid membrane is located between the thyroid and cricoid cartilages. The cricoid cartilage is the only complete ring and connects the trachea to the larynx.

The trachea is a pipe consisting of semicircular cartilaginous rings that connect the pharynx and larynx to the main bronchi. The trachealis muscle forms the posterior wall of the trachea. The tracheal semicircular rings are joined by horizontal bands of fibrous connective tissue known as the annular ligaments of the trachea. The epiglottis is composed of elastic cartilage covered anteriorly by non-keratinized stratified squamous epithelium (consistent with the pharynx) and posteriorly by pseudo-stratified columnar epithelium (consistent with the larynx). Under the epithelial layer is a thin layer of areolar connective tissue that provides a loose attachment for the epithelium and supplies it with blood vessels and nerve fibres. During swallowing, the pharynx, hyoid, and larynx move superiorly. This movement of the hyoid allows the epiglottis to fold down over the glottis and prevents aspiration.

The thyroid gland lies anterior to the trachea and its isthmus usually crosses the trachea at the level of the second and third tracheal rings. The innominate artery crosses the mid-trachea but may be in a higher position at the base of the neck. In this position catastrophic postoperative bleeding may occur from a trachea–vascular fistula when a tracheostomy tube erodes into the artery over time (discussed in detail in Chapter 16).

Posteriorly, the oesophagus contacts the trachea on the left and vertebral bodies on the right. The carotid artery and internal jugular veins are located laterally.

Elective tracheostomy

This can be performed either percutaneously or as an open surgical technique and may be either temporary or permanent. Generally, an open surgical technique may be performed in either an elective or emergency setting, whereas the percutaneous approach is usually performed semi-electively. The percutaneous dilatational tracheostomy is often a Seldinger-based technique with dilatation of the space between the tracheal rings compared to surgical dissection and placement under direct vision.

The indications for tracheostomy include the following:

1. Bypass of an obstructed upper airway due to varying pathologies such as tumour, infection, oedema, trauma, or congenital malformations.
2. Protracted intubation and ventilation, that is, high cervical spine injuries or neuromuscular diseases and mechanical ventilation where tracheostomy facilitates weaning.
3. Potential airway protection in patients with long-term reduced conscious states or bulbar disorders.

The advantages of a tracheostomy over tracheal intubation in the critically ill population who require prolonged intubation include patient comfort, reduced sedation requirements, reduced resistance to breathing, improved tracheal toilet so improving oropharyngeal hygiene, and early patient mobilization. Early use over late tracheostomy insertion may reduce the duration of mechanical ventilation but without mortality benefit.[3]

There are few absolute contraindications for tracheostomy other than patient refusal. In addition, percutaneous tracheostomy is generally not recommended for emergency airway access or in children. Relative contraindications for tracheostomy may include morbid obesity, malignancy, radiotherapy, limited neck extension, kyphoscoliosis, unstable cervical spine, large goitres, coagulopathies, high ventilatory support (high risk of significant desaturation during procedure), and infection at the insertion site. Where tracheostomy is deemed necessary in the above-mentioned conditions, an open surgical technique is generally preferred.

Percutaneous techniques are associated with a lower incidence of infections compared to the open surgical approach.[4–6] Originally, it was suggested that the mortality rate and cardio-respiratory complications were higher with the percutaneous route.[7] However, recent reviews showed that there were no significant statistical differences in haemorrhagic events, mortality, stenosis rate, or false passage complications.[5,6] The higher infection rate could be related to the more complex cases being performed as a surgical technique. The cost benefit of the percutaneous technique is probably more related to it being performed in an ICU setting rather than the operating theatre.

A surgical tracheostomy performed in ICU is probably also more cost-effective than if it were performed in the operating theatre.[8] Finally, there may be better cosmetic results with a percutaneous approach.[5]

Training and education utilizing either manikins or biological models is encouraged to enhance the effective and safe performance of these techniques. Both the UK National Tracheostomy Safety project (NTSP—https://www.tracheostomy.org.uk/) and Australasian Tracheostomy Review and Management Services (TRAMS—https://www.tracheostomyteam.org/) aim to enhance patient safety with improvement in skills, knowledge, and competencies of clinical staff in dealing with tracheostomies.[9]

Percutaneous dilatational tracheostomy

These techniques may be used as part of the postoperative surgical airway management of oral and maxillofacial surgical patients. Percutaneous dilatational tracheostomy may be performed in ICU at the patient's bedside (Table 3.1). This procedure may be quicker to perform than the open technique[6] by avoiding the logistics of returning the patient to the operating theatre.

The earliest dilatational tracheostomies were performed by a serial dilatational method developed by Ciaglia.[10] Several other dilatational techniques have also been described, including a modification of the Ciaglia method employing a single dilator such as the Ciaglia Blue Rhino™ (Cook Critical Care, Bloomington, IL, USA),[11,12] Griggs dilatational forceps approach (Portex®, Smiths Medical International Ltd., Hythe, Kent, UK)[13], PercuTwist™ screw-action dilator technique (Rüsch, Kernen, Germany),[14] and Fantoni's translaryngeal method[15] of placement.

Serial dilatational technique

Ciaglia described this technique in 1985. The procedure requires a series of dilators of gradually increasing gauge to create the stoma. It is considered to be easier to perform and associated with less complications at 24 hours[16] compared to the Griggs dilatational forceps method.

Balloon dilatational technique

This technique is slower, more challenging, and has a higher incidence of minor bleeding complications than the single dilator technique.[17]

Forceps dilatational technique

One version was developed by Griggs in 1990[13] using modified Howard–Kelly forceps. A Seldinger technique is used to locate and pass a guide wire into the trachea. A pair of customized forceps is then threaded over the wire, firstly through the skin and subcutaneous tissue. The forceps are then opened to stretch up these tissues. The forceps are advanced further along the wire into the trachea itself and opened a second time to stretch up a hole in the tracheal wall. A tracheostomy tube is then passed over the wire through the passage created. This technique tends to cause more bleeding and is perceived to be more difficult to perform than the single dilator technique. However, less tracheal cartilage damage may occur.[18,19]

Table 3.1 A stepwise approach to percutaneous dilatational tracheostomy

1	The checklist must be completed and the team brief undertaken. Appropriate monitoring should be applied A minimum of three skilled people are required: operator (performing the tracheostomy—OP), airway doctor (performing the supraglottic airway management—AD), and an assistant *The FiO₂ should be increased to 1.0 to minimize the risk of desaturation during the procedure* Depth of sedation should be increased to minimize the risk of awareness A neuromuscular blocking agent should be administered
2	The patient position should be optimized by extending the neck Ultrasound should be used to identify and mark landmark anatomy
3	The AD should check the tracheal tube with a laryngoscope (videolaryngoscopy or direct laryngoscopy) and suction supraglottic secretions If reintubation is considered to be difficult (difficult laryngoscopy and/or intubation), consider expert help
4	The pilot balloon should be deflated, and AD should withdraw the tracheal tube under direct vision or fibrescopic guidance, so that the cuff remains at or just below the vocal cords *Ensure that the tracheal tube is not dislodged from the trachea and re-inflate the pilot balloon.* A Bodai Swivel adaptor (Sontek Medical, Inc., Hingham, MA, USA) should be used with the fibrescope
5	The OP should prepare the neck using a strict aseptic technique and infiltrate local anaesthetic with adrenaline subcutaneously (to reduce bleeding) All staff must be wearing *appropriate personal protective equipment*, including eye protection
6	A 2 cm horizontal incision should be made midway between the sternal notch and the cricoid cartilage
7	Blunt dissection should be undertaken to allow palpation of the trachea The cannula should be inserted into the trachea while aspirating for air. The ideal location is between second and third tracheal rings The fibrescope can be used for internal visualization of the cannula passing into the trachea and optimization of the cannula position
8	A Seldinger technique should then be undertaken, finally placing the tracheostomy tube into the trachea. Placement should be confirmed with capnography
9	The tracheostomy tube should be secured carefully. The tracheal tube can then be removed

Note: there are many different ways of performing the technique—including a different approach to the timing of the steps for skin incision and tracheal puncture. The exact method should be determined by local policy and expertise.

Screw-action dilatation technique

A technique developed by Rusch known as PercuTwist™[14] involves a single-step dilatation of the tracheal wall. In this device, the screw-like dilator lifts the anterior wall of the trachea during its insertion. This contrasts with the posterior displacement of the anterior tracheal wall commonly observed with the use of the Blue Rhino™ dilator. This has the advantage of ensuring an unobstructed bronchoscopic view of the procedure. However, serious posterior laryngeal wall injuries have been reported.[20]

Translaryngeal technique

This technique was developed by Fantoni in 1993.[15] In this method, the guide wire placed in the trachea is directed superiorly through the larynx. A specially designed tracheostomy tube is then threaded over the guide wire and passed first through the larynx and then through the anterior tracheal wall. This technique may theoretically reduce the risk of damage to the posterior tracheal wall but is more complicated than other techniques. It is associated with a high incidence of technical difficulties, a higher rate of serious complications, higher conversion rate to other techniques, and takes longer than the Griggs technique.[21]

Single dilator technique

This technique is generally faster than the serial dilatational technique[22,23] and is perceived to be among the safer approaches.[24]

An airway assessment should be performed prior to any percutaneous technique to identify any potential difficulties and may include the use of an ultrasound scan to help locate the trachea (and prominent blood vessels). A locally developed checklist is of benefit to ensure all the appropriate monitoring including capnography, emergency airway equipment, bronchoscopic equipment, fasting status, coagulation profile, ventilation parameters, consent, sedation medication, neuromuscular agents, adequate assistance, and appropriate skill mix are met, prior to embarking on the procedure. Ultrasound has been shown to improve the accuracy of identifying anatomical landmarks.[25]

The surgeons should be made aware that a percutaneous tracheostomy is being performed and should be available in the event of a serious complication. As it is a planned procedure, it should be performed during normal working hours.

Surgical tracheostomy

A surgical or open tracheostomy is most commonly performed in the operating theatre, although occasionally it is undertaken in the ICU. It is considered the gold standard for patients with difficult anatomy and provides better exposure to ensure haemostatic control and management of bleeding complications compared to the percutaneous approach (Table 3.2).

Ideally, the patient is positioned supine with the shoulders elevated and the neck extended. This position will maximally expose the trachea and may be facilitated by placing a shoulder roll between the scapulae, or a pillow behind the patient's shoulders. Although neck extension facilitates the procedure, overextension should be avoided, as it firstly tends to narrow the airway, and secondly may encourage the operator to place the stoma in too caudal a position, particularly in the paediatric patient with a very small and mobile trachea.

Table 3.2 A stepwise approach to surgical tracheostomy in the operating theatre with an anaesthetized patient

1	Ensure checklist and World Health Organization timeout procedure has been completed, team brief undertaken, and appropriate monitoring applied
2	Optimize the patient position, extend the neck (if appropriate), and elevate the shoulders
3	Provide a sterile field between the chin to below the clavicles. The skin overlying the second tracheal ring should be identified and infiltrated with a lidocaine and adrenaline mixture
4	A midline 2–3 cm vertical skin incision should be made (a horizontal incision may provide a better long-term cosmetic outcome but traps more secretions)
5	Sharp dissection should be used to divide the platysma muscle. Any vessels (such as aberrant anterior jugular veins) should be cauterized or ligated. Haemostasis must be meticulous
6	Midline blunt dissection should then be used to divide the strap muscles. These are retracted laterally to expose the thyroid isthmus. If the isthmus lies superior to the third tracheal cartilage, it may simply be mobilized superiorly to gain access to the trachea. More commonly, however, the isthmus overlies the second and third rings—it must be incised or even completely divided to gain suitable access to the trachea
7	The anaesthetist should be informed that the trachea is about to be entered. The oropharynx should be aspirated of all secretions prior to surgical incision of the trachea. Access to the tracheal lumen is often associated with inadvertent puncture of the underlying tracheal tube cuff, resulting in a leak with ventilation. There is the option to insert the tracheal tube further into the trachea, which may avoid this occurring
8	Tracheal lumen access can be achieved in one of three ways, as described below: a. Anterior tracheal ring removal b. T-shaped tracheal opening c. U- or H-shaped tracheal opening
9	Once the tracheal stoma has been created, the tracheal tube should be withdrawn slowly under direct vision, such that the tracheal tube tip lies just proximal to the upper border of the stoma. Any secretions or blood within the trachea should be suctioned
10	The tracheostomy tube is then inserted through the stoma under direct vision, usually with an obturator *in situ* to guide it into place
11	Once the tracheostomy tube placement has been confirmed by capnography, the tracheal tube may be removed, and the tracheostomy tube secured
12	The skin should be left open to avoid the risk of complications such as subcutaneous emphysema and pneumomediastinum

A low position may result in a tube encroaching on the carina, or very close to the innominate artery. In the patient with a cervical spine injury, however, neck extension should be avoided, and inline immobilization maintained.

If the procedure is being performed in the awake patient under local anaesthesia, the positioning may have to be compromised to minimize patient distress, and it may be necessary to have the patient sitting or semi-recumbent.

Anterior tracheal ring removal technique

The anterior portion of one or more of the tracheal rings is removed to create a rectangular stoma. Stay sutures are placed in the tracheal wall at either side of the stoma and left uncut. These sutures are used to provide countertraction during the insertion of the tracheostomy tube but are also usually left *in situ* following the procedure to

facilitate reinsertion of an accidentally displaced tracheostomy tube (Fig. 3.1). This technique is associated with subsequent tracheal stenosis and should probably be reserved for permanent stomas.

T-shaped tracheal opening technique

A 2 cm incision is made horizontally through the tracheal wall between the second and third tracheal rings, or the third and fourth rings. A vertical incision is then made perpendicular to the first incision in the midline through the distal one or two tracheal rings using heavy scissors. Stay sutures are then inserted into each flap and taped to either side of the neck or upper chest.

U- or H-shaped tracheal opening technique

This method, described by Björk,[26] involves the creation of an inverted U-shaped tracheal wall flap. The flap is made at the level of the

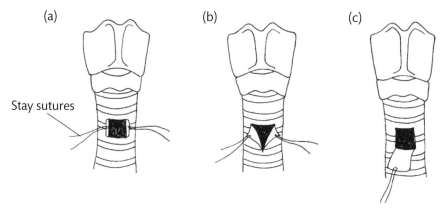

(a)   (b)   (c)

Stay sutures

Fig. 3.1 Approaches to surgical tracheostomy. (a) Ring removal. (b) T-shaped incision. (c) Inverted U-shaped incision.
Reproduced with permission from Shaw et al, The Oxford textbook of anaesthesia for oral and maxillofacial surgery, First Edition, Oxford University Press, UK.

second to fourth tracheal rings, and reflected downwards, with its upper border sutured to the skin, creating a bridge of tracheal tissue that assists with tube placement. In the emergency replacement of the displaced tube, the flap will not only assist in guiding the tracheal tube into the trachea lumen, but will also help to prevent the creation of a false passage through pre-tracheal tissues. A modification of this method involves the creation of an H-shaped flap in which the tracheal flaps are reflected and secured to skin both superiorly and inferiorly.

Complications of surgical and percutaneous tracheostomy

There are many potential complications associated with both surgical and percutaneous tracheostomy (Table 3.3), and so the risk:benefit ratio must be carefully considered in every patient before proceeding, particularly in the critical care setting. The complications may be divided into immediate (procedural), early, and late. The periprocedural complication rate is between 4% and 9% (Australian New Zealand Intensive Care Society—https://www. anzics.com.au/wp-content/uploads/2018/08/2014-The-ANZICS-Percutaneous-Dilatational-Tracheostomy-Consensus-Statement.pdf).

Bleeding

Bleeding within the first 48 hours is most often the result of venous injury (anterior jugular or inferior thyroid veins). The

Table 3.3 Complications of surgical and percutaneous tracheostomy

Immediate	Bleeding Damage to tissues during procedure: • Puncture of adjacent structures: nerves, arteries, veins, oesophagus • Damage to the posterior tracheal wall • Cartilage fracture • Misplacement of tracheostomy tube: pretracheal, endobronchial, perforation of the posterior tracheal wall Hypoxia and alveolar collapse Hypercapnia owing to inadequate ventilation Loss of airway and apnoea Pneumomediastinum Pneumothorax Surgical emphysema Type 2 post-obstructive pulmonary oedema
Early	Bleeding trachea-innominate artery fistulae Blockage of the tracheostomy tube with secretions, mucous, or blood Displacement of the tracheostomy tube Endobronchial or main stem bronchus intubation Erosion of tissue due to pressure from the tracheostomy tube or cuff Infection: cellulitis, mediastinitis, tracheitis Mucosal ulceration Subcutaneous emphysema Tracheo-oesophageal fistula
Late	Bleeding: tracheo-innominate artery fistulae Stoma scarring Tracheal granulomas Tracheal stenosis Tracheo-cutaneous fistula Tracheo-oesophageal fistula Tracheomalacia

wound should be carefully explored and the source of the bleeding addressed by either the intensive care specialist or surgeon. Granulation tissue may be treated by excision or cautery. Pressure from the tracheostomy tube or cuff may erode the trachea. Haemorrhage more than 48 hours postoperatively may be due to secondary haemorrhage, granulation tissue, or possibly a tracheo-innominate artery fistula (TIF).[27] The latter is an uncommon complication (0.1–1%) and may present at any time following tracheostomy. A 'sentinel' bleed (brief episode of brisk, bright red blood from the tracheostomy site) often precedes catastrophic haemorrhage by hours or days. It is therefore essential that the source of any tracheostomy bleeding should be carefully examined to ensure that the cause is not a TIF.

Tracheostomy tube designs often incorporate a gentle curve and compliant, low-pressure tracheal cuffs which have reduced the incidence of TIF. Other factors implicated in causing TIF include low tracheostomy tube placement, a malpositioned cannula tip, excessive neck movement, prior radiation, steroid use, and prolonged intubation. Management of catastrophic bleeding includes hyperinflation of the tracheostomy cuff or replacement of the tracheostomy tube with a tracheal tube. If unsuccessful, the 'Utley manoeuvre' may be used where digital pressure is applied to compress the innominate artery against the posterior wall of the manubrium.[28]

Emergency airway rescue of a tracheostomy or laryngostomy

The multidisciplinary guidelines for the management of tracheostomy and laryngectomy airway emergencies are essential reading.[29] They highlight that patients with a tracheostomy have a potentially patent upper airway while laryngectomy patients do not. This alters the emergency management and requires oxygenation to be attempted via the laryngectomy stoma. This can be accomplished by using a laryngeal or paediatric face mask applied over the stoma or a tracheal tube through the stoma.

The website for the guidelines is http://www.tracheostomy.org.uk.

Submental tracheal intubation

This technique was first described in 1986 by Francisco Hernandez Altemir.[30] It involves the passing of a tracheal tube through the anterior floor of the mouth (Table 3.4). It is useful by allowing intraoperative access to the oral, nasal, and base of skull regions, as well as permitting assessment of dental occlusion.[31] It is beneficial in complex cranio-maxillofacial trauma[32,33] and cancer surgery and may avoid the need for a tracheostomy and its inherent complications.[34] Another advantage is the cosmetic effect of making the scar less visible than that of a tracheostomy. (This technique is also discussed in Chapters 2 and 10).

The complications of this procedure include bleeding, infection, mucocele or fistula formation, hypertrophy of the scar, and damage to the lingual nerve, salivary ducts, and glands. The immediate concerns for the anaesthetist are tracheal tube obstruction, a main stem intubation, and accidental extubation. Therefore, a plan for emergency reintubation should be delineated with the entire surgical and anaesthetic team prior to embarking on this procedure.

Table 3.4 A stepwise approach to submental tracheal intubation

1	After conventional orotracheal intubation with a reinforced tracheal tube, a 2 cm skin incision is made in the submental area adjacent to the lower border of the mandible. A passage is created into the floor of the mouth by blunt dissection from the submental incision close to the lingual cortex of mandible, anterior to the sublingual caruncle *The FiO₂ should be increased to minimize the risk of desaturation during the procedure* *The anaesthetist must check that the universal connector can be removed from the tracheal tube prior to starting the procedure (some reinforced tracheal tubes do not have removable connectors)*
2	The pilot balloon of the tracheal tube should be deflated and then brought through the newly formed tunnel *Care must be taken so the pilot balloon is not ruptured*
3	The pilot balloon should be re-inflated The patient is then disconnected from the ventilator, the universal connector removed from the tracheal tube, and the proximal end of the tube drawn through the tunnel to emerge through the skin of the submental region *Care must be taken to ensure that the tracheal tube is not dislodged from the trachea*
4	The inner surface of the tracheal tube should be cleaned of any blood or tissue
5	The universal connector should be reattached and the patient connected to the breathing circuit and ventilator *There may be some difficulty in reattaching the connector to the tracheal tube*
6	Once the tracheal tube position is satisfactory, it should then be sutured in place *Care must be taken not to advance the tracheal tube excessively into a main stem bronchus or to cause inadvertent extubation*

Emergency front of neck airway

Patient positioning

The ideal position for all front of neck airway (FONA) procedures is the same as that for an elective surgical tracheostomy, that is, pillow removed, head ring, and sandbag under the shoulders to extend the neck. This may be very difficult to achieve during an emergency CICO scenario due to time pressures. Sliding the patient up the bed or operating table and allowing the head to gently hang over the top edge will provide moderate neck extension and improve access to the front of the neck, especially in the morbidly obese patient. This manoeuvre should be avoided when cervical spine injuries are suspected.

Needle versus scalpel cricothyroidotomy

The debate continues regarding the most appropriate method for anaesthetists to facilitate oxygenation during CICO while a definitive airway is secured. Emergency front-of-neck airway (eFONA) courses in some parts of the world encourage teaching both scalpel and cannula techniques.[35] However, opinions are divided concerning the high failure rate of cannula cricothyroidotomy in CICO management when compared to surgical access.[36–39] Criticism of the needle cricothyroidotomy is based largely on the Royal College of Anaesthetists' Fourth National Audit Project (NAP4) data.[40] In NAP4, there were 58 anaesthetic cases (of the estimated 2.9 million annual general anaesthetics) where attempts at emergency reoxygenation were undertaken. In 25 of these cases, the anaesthetist initiated the primary rescue attempt and was successful in nine cases. Eleven cases were subsequently rescued by a surgical tracheostomy, three by tracheal intubation, one by a percutaneous tracheostomy performed by an anaesthetist, and one patient died.

Anaesthetists in this study tended to use cannula-based techniques, with a narrow-bore cannula being used in 19 cases, with 12 failures. Anaesthetists were therefore successful in only 33% with other techniques (two successes out of six cases). Conclusions that may be logically drawn suggest that anaesthetists untrained in CICO techniques exhibited a high failure rate with both cannula and scalpel techniques (63% and 67%, respectively).[41] In contrast, surgeons achieved a high success rate using a scalpel but were slow in achieving a definitive airway under extreme pressure. Although rare, over half of experienced anaesthetists report encountering CICO at least once during their career.[42]

Before commencing eFONA rescue airway techniques, it is assumed that all oxygenation attempts via the upper airway have been considered, performed, and exhausted (https://www.das.uk.com/guidelines/das_intubation_guidelines). No patient should undergo percutaneous emergency oxygenation without having first undergone oxygenation attempts through facemask ventilation, supraglottic airway device insertion, and tracheal intubation via the upper airway. Where possible, oxygen and airway manoeuvres should continue to be administered via the upper airway (facemask or supraglottic airway device) at all times. Apnoeic oxygenation may occur if there is a patent aperture between the upper and lower airways and this may also importantly provide an expiratory pathway.

Needle cricothyroidotomy

This is also referred to as needle cricothyroid puncture or needle cricothyrotomy. Simulating crisis in a live, anaesthetized animal model is arguably the closest method of reproducing the stressful conditions of CICO in humans. The Royal Perth Hospital group in Australia have observed over 10,000 CICO rescue attempts in anaesthetized sheep by practitioners and refined their approach over time. The rationale for using a cannula as a conduit for reoxygenation includes a high success rate with training, its potential for conversion by Seldinger technique to a cuffed airway, anaesthetists' familiarity and confidence with the cannula, limited tissue destruction, and an attempt does not significantly impair subsequent attempts with either cannula or scalpel. The procedure may also be rapidly performed. The 14 G Insyte™ cannula (BD Medical Systems, Oakville, Canada) is cheap and widely available, enabling anaesthetists to practise transtracheal access. The cannula and the Rapid-O2™ (Meditech Systems Ltd, Dorset, UK) oxygen insufflation device is an affordable combination as basic oxygenation equipment in all clinical areas. The cannula provides a temporary conduit to provide rescue oxygenation allowing the patient to resume spontaneous respiration and be woken up or failing which a definitive airway may be obtained using either more complex airway manoeuvres (e.g.

fibreoptic intubation) or converting to a surgical airway. If immediately available, a competent surgeon may perform a tracheostomy or alternatively the cannula may be used to insert a Melker™ size 5.0 mm cuffed airway (Cook Medical Inc., Bloomington, IN, USA).

Indications

Needle or cannula cricothyroidotomy may be performed as an elective part of the anaesthetic technique for oral and maxillofacial surgical procedures. Needle or cannula cricothyroidotomy may be used to topicalize the airway in preparation for awake fibreoptic intubation. The cannula may be favoured over the needle here as this may remain in the airway and allow for rescue in the event of a failed awake fibreoptic intubation or sudden patient deterioration. Similarly, the cannula may be inserted prophylactically in a patient where difficulty in securing the airway is anticipated and access to the infraglottic airway is likely. However, it is most commonly associated with the CICO scenario. Therefore, it is commonly indicated for patients with impending or actual complete airway obstruction that may result from severe facial trauma, anaphylaxis, infection (e.g. submandibular abscess and epiglottitis), and laryngeal pathology (e.g. tumour).

Contraindications

In the elective scenario, relative contraindications include lack of adequate training, an uncooperative patient, and laryngeal human papillomavirus or carcinoma where virus and tumour cells may spread along the needle track and seed in the submandibular tissues. In the emergency CICO scenario, there are no absolute contraindications to cannula cricothyroidotomy or tracheotomy. Conditions such as previous neck surgery, radiotherapy to the neck with scar tissue, overlying infection, coagulopathy, and neck trauma may all serve to make all FONA procedures challenging, including cannula techniques.

Technique

If time allows, the skin should be prepared with an antiseptic solution such as 2% chlorhexidine in alcohol and the skin should be anaesthetized using a local anaesthetic solution, most commonly lidocaine and adrenaline. Frerk and colleagues,[43] in the Difficult Airway Society 2015 guidelines for management of unanticipated difficult intubation in adults, recommended Levitan's 'laryngeal handshake' (**Fig. 3.2**) using the non-dominant hand to recognize the three-dimensional anatomy of the laryngeal structures. The

larynx is stabilized between thumb and middle finger, and the index finger moves down the neck to palpate the cricothyroid membrane (**Table 3.5**).

Limitations

The cannula technique may fail because of kinking, blood, or vomitus in the airway and because of difficult anatomy. There may also be no obvious reason and after three attempts at cannula cricothyroidotomy in the hypoxic patient, the practitioner is encouraged to move on to prevent fixation error. In the patient with impalpable anterior neck anatomy, the first cannulation attempt should be performed in the apparent midline unless there is information suggesting a laterally located trachea. If the first cannula attempt fails then the second attempt should be performed lateral (approximately 1 cm) to the first, that is, horizontally across the neck. The insertion attempts should remain vertical and parallel to the first insertion. A maximum of three blind attempts to cannulate the trachea should be considered before moving to the scalpel–finger–cannula technique described below.[44]

Scalpel–bougie cricothyroidotomy

Indications

These include failed cannula cricothyroidotomy in the patient with palpable anterior neck anatomy. Anaesthetists are familiar with the bougie and the deliberate stab incision reduces scalpel manipulation. The hollow bougie also has the advantage of enabling oxygenation, via a Rapi-Fit™ connector (Cook Medical Inc., Bloomington, IN, USA), prior to securing a cuffed airway. It must be emphasized that when inserted percutaneously, the tip of the bougie may be inadvertently placed more distally in the airway than intended (i.e. below the carina). High-pressure oxygenating devices should be used with extreme caution in these circumstances as this may result in barotrauma. Oxygenating using a self-inflating bag or anaesthetic circuit via the standard 15 mm Rapi-Fit™ connector minimizes this risk.

Technique

See **Table 3.6** and **Fig. 3.4**.

Scalpel–finger–cannula cricothyroidotomy

Indications

These include the CICO scenario with failed cannula cricothyroidotomy due to impalpable anterior neck anatomy and failed

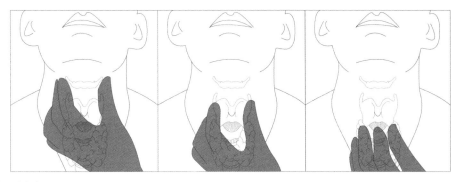

Fig. 3.2 The laryngeal handshake.

Reproduced with Permission from H. G. Ryu, J. Lee, H. Lee, et al, Utility of the laryngeal handshake method for identifying the cricothyroid membrane, Acta Anaesthesiologica Scandinavica, Jun 21, 2018, 62(9) p.6, John Wiley and Sons.

Table 3.5 Stepwise approach to needle cricothyroidotomy

1	Stand on the patient's left-hand side (if you are right hand dominant, and vice versa if left-hand dominant)
2	Connect a 5 mL syringe containing 2 mL saline to the 14 G Insyte™ needle-cannula, aligning the bevel of the needle with the graduation markings on the syringe to allow easy identification of bevel position. Hold this in the dominant hand with fingers between the barrel flange and plunger, enabling an 'aspirate as you go' technique
3	Identify and stabilize the cricothyroid membrane or trachea using the non-dominant hand. Place the thumb and middle finger on either side of the thyroid cartilage with the index finger resting over the cricothyroid membrane
4	Insert the tip of the needle through the skin and advance in a caudal direction while continually aspirating (Fig. 3.3). Insertion angle should be as shallow as practical. Aspirate while advancing. Never aspirate while withdrawing as the cannula may inadvertently be separated from the needle creating an air leak between the needle and cannula. This enables air to be aspirated between the inner surface of the cannula and outer surface of the needle. This explains how air may be inadvertently 'aspirated' despite the needle not being in the trachea. This is known as a false-positive aspiration of air. Similarly, pre-loosening the cannula off the needle is discouraged for the same reason
5	Successful free aspiration of air to the full length of the syringe barrel and then releasing it without recoil confirms intratracheal placement ('check' aspiration)
6	The non-dominant hand should stabilize the cannula at the hub. The dominant hand should move to hold the needle. The non-dominant hand is used to advance the cannula off the needle into the tracheal lumen
7	Grip the cannula hub with the non-dominant hand and remove the syringe and needle
8	Expel the air from the 5 mL syringe containing 2 mL saline and reconnect to the cannula. Repeat the 'check' aspiration prior to jet oxygenation. If the re-check fails, the cannula should be withdrawn slightly while aspiration is continued. If the cannula is kinked or tip impacted on the posterior pharyngeal wall, this will be easily corrected

scalpel–bougie technique in the patient with palpable anterior neck anatomy.

Technique

See Table 3.7.

Complications of eFONA techniques

Complications can be divided into immediate, intermediate, and late:

Immediate

These include failure to locate the trachea, misplacement of the tracheal tube including endobronchial intubation, haemorrhage, and prolonged time to oxygenation resulting in significant morbidity and mortality.[46–48] Other potential complications include:

- Pulmonary aspiration.
- Kinking and obstruction of the cannula with inability to oxygenate the patient or inability passing the guide wire of the Melker™ airway.

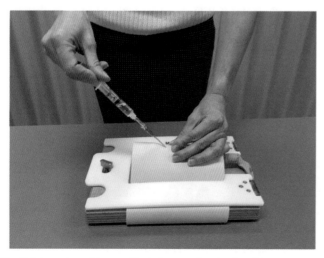

Fig. 3.3 Insertion of the needle during needle cricothyroidotomy.

- Haemorrhage.
- Trauma to trachea and surrounding structures.
- Misplacement of the cannula leading to subcutaneous emphysema, pneumothorax with attempted insufflation.
- Barotrauma and volutrauma due to overzealous attempts at oxygenation.
- Creation of a false passage leading to subcutaneous emphysema, mediastinal emphysema, and pneumothorax with attempted insufflation.
- Progressive hypercapnia and acidosis with limited ventilation.
- Reflex coughing on insufflation. This may be treated with injection of lidocaine down the cannula.

Intermediate complications

These include bleeding, infection, oesophageal perforation and tracheo-oesophageal fistula, recurrent laryngeal nerve injury, and dysphonia due to laryngeal trauma.

Late complications

The most significant delayed complication is subglottic stenosis.

Use of ultrasound

Ultrasound has been used to rapidly identify the cricothyroid membrane.[49] Ultrasound may also help in assessing the location of the trachea in patients with impalpable anterior neck anatomy because of deep tissue neck infections, tumours, and dysmorphia. Knowledge regarding the depth and deviation of the trachea may serve to fine-tune the percutaneous approach to the airway. The presence and location of major vessels can also be identified and avoided. An ultrasound machine, if immediately available, may be useful even in the CICO situation in patients with impalpable anterior neck anatomy—improving accuracy and efficiency.[33] If progression to a scalpel technique is required, the incision depth and position can be elucidated in

Table 3.6 Stepwise approach to scalpel–bougie cricothyroidotomy

1	Operator stands on the patient's left-hand side (if right hand dominant, and vice versa if left hand dominant)
2	Identify and stabilize the cricothyroid membrane or anterior trachea using the non-dominant hand (as described in Table 3.5)
3	Make a horizontal stab incision through the cricothyroid membrane or anterior trachea with the cutting edge of the size 10 scalpel blade facing towards the operator
4	The operator should apply gentle traction towards them and then rotate the blade 90° so that the cutting edge of the blade points caudally. This is to reduce the risk of trauma to the vocal cords
5	Keeping the scalpel vertical, the operator should now gently pull the scalpel towards them. This creates a triangular hole with the blade of the scalpel forming the base
6	Swap hands to hold the scalpel with the non-dominant hand
7	The dominant hand now holds the bougie parallel to the floor with the coudé tip pointing towards the operator and inferiorly, i.e. the bougie is parallel to the floor and perpendicular to the patient (Fig. 3.4). Using the scalpel blade as a guide, slide the bougie tip down the scalpel blade until it lies within the trachea. The triangular hole created by the combination of incision, rotation, and gentle traction of the blade is often crucially underappreciated when practising on manikins or cadavers. Significant bleeding, which commonly occurs at this point, will obscure the incision. This not only makes insertion of the bougie difficult but also risks the inadvertent creation of a false passage
8	Rotate and align the bougie to allow gentle insertion observing the characteristic feel of tracheal rings (clicks); 'hold up' may be encountered
9	The scalpel blade may now be carefully removed
10	Oxygenate via the hollow oxygenating bougie (if used) using the Rapi-Fit™ 15 mm standard connector and self-inflating bag or anaesthetic circuit if immediately available. Confirm placement of the bougie within the trachea using capnography
11	Remove the Rapi-Fit™ connector if this is being used and railroad a lubricated size 6.0 cuffed tracheal tube over the bougie. Continual rotation of the tracheal tube starting as it is advanced down the bougie prevents 'hold up' of the tube tip at the skin. A size 5.0 cuffed Melker™ airway may also be 'railroaded' over the bougie. The Melker™ airway sits snuggly over the bougie eliminating the need for the Melker™ introducer[45]
12	Remove the bougie, inflate the cuff, and ventilate via the tracheal tube or Melker™. Confirm using capnography. Insertion of a tracheal tube through the anterior neck is prone to endobronchial intubation. Prior to securing the tracheal tube, ensure to exclude this complication
13	Secure the tube or Melker™ in position

advance. This leads to a safer and more confident approach. However, task fixation and delays using ultrasound should be avoided.

Conversion techniques

One such technique involves the use of the Melker™ Emergency Cricothyrotomy Catheter set (Cook Medical Inc., Bloomington, IN, USA). The set contains a scalpel, needle, guide wire, and the cuffed airway with dilating introducer.

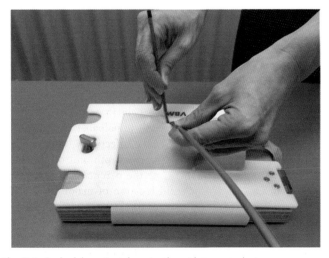

Fig. 3.4 Scalpel–bougie–tube cricothyroidotomy technique.

Technique

See Table 3.8 for a stepwise approach to using a Melker™ Emergency Cricothyrotomy set. The commonest reason for difficulty when advancing the Melker™ airway is that the dilator slips back within the Melker™ airway creating a 'step' between the dilator and the tip

Table 3.7 A stepwise approach to scalpel–finger–cannula cricothyroidotomy

1	Stabilize the skin of the neck with the non-dominant hand. With a size 10 scalpel blade make a generous, vertical, midline incision. For the right-handed practitioner standing on the patient's left-hand side, the incision should be made in a caudad to cephalad direction. If time allows, the right-handed operator would be best making an incision from cephalad to caudal by standing on the patient's right-hand side (the opposite would be advised for a left-handed practitioner). The incision should be performed in the midline to avoid vascular structures located laterally unless it is suspected that the airway is laterally displaced. The incision should be superficial, passing through skin and subcutaneous tissue and down to the strap muscles
2	Insert the fingers of both hands into the incision to separate the strap muscles by blunt dissection and therefore avoiding damage caused by a more significant scalpel incision
3	The non-dominant hand should be used to identify the airway. The trachea is mobile, has tracheal cartilage rings, and the ability to get behind it with the fingers
4	Stabilize the airway with the non-dominant hand. Insert a 14 G Insyte™ cannula directly into the trachea as described previously
5	Jet oxygenation may then be performed via the cannula
6	Following rescue oxygenation, a wire may be passed down the cannula, followed by insertion of a size 5.0 cuffed Melker™ using the Seldinger technique. When inserting the Melker™ airway directly into the trachea, no further incision is required

Table 3.8 A stepwise approach to use of the Melker™ Emergency Cricothyrotomy set

1	Stand on the left-hand side of patient (if right hand dominant, and vice versa if left hand dominant). Insert the soft flexible tip of the wire through the cannula. Kinking of the cannula may lead to difficulty passing the guide wire. Withdrawing the cannula slightly should allow the guide wire to pass
2	Withdraw the cannula over the guide wire. If desaturation occurs prior to successful Melker™ insertion, the cannula may be passed back over the guide wire and jet oxygenation recommended
3	Make an incision along the guide wire with the cutting edge of the scalpel blade pointing caudally to a depth sufficient to enter the airway. Ensure the incision is continuous with the guide wire
4	Grip the dilator and cuffed Melker airway to ensure that the dilator and Melker™ airway remains fully engaged. The 'Vulcan hand grip' (Fig. 3.5) is one way of gripping the dilator and Melker™ airway in the dominant hand to ensure there is no disengagement. It minimizes the risk of the wire injuring the operator and allows a fluid insertion motion, while avoiding hang up on the chin
5	Pass the guide wire through the tip of the dilator Melker™ airway
6	Continuously advance the Melker™ dilator airway over the guide wire. With the non-dominant hand stabilizing the trachea, the dominant hand advances the Melker™ airway in a caudal direction. Moderate force is required
7	Once the airway is fully inserted, securely hold the 15 mm connector, remove the guide wire and dilator, inflate the cuff, and ventilate via a self-inflating bag or anaesthetic circuit. Check for end-tidal carbon dioxide, look for chest movement, and observe the anterior neck for swelling

of the airway. Ensure that the dilator Melker™ airway unit is always properly engaged. Check the incision is continuous with the wire and extend the incision as necessary. The wire may become kinked from an overly forceful attempt at insertion. A wire from a 'central venous catheter' set may be used as an alternative if required. Re-passing the cannula back over the wire and further jet oxygenation may be required.

Retrograde intubation

Retrograde intubation refers to a translaryngeal-guided tracheal intubation technique. First described in 1960 by Butler and Cirillo,[50] the approach outlined by Waters in 1963[51] is most commonly used today (retrograde intubation is also discussed in Chapter 2).

Indications

Its use tends to be limited to adults and children in whom semi-urgent intubation is required and where other airway techniques have failed because of anatomical abnormalities such as limited mouth opening, unstable cervical spine injuries, and/or the presence of blood or secretions in the supraglottic airway (e.g. in oromaxillofacial trauma). Other indications include patients with impending airway obstruction in whom an awake fibreoptic intubation is not feasible and a tracheostomy is not desirable.

Complications

Retrograde intubation is more complex, time-consuming, and has potentially more complications than other surgical airway techniques. Bleeding, subcutaneous emphysema, pneumothorax, pneumomediastinum, and trigeminal nerve trauma have all been described.[52]

Technique

Using the Cook retrograde intubation set (Cook Critical Care, Bloomington, IN, USA), the technique is described in **Table 3.9**.

It is important to select a tracheal tube with a diameter just slightly larger than that of the guide wire catheter, as this helps to reduce the incidence of 'hold-up' at the glottis.

Given the proximity of the cricothyroid membrane to the glottis, unsurprisingly the guide wire–catheter tends to 'flick' or 'flip' out of the airway while advancing the tracheal tube and withdrawing the wire and catheter resulting in an oesophageal intubation. Modifications of the above technique have attempted to reduce this occurring and so improve the success rates. These techniques include:

- Removing the J guide wire and advancing the catheter distally into the airway before passing the tracheal tube.[53]
- Inserting the guide wire through the Murphy's eye of the tracheal tube.[54]
- Inserting the needle into the trachea well below the level of the cricothyroid membrane, using a pulling technique and a multi-lumen catheter.[55–57]
- Fibreoptic-assisted techniques that allow visual verification and confirmation of intratracheal placement (i.e. retrograde-guided fibreoptic intubation or oral fibreoptic intubation over a retrograde wire).[58,59] The guide wire may be passed through the distal opening of the fibreoptic scope's suction port, guided through the glottis and into the airway. Success rates are further improved if the tracheal tube is passed over the guide wire and the fibreoptic scope is then passed through the lumen of the tracheal tube adjacent to the wire. The tracheal tube may be followed and seen to be abutting the cricothyroid membrane. The fibreoptic scope is then advanced into the airway towards the carina. The guide wire is removed at this point and the tracheal tube passed over the fibreoptic scope and into the trachea.[60]

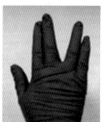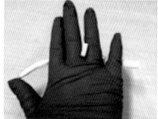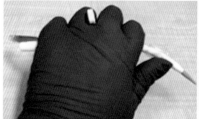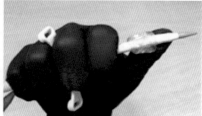

Fig. 3.5 The 'Vulcan hand grip'.

Table 3.9 Stepwise approach to retrograde intubation

1	A cricothyroid membrane puncture is made using the 18 G introducer needle
2	The guide wire is advanced cephalad through the introducer until it can be retrieved from the naso- or oropharynx using Magill's forceps
3	The wire is withdrawn through the mouth or nose until the neck positioning mark draws level with the skin. The guide wire is then anchored with artery forceps
4	The tapered catheter is then inserted over the guide wire from above until it abuts the cricothyroid membrane
5	The tracheal tube is then advanced over the catheter and into the airway as the guide wire and catheter are removed

- The use of a lightwand to facilitate the retrograde intubation procedure has also been described.[61]

Jet oxygenation

Oxygenation does not require the correct identification of the cricothyroid membrane. Whether eFONA is performed through the cricothyroid membrane or anterior wall of the trachea is not likely to be important.[62] Retrospective analysis of emergency cricothyrotomies and tracheotomies undertaken in a trauma centre in the US found no complications in either group.[63]

Transtracheal jet ventilation has, justifiably, been implicated in secondary barotrauma and highlights the pitfalls of attempting to achieve minute volume ventilation via a fine bore cannula without sufficient training. The use of a cannula may be inappropriate without an appropriate jet oxygenation device and suitable training. CICO prioritizes oxygenation over ventilation and carbon dioxide elimination. Ventilation in the obstructed airway may in fact be harmful. The preferred term in these circumstances is therefore 'jet oxygenation'. Oxygen delivery is aimed at preventing cardiac arrest and limiting hypoxic consequences, before rapidly moving on to secure the airway or waking the patient up (depending on the circumstances).

Ideal features of a jet oxygenation device

- Affordable, so it may be used for training and be stocked at all anaesthesia locations.
- Easily transportable.
- Intuitive function.
- Quick and easy to set up.
- High safety rating.
- True on–off device.
- Delivers a known and accurate oxygen flow rate:
  - Wall supply at 15 L/min, or cylinder supply at 250 mL/sec.
  - For example, the Manujet™, set at 0.5–1 bar, can deliver flow rates in the region of 250–300 mL/sec.[64,65]
- Allows passive expiration.
- If flow is not delivered, the device should provide feedback to the operator.

Between jets, the device should enable expiration and, more importantly, pressure relief via the cannula. Users should be aware that a significant disadvantage of the Manujet™ is the complete lack of an expiratory pathway and hence pressure relief via the device during expiration when it is connected directly to a cannula.[65]

Jet oxygenation plan

In the elective scenario, jet ventilation may be modified as considered clinically relevant.

In CICO, however, it is not how frequently one should provide jet oxygenation, but how infrequently. The focus is to provide oxygenation for only as long as it takes to either wake the patient up or to secure the airway.

A suggested technique might be as follows:

1. Four-second initial jet delivering 1000 mL of oxygen (e.g. using Rapid-O2 oxygen insufflation device connected to oxygen flow meter at 15 L/min).
2. Wait for peak in oxygen saturation (SpO$_2$) response and then wait for drop by 5% from peak.
3. Subsequent jets of 500 mL (2 seconds), waiting for each peak and drop by 5% and repeat.
4. If there is no response to first jet within 20 seconds, then immediately deliver second jet of 500 mL.
5. If no SpO$_2$ reading is available to guide the jetting rate, deliver 500 mL jets every 30 seconds after the initial 1000 mL.
6. Move as quickly as practical to secure a definitive airway.
7. If poor response and obviously patent expiratory pathway, consider Manujet™ at 4.0 bar delivering 1-second insufflations. Again, secure a definitive airway as quickly as possible.

Jet oxygenation devices

There are a number of jet oxygenation devices currently available. Training in the device is essential for safe usage, as each have their nuances:

Cook® Enk oxygen flow modulator (Cook Medical Inc., Bloomington, IN, USA)

This device (**Fig. 3.6a**) has an oxygen supply connector at one end and a Luer-lock connection for attachment to a needle/cannula cricothyroidotomy at the other. Intermittently covering and

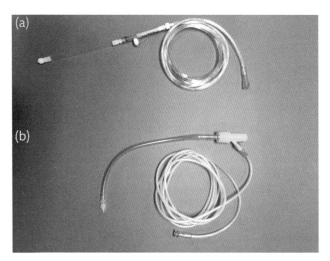

Fig. 3.6 (a) Cook® Enk oxygen flow modulator and (b) Rapid-O2™ cricothyroidotomy insufflation device.

releasing the five holes (by pressing thumb and index finger together) allows control of oxygen delivery and acts as pressure and flow relief vents. When the holes are occluded, oxygen is delivered and when uncovered, passive expiration occurs. The device has a side-port for drug administration. The side-port cap should remain closed to ensure oxygen delivery. The device usually comes with an Emergency Transtracheal Airway Catheter™, which is wire reinforced to prevent kinking or collapsing once inserted over its needle.

Rapid-O2™ cricothyroidotomy insufflation device (previously known as the 'Leroy'—Meditech Systems Ltd., Dorset, UK)

This device (**Fig. 3.6b**)[66] is sold through GE Healthcare. This modified T-piece is affordable, simple, and easy to use, and allows jet oxygenation as soon as the transtracheal cannula has been sited. It is a true on–off device, provides feedback, and also affords an expiratory pathway. Expiration is possible through the cannula.

Manujet™ (VBM Medizintechnik GmbH, Sulz am Neckar, Germany)

This is a pressure-regulated jet ventilation device designed for use with either oxygen or compressed air and comes supplied with a pressure hose attached. The device requires a working pressure of >4 bar. The device may be attached via a Luer-lock connecting tube to the cannula (VBM Ravussin 13-gauge needle). The pressure regulator knob needs to be pulled out to allow adjustment prior to use. Turning the black knob of the pressure regulator enables the respiration pressure to be decreased or increased as appropriate. Once set, the knob should be pushed back into position prior to use. Once connected to the cannula, the device itself affords no expiratory option. It is important to observe the patient at all times. The rise and subsequent fall of the patient's chest indicates successful respiration, but the operator should closely monitor the patient for barotrauma and inadvertent cannula displacement.

Ventrain™ (Dolphys Medical B.V., Eindhoven, The Netherlands)

This device offers the possibility of suction-generated, assisted expiration designed to achieve physiological minute ventilation in CICO. It is supplied together with a flexible 2 mm needle cricothyrotomy catheter, Cricath™. It is recommended that the device only be used together with the Cricath™ as the negative pressure generated during expiration may be sufficient to cause collapse of the cannula lumen if using other devices. Timing of inspiration and expiration need to be matched to avoid excessive flow in one direction.

Three-way tap and oxygen tubing

Bulk oxygen gas supply and cylinder oxygen are delivered at 4 bar (345–380 kPa or 50–55 psi). Unsurprisingly, there is a high risk of barotrauma when oxygen is delivered from a flow meter through a rudimentary three-way tap and oxygen-tubing device if the side port is not occluded, as there is neither pressure nor flow relief.[65,67,68] During supposed 'expiration' (i.e. no active jetting), flow will continue into the trachea and dangerously high intrathoracic pressures may be generated. The same situation may arise with the use of oxygen tubing with a hole cut into the sidewall. These techniques are often taught and tested in manikins and bench top models with a patent expiratory pathway. However, under CICO conditions with an obstructed upper airway, the risk of barotrauma becomes obvious. This method of oxygen delivery should not be used in contemporary practice.

Conclusion

Anaesthetists should make every effort to anticipate the difficult airway through a thorough history, examination, and review of special investigations. The preoperative assessment should inform the airway plan. However, reality dictates that despite rigorous assessment, unexpected difficulty may be encountered, and the practitioner should be equipped to deal with the CICO scenario should this arise. Surgical airways, whether elective or urgent, are always potentially hazardous interventions. Understanding the dangers and pitfalls associated with the various procedures should enable the anaesthetist to anticipate problems and make every effort to minimize risks.

Acknowledgements

The authors would like to thank Dr Kaye Cantlay, Consultant in Anaesthesia and Critical Care, Royal Victoria Infirmary, Newcastle Upon Tyne—for her valued contribution as author of *The surgical airway* in the *Oxford Textbook of Anaesthesia for Oral and Maxillofacial Surgery First Edition*.

REFERENCES

1. Kheterpal S, Martin L, Shanks AM, Tremper KK. Prediction and outcomes of impossible mask ventilation: a review of 50,000 anesthetics. *Anesthesiology*. 2009;**110**(4):891–897.
2. Nagaro T, Yorozuya T, Sotani M, Adachi N, Tabo E, Arai T, et al. Survey of patients whose lungs could not be ventilated and whose trachea could not be intubated in university hospitals in Japan. *J Anesth*. 2003;**17**(4):232–240.
3. Young D, Harrison DA, Cuthbertson BH, Rowan K, TracMan C. Effect of early vs late tracheostomy placement on survival in patients receiving mechanical ventilation: the TracMan randomized trial. *JAMA*. 2013;**309**(20):2121–2129.
4. Delaney A, Bagshaw SM, Nalos M. Percutaneous dilatational tracheostomy versus surgical tracheostomy in critically ill patients: a systematic review and meta-analysis. *Crit Care*. 2006;**10**(2):R55.
5. Higgins KM, Punthakee X. Meta-analysis comparison of open versus percutaneous tracheostomy. *Laryngoscope*. 2007;**117**(3):447–454.
6. Johnson-Obaseki S, Veljkovic A, Javidnia H. Complication rates of open surgical versus percutaneous tracheostomy in critically ill patients. *Laryngoscope*. 2016;**126**(11):2459–2467.
7. Dulguerov P, Gysin C, Perneger TV, Chevrolet JC. Percutaneous or surgical tracheostomy: a meta-analysis. *Crit Care Med*. 1999;**27**(8):1617–1625.
8. Grover A, Robbins J, Bendick P, Gibson M, Villalba M. Open versus percutaneous dilatational tracheostomy: efficacy and cost analysis. *Am Surg*. 2001;**67**(4):297–301.
9. Cameron TS, McKinstry A, Burt SK, Howard ME, Bellomo R, Brown DJ, et al. Outcomes of patients with spinal cord injury

before and after introduction of an interdisciplinary tracheostomy team. *Crit Care Resusc.* 2009;**11**(1):14–19.

10. Ciaglia P, Firsching R, Syniec C. Elective percutaneous dilatational tracheostomy. A new simple bedside procedure; preliminary report. *Chest.* 1985;**87**(6):715–719.

11. Byhahn C, Lischke V, Halbig S, Scheifler G, Westphal K. [Ciaglia blue rhino: a modified technique for percutaneous dilatation tracheostomy. Technique and early clinical results]. *Der Anaesthesist.* 2000;**49**(3):202–206.

12. Byhahn C, Zgoda M, Birkelbach O, Hofstetter C, Gromann T. Ciaglia Blue Dolphin: a new technique for percutaneous tracheostomy using balloon dilation. *Crit Care.* 2008;**12** Suppl 2;P333.

13. Griggs WM, Worthley LI, Gilligan JE, Thomas PD, Myburg JA. A simple percutaneous tracheostomy technique. *Surg Gynecol Obstet.* 1990;**170**(6):543–545.

14. Westphal K, Maeser D, Scheifler G, Lischke V, Byhahn C. PercuTwist: a new single-dilator technique for percutaneous tracheostomy. *Anesth Analg.* 2003;**96**(1):229–232.

15. Fantoni A, Ripamonti D. A non-derivative, non-surgical tracheostomy: the translaryngeal method. *Intensive Care Med.* 1997;**23**(4):386–392.

16. Nates JL, Cooper DJ, Myles PS, Scheinkestel CD, Tuxen DV. Percutaneous tracheostomy in critically ill patients: a prospective, randomized comparison of two techniques. *Crit Care Med.* 2000;**28**(11):3734–3739.

17. Cianchi G, Zagli G, Bonizzoli M, Batacchi S, Cammelli R, Biondi S, et al. Comparison between single-step and balloon dilatational tracheostomy in intensive care unit: a single-centre, randomized controlled study. *Br J Anaesth.* 2010;**104**(6):728–732.

18. Ambesh SP, Pandey CK, Srivastava S, Agarwal A, Singh DK. Percutaneous tracheostomy with single dilatation technique: a prospective, randomized comparison of Ciaglia blue rhino versus Griggs' guidewire dilating forceps. *Anesth Analg.* 2002;**95**(6):1739–1745.

19. Añón JM, Escuela MP, Gómez V, Moreno A, López J, Díaz R, et al. Percutaneous tracheostomy: Ciaglia Blue Rhino versus Griggs' guide wire dilating forceps. A prospective randomized trial. *Acta Anaesthesiol Scand.* 2004;**48**(4):451–46.

20. Byhahn C, Westphal K, Meininger D, Gurke B, Kessler P, Lischke V. Single-dilator percutaneous tracheostomy: a comparison of PercuTwist and Ciaglia Blue Rhino techniques. *Intensive Care Med.* 2002;**28**(9):1262–1266.

21. Cantais E, Kaiser E, Le-Goff Y, Palmier B. Percutaneous tracheostomy: prospective comparison of the translaryngeal technique versus the forceps-dilational technique in 100 critically ill adults. *Crit Care Med.* 2002;**30**(4):815–819.

22. Johnson JL, Cheatham ML, Sagraves SG, Block EF, Nelson LD. Percutaneous dilational tracheostomy: a comparison of single- versus multiple-dilator techniques. *Crit Care Med.* 2001;**29**(6):1251–1254.

23. Byhahn C, Wilke HJ, Halbig S, Lischke V, Westphal K. Percutaneous tracheostomy: Ciaglia Blue Rhino versus the basic Ciaglia technique of percutaneous dilational tracheostomy. *Anesth Analg.* 2000;**91**(4):882–886.

24. Cabrini L, Monti G, Landoni G, Biondi-Zoccai G, Boroli F, Mamo D, et al. Percutaneous tracheostomy, a systematic review. *Acta Anaesthesiol Scand.* 2012;**56**(3):270–281.

25. Rudas M, Seppelt I, Herkes R, Hislop R, Rajbhandari D, Weisbrodt L. Traditional landmark versus ultrasound guided tracheal puncture during percutaneous dilatational tracheostomy

in adult intensive care patients: a randomised controlled trial. *Crit Care.* 2014;**18**(5):14.

26. Bjork VO. Partial resection of the only remaining lung with the aid of respirator treatment. *J Thorac Cardiovasc Surg.* 1960;**39**:179–288.

27. Grant CA, Dempsey G, Harrison J, Jones T. Tracheo-innominate artery fistula after percutaneous tracheostomy: three case reports and a clinical review. *Br J Anaesth.* 2006;**96**(1):127–131.

28. Utley JR, Singer MM, Roe BB, Fraser DG, Dedo HH. Definitive management of innominate artery hemorrhage complicating tracheostomy. *JAMA.* 1972;**220**(4):577–579.

29. McGrath BA, Bates L, Atkinson D, Moore JA; National Tracheostomy Safety Project. Multidisciplinary guidelines for the management of tracheostomy and laryngectomy airway emergencies. *Anaesthesia.* 2012;**67**(9):1025–1041.

30. Hernandez Altemir F. The submental route for endotracheal intubation. A new technique. *J Maxillofac Surg.* 1986;**14**(1):64–65.

31. Amin M, Dill-Russell P, Manisali M, Lee R, Sinton I. Facial fractures and submental tracheal intubation. *Anaesthesia.* 2002;**57**(12):1195–1199.

32. Caron G, Paquin R, Lessard MR, Trepanier CA, Landry PE. Submental endotracheal intubation: an alternative to tracheotomy in patients with midfacial and panfacial fractures. *J Trauma.* 2000;**48**(2):235–240.

33. Biglioli F, Mortini P, Goisis M, Bardazzi A, Boari N. Submental orotracheal intubation: an alternative to tracheotomy in transfacial cranial base surgery. *Skull Base.* 2003;**13**(4):189–195.

34. Malhotra N, Bhardwaj N, Chari P. Submental endotracheal intubation: a useful alternative to tracheostomy. *Indian J Anaesth.* 2002;**46**(5):400–402.

35. Heard AMB, Green RJ, Eakins P. The formulation and introduction of the 'can't intubate, can't ventilate' algorithm into clinical practice. *Anaesthesia.* 2009;**64**(6):601–608.

36. Baker PA, O'Sullivan EP, Kristensen MS, Lockey D. The great airway debate: is the scalpel mightier than the cannula? *Br J Anaesth.* 2016;**117** Suppl 1:i17–i19.

37. Duggan LV, Ballantyne Scott B, Law JA, Morris IR, Murphy MF, Griesdale DE. Transtracheal jet ventilation in the 'can't intubate can't oxygenate' emergency: a systematic review. *Br J Anaesth.* 2016;**117** Suppl 1:i28–i38.

38. Pracy JP, Brennan L, Cook TM, Hartle AJ, Marks RJ, McGrath BA, et al. Surgical intervention during a can't intubate can't oxygenate (CICO) event: emergency front-of-neck airway (FONA)? *Br J Anaesth* 2016;**117**(4):426–428.

39. Kristensen MS, Teoh WH, Baker PA. Percutaneous emergency airway access; prevention, preparation, technique and training. *Br J Anaesth.* 2015;**114**(3):357–361.

40. Cook TM, Woodall N, Frerk C; Fourth National Audit Project. Major complications of airway management in the UK: results of the Fourth National Audit Project of the Royal College of Anaesthetists and the Difficult Airway Society. Part 1: anaesthesia. *Br J Anaesth.* 2011;**106**(5):617–631.

41. Bradley P. Continued provision of cannula cricothyroidotomy equipment. *Anaesthesia.* 2016;**71**(7):854–855.

42. Wong DT, Lai K, Chung FF, Ho RY. Cannot intubate-cannot ventilate and difficult intubation strategies: results of a Canadian national survey. *Anesth Analg.* 2005;**100**(5):1439–1446.

43. Freck CM, Mitchell V, McNarry A, Mendonca C, Bhagrath R, Patel A, et al. Difficult Airway Society 2015 guidelines for the management of unanticipated difficult intubation in adults. *Br J Anaesth.* 2015;**115**(6):827–848.

44. Heard A. Instructor check-lists for percutaneous emergency oxygenation strategies in the 'can't intubate, can't oxygenate' scenario. 2014. https://www.smashwords.com/books/view/494739

45. Parameswaran A, Beckmann L, Nadarajah P. Scalpel-bougie cricothyroidotomy. *Anaesthesia.* 2014;**69**(5):517–518.

46. McGill J, Clinton JE, Ruiz E. Cricothyrotomy in the emergency department. *Ann Emerg Med.* 1982;**11**(7):361–4.

47. Erlandson MJ, Clinton JE, Ruiz E, Cohen J. Cricothyrotomy in the emergency department revisited. *J Emerg Med.* 1989;**7**(2):115–118.

48. Schillaci CR, Iacovoni VF, Conte RS. Transtracheal aspiration complicated by fatal endotracheal hemorrhage. *N Engl J Med.* 1976;**295**(9):488–490.

49. Nicholls SE, Sweeney TW, Ferre RM, Strout TD. Bedside sonography by emergency physicians for the rapid identification of landmarks relevant to cricothyrotomy. *Am J Emerg Med.* 2008;**26**(8):852–856.

50. Butler FS, Cirillo AA. Retrograde tracheal intubation. *Anesth Analg.* 1960;**39**:333–338.

51. Waters DJ. Guided blind endotracheal intubation. For patients with deformities of the upper airway. *Anaesthesia.* 1963;**18**:158–162.

52. Dhara SS. Retrograde tracheal intubation. *Anaesthesia.* 2009;**64**(10):1094–1104.

53. King HK, Wang LF, Khan AK, Wooten DJ. Translaryngeal guided intubation for difficult intubation. *Crit Care Med.* 1987;**15**(9):869–871.

54. Bourke D, Levesque PR. Modification of retrograde guide for endotracheal intubation. *Anesth Analg.* 1974;**53**(6):1013–1014.

55. Abou-Madi MN, Trop D. Pulling versus guiding: a modification of retrograde guided intubation. *Can J Anaesth.* 1989;**36**(3, Pt 1):336–339.

56. Dhara SS. Retrograde intubation—a facilitated approach. *Br J Anaesth.* 1992;**69**(6):631–633.

57. Shantha TR. Retrograde intubation using the subcricoid region. *Br J Anaesth.* 1992;**68**(1):109–112.

58. Bissinger U, Guggenberger H, Lenz G. Retrograde-guided fiberoptic intubation in patients with laryngeal carcinoma. *Anesth Analg.* 1995;**81**(2):408–410.

59. Gupta B, McDonald JS, Brooks JH, Mendenhall J. Oral fiberoptic intubation over a retrograde guidewire. *Anesth Analg.* 1989;**68**(4):517–519.

60. Lenfant F, Benkhadra M, Trouilloud P, Freysz M. Comparison of two techniques for retrograde tracheal intubation in human fresh cadavers. *Anesthesiology.* 2006;**104**(1):48–51.

61. Hung OR, al-Qatari M. Light-guided retrograde intubation. *Can J Anaesth.* 1997;**44**(8):877–882.

62. Law JA. Deficiencies in locating the cricothyroid membrane by palpation: We can't and the surgeons can't, so what now for the emergency surgical airway? *Can J Anaesth.* 2016;**63**(7):791–796.

63. Dillon JK, Christensen B, Fairbanks T, Jurkovich G, Moe KS. The emergent surgical airway: cricothyrotomy vs. tracheotomy. *Int J Oral Maxillofac Surg.* 2013;**42**(2):204–208.

64. Bould MD, Bearfield P. Techniques for emergency ventilation through a needle cricothyroidotomy. *Anaesthesia.* 2008;**63**(5):535–539.

65. Abstracts presented at the Difficult Airway Society's Annual Meeting in Nottingham, November 2011. *Anaesthesia.* 2012;**67**(5):558–561.

66. Frerk C, Mitchell VS, McNarry AF, Mendonca C, Bhagrath R, Patel A, et al. Reply. *Br J Anaesth.* 2016;**117**(4):535–536.

67. Hamaekers A, Borg P, Enk D. The importance of flow and pressure release in emergency jet ventilation devices. *Paediatr Anaesth.* 2009;**19**(5):452–457.

68. Hamaekers AE, Borg PA, Enk D. A bench study of ventilation via two self-assembled jet devices and the Oxygen Flow Modulator in simulated upper airway obstruction. *Anaesthesia.* 2009;**64**(12):1353–1358.

4

Regional anaesthesia

Shona Love and Ian Bailes

Introduction

Regional anaesthesia is a fundamental and valuable technique in the armamentarium of any anaesthetist. Deployed correctly, it can allow many surgical procedures to be undertaken without the need for general anaesthesia, or when employed as an adjunct, it can improve patient experience, reduce systemic analgesia (and the associated side effects), and reduce recovery time.

Oromaxillofacial surgery is no exception. However, the application of regional anaesthesia to this particular anatomical area differs greatly from lower limb anaesthesia, for instance, where the nerves supplying the affected area are relatively superficial and often clearly identifiable on ultrasound. Instead, sensation to the head and neck is supplied by the cranial nerves (CNs) and upper cervical nerve roots. The paired CNs arise deep within the brainstem and have torturous paths through the bony skull base before emerging as multiple small terminal branches with short courses, each supplying sensation to small, often variable, areas of the skin or mucosa. This anatomical distribution renders oromaxillofacial surgery less amenable to the targeted nerve blocks traditionally associated with regional anaesthesia. There are, however, some notable exceptions, for example, the inferior alveolar nerve block used in dental procedures.

The multiplicity of small nerves means the superficial tissues of the head and neck are generally amenable to a field block. Local subcutaneous or submucosal infiltration of local anaesthetic agents often provides very good anaesthesia. When combined with vasoconstrictors this also helps prepare the surgical field and reduce bleeding.

Unlike other parts of the body, where regional anaesthesia techniques are principally undertaken to facilitate surgical operations, regional anaesthesia of the airway may be performed solely to facilitate anaesthetic interventions. The obvious example is awake tracheal intubation, in which anaesthesia of the oral or nasal cavity, the pharynx, and the larynx may be undertaken to aid passage of an oral or nasal tracheal tube.

Rather than proffering an exhaustive description of head and neck and oromaxillofacial anatomy, this chapter focuses on areas of particular relevance to the anaesthetist. The head and neck may be considered as six functional units, consisting of the face, the scalp, the nasal cavity, the oral cavity, the pharynx, and the larynx. Each functional unit is considered in turn, with a practical approach to the anatomy and innervation, to enable sufficient knowledge and understanding to safely anaesthetize selected tissues.

The face

The face is the anterior part of the head, bounded superiorly by the hairline, inferiorly by the chin, and laterally by the pinnae of the ears. The main sensory supply to the face is derived from the fifth CN, the trigeminal nerve (CN V). Since this is the dominant sensory nerve in the head and neck, its anatomy and branches will be described in detail.

The trigeminal nerve emerges from the pons as a large sensory and small motor root. Prior to exiting the skull, at the trigeminal (Gasserian) ganglion, the nerve divides into three primary divisions named according to the area of the face that they supply: the ophthalmic (CN V_1), maxillary (CN V_2), and mandibular (CN V_3) branches of the trigeminal nerve (**Figs 4.1 and 4.2**).[1]

The ophthalmic division (CN V_1)

Just prior to reaching the superior orbital fissure, the ophthalmic division of the trigeminal nerve divides into three major branches (the frontal, nasociliary, and lacrimal nerves).[2] The major branches then divide further. All of the branches have sensory function. Those providing cutaneous supply to the face are outlined below. The area covered includes the skin of the forehead, upper eyelid, and most of the surface of the nose.

The frontal nerve

The frontal nerve has two branches, both providing facial sensation[1,3]:

- The supraorbital nerve runs in the superior aspect of the orbit, in the extraconal space, and exits the orbit through the supraorbital foramen. It supplies the skin of the forehead and scalp, and the conjunctivae of the upper eyelid.
- The supratrochlear nerve runs in the superomedial aspect of the orbit, passes over the trochlea, and exits the orbit more medially

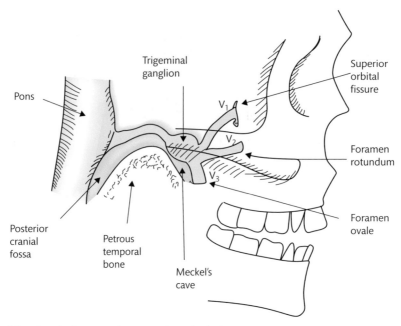

Fig. 4.1 Anatomical relations of the trigeminal nerve as it emerges from the brainstem.

via the frontal notch. It supplies the skin of the medial forehead, the medial upper eyelid, and medial canthus.

The nasociliary nerve

The nasociliary nerve has five branches. Two of these provide facial sensation[1]:

- The infratrochlear nerve runs in the medial aspect of the orbit, in the extraconal space, and emerges from the orbit below the

trochlea. It supplies sensation to the inner canthus, and the skin of the bridge of the nose.[4]
- The anterior ethmoid nerve terminates as the external nasal nerve. This terminal branch pierces the nasal cartilage and supplies the skin of the dorsal aspect of the nose.

The other branches of the nasociliary nerve provide sensation to the sinuses, the globe, and the dura of the anterior cranial fossa.[5]

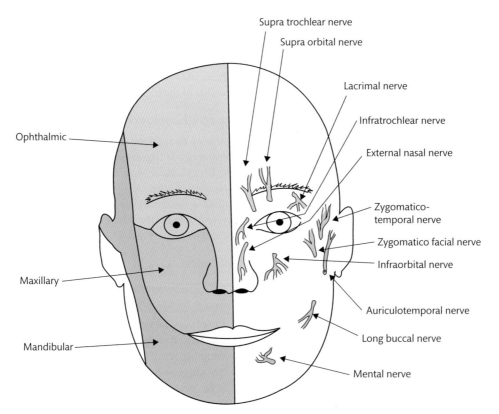

Fig. 4.2 The sensory supply to the face and anterior scalp from the three divisions of the trigeminal nerve. The right half of the diagram shows some of the major branches of the trigeminal nerve as they emerge from the skull.

The lacrimal nerve

The lacrimal nerve runs in the lateral aspect of the orbit, and exits the orbit under the lateral part of the superior orbital margin. It supplies the skin of the lateral part of the upper eyelid.[6]

The maxillary division (CN V₂)

The maxillary division of the trigeminal nerve exits the skull via the foramen rotundum, then divides into its various branches.[1] Two of these branches provide sensory supply to the face. The area covered includes the skin of the lower eyelid, the most lateral part of the external nose, the upper lip, the skin over the zygomatic arch, and the anterior part of the temple.

The infraorbital nerve

The infraorbital nerve enters the orbit through the inferior orbital fissure, then runs on the inferior aspect of the orbit in the infraorbital groove. As it runs in the groove, it gives off sensory branches to the teeth and the maxillary sinus.[1] The nerve then passes through the infraorbital foramen to emerge onto the face. Once through the infraorbital foramen, the infraorbital nerve separates into a number of terminal branches:

- Palpebral branches, that supply the lower eyelid and cheek.
- Nasal branches, that supply the lateral side of the nose.
- Superior labial branches, that supply the upper lip.

The zygomatic nerve

The zygomatic nerve divides in the lateral wall of the orbit to become two nerves with sensory function[5]:

- The zygomaticotemporal nerve, which emerges through the zygomaticotemporal foramen and supplies the skin over the anterior temporal region.
- The zygomaticofacial nerve, which emerges onto the face through the zygomaticofacial foramen, and supplies the skin over the zygomatic arch.

The mandibular division (CN V₃)

The mandibular division of the trigeminal nerve is the largest branch and has both sensory and motor components (**Fig. 4.3**). The sensory nerve is larger and arises from the trigeminal ganglion, while the smaller motor root arises in the motor nucleus in the pons. These roots unite to become the main trunk of the mandibular nerve. The nerve passes through the foramen ovale into the infratemporal fossa where it then divides.[2] The main branches are the anterior and posterior divisions. These have both sensory and motor components. The sensory supply of the mandibular division is to the skin of the tragus of the ear, the skin anterior to the ear, the temple region, the lateral part of the cheek, the chin, and the lower lip.[1]

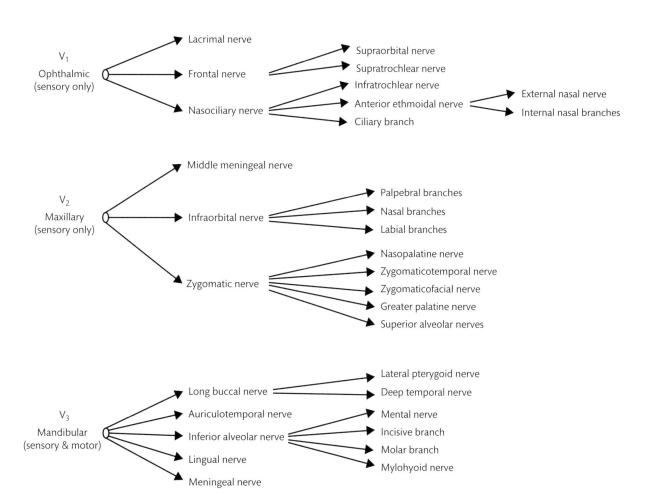

Fig. 4.3 Schematic showing branches and divisions of the trigeminal nerve.

The anterior division

The anterior branch of the mandibular nerve has one sensory branch, and three motor branches. The buccal nerve is the sensory branch. It provides cutaneous supply to an area of skin inferior to the lateral part of the cheek. It also provides sensation to some of the molar teeth, the inner cheek, and the gums.[5]

The posterior division

The posterior division has two sensory branches, and one branch with mixed motor and sensory function. Two of these supply sensation to the face:

- The auriculotemporal nerve, which emerges behind the temporomandibular joint. It supplies the skin of the posterior part of the temple, and the tragus, concha, and external acoustic meatus of the ear.[1]
- The inferior alveolar nerve, which branches to become the mental nerve. This terminal branch emerges from the mental foramen and supplies the skin of the chin and the lower lip.[3]

Anaesthetizing the face

Anaesthetists rarely perform local anaesthetic blocks of the face; however, a working knowledge of the most common regional techniques performed during surgical practice is useful.

Field blocks

Field blocks can be used to provide anaesthesia for operative procedures performed under local anaesthesia alone, or as an adjunct in more extensive surgery performed under general anaesthesia. Local anaesthetic is frequently combined with adrenaline to provide vasoconstriction and so aid haemostasis in the operative field. Any area of facial tissue can be anaesthetized by infiltrating local anaesthetic around its margins. Examples of procedures that can be performed under field block include excision of small lesions of the skin and subcutaneous tissues, and cosmetic procedures such as blepharoplasty.

Nerve blocks

Superficial nerve blocks of the face are commonly used by oromaxillofacial and plastic surgeons when repairing superficial lacerations of the face, without the need for general anaesthesia. In the paediatric population they also serve as a useful adjunct to cleft lip surgery.[7] Nerve blocks of the face involve anaesthetizing the major branches of the trigeminal nerve at the point where they emerge either from the cranium, or more superficially where they emerge from foramen in the facial bones.[3,8]

Supraorbital nerve block (CN V$_1$)

Palpate the supraorbital foramen, found at the junction of the medial one-third and lateral two-thirds of the supraorbital ridge, and generally in line with the ipsilateral pupil. Insert a short 27 G needle just below this landmark and perform a test aspiration (the nerve lies in close proximity to the supraorbital vessels). Inject up to 1 mL of local anaesthetic solution, then apply pressure to encourage spread.[3,9] Ultrasound can add accuracy to the landmark technique, by identifying the foramen.

Supratrochlear nerve block (CN V$_1$)

This can be performed through the same injection point as the supraorbital nerve block, with the needle being directed slightly more medially. Alternatively, insert the needle just medial to the supraorbital foramen, and superior to the level of the eyebrow. Inject 0.5–1 mL of local anaesthetic solution, then apply pressure to encourage spread.[3,9]

Lacrimal nerve block (CN V$_1$)

The lacrimal nerve can be blocked by depositing 1–2 mL of local anaesthetic behind the lacrimal gland. The entry point for the needle is just below the superolateral orbital rim, at a depth of approximately 2 cm.[9]

Maxillary nerve block (CN V$_2$)

Complete maxillary nerve block can be performed to achieve a larger field of anaesthesia, for instance, in cancer resection surgery involving the maxilla or hard palate. The maxillary nerve can be accessed in the pterygopalatine fossa using a percutaneous technique. The suprazygomatic approach is preferred, as the risk of complications is lower. A long 25 G needle is inserted at the angle formed by the posterior orbital ridge and the upper aspect of the zygomatic arch, and directed towards the sphenoid wing. It is then redirected, and advanced towards the pterygopalatine fossa, where 3–5 mL of local anaesthetic is injected.[3,8] Ultrasound guidance can prove very useful in this block, allowing both the pterygopalatine fossa, and the maxillary artery to be identified. The probe is placed in the infrazygomatic position (out of plane with the needle) such that the pterygopalatine fossa can be visualized between the maxilla and the sphenoid.

The maxillary nerve can also be anaesthetized using two different intraoral approaches: via the greater palatine canal, and via an infrazygomatic approach to the pterygopalatine fossa. The latter carries a significant risk of injury to the maxillary artery.[3]

Infraorbital nerve block (CN V$_2$)

Two approaches have been described to anaesthetize this terminal branch of the maxillary nerve.[3,8,9] Both involve deposition of local anaesthetic near the infraorbital foramen, taking care not to enter it. The foramen is sometimes palpable, located 0.5–1 cm below the mid-point of the inferior border of the orbit, in line with the pupil. Ultrasound can be used to identify the foramen.

In the external approach, a 27 G needle is inserted percutaneously in the vicinity of the infraorbital foramen until bony resistance is encountered, and 1–3 mL of local anaesthetic is injected. An alternative approach is the intraoral route, passing the needle through topicalized buccal mucosa, in line with the first canine tooth and upwards towards the infraorbital foramen. In both instances, a finger should be placed in the foramen to ensure the injection is not inadvertently intraorbital.

Mental nerve block (CN V$_3$)

The mental foramen is located in line with the lower canine on the mental protrusion of the mandible. Ultrasound can be used to identify the foramen with greater accuracy. A 27 G needle is inserted lateral to the foramen and advanced towards the midline, with 1–3 mL of local anaesthetic deposited outside the foramen.[1] An alternative approach is the intraoral route, passing the needle inferiorly through topicalized mucosa alongside the lower canine tooth, and towards the foramen.[3,8]

The scalp

The scalp is bounded posteriorly by the superior nuchal lines of the occipital bone, anteriorly by the supraorbital margin of the frontal bone, and laterally by the zygomatic arches.

Sensory innervation of the scalp

Sensory innervation anterior to the auricle of the ear is from all three branches of the trigeminal nerve. The course of these nerves has been described previously and is illustrated in **Figs 4.1 and 4.2.** Sensory innervation posterior to the auricle of the ear is from the spinal cutaneous nerves of the second (C2) and third (C3) cervical nerves.[10]

The lesser occipital nerve

The lesser occipital nerve arises from the primary ventral rami of C2 and C3 and travels along the posterior border of the sternocleidomastoid muscle. It supplies the lateral portion of the posterior scalp, and the cranial surface of the pinna of the ear.

The greater occipital nerve

The greater occipital nerve arises from the dorsal rami of C2 and emerges at the back of the head above the superior nuchal line, and approximately two-thirds of the distance between the mastoid process and the external occipital protuberance. It lies medial to the occipital artery. It supplies sensation to the posterior part of the scalp and the cranial vertex.

The great auricular nerve

The great auricular nerve arises from C2 and C3 and travels along the posterior border of the sternocleidomastoid muscle. It divides into an anterior and a posterior branch. The posterior branch supplies the skin overlying the mastoid process, and part of the lobule of the ear. The anterior part supplies the skin overlying the parotid gland.

Anaesthetizing the scalp

Local anaesthetic field blocks can be used to anaesthetize small parts of the scalp. Full anaesthesia of the scalp can be achieved using a 'scalp block'.[11,12]

Scalp block

The nerves of the scalp may be anaesthetized for a variety of reasons. These include chronic pain procedures, and the treatment of some varieties of migraine. Additionally, blocking these nerves may be used to augment postoperative pain relief following coronal incision. A complete scalp block involves anaesthetizing seven nerves on each side.[3,11] The amount of local anaesthetic used must be carefully calculated for each patient. Infiltration of the scalp has been shown to result in a more rapid rise in plasma concentrations of local anaesthesia than other regional techniques.[13,14]

The supraorbital nerve (CN V_1)

As described in the section on nerve blocks of the face.

The supratrochlear nerve (CN V_1)

As described in the section on nerve blocks of the face.

The zygomaticotemporal nerve (CN V_2)

Infiltrate from the lateral margin of the supraorbital ridge to the distal portion of the zygomatic arch. The local anaesthetic must be infiltrated both superficially and deep to the temporalis muscle.

The auriculotemporal nerve (CN V_3)

Insert a 25 or 27 G needle approximately 1 cm anterior to the tragus of the ear, above the level of the temporomandibular joint. Care should be taken to avoid the superficial temporal artery.

The greater auricular nerve (C2–C3)

Insert a 25 or 27 G needle at the level of the tragus, and approximately 1.5 cm posterior to the auricle of the ear.

The lesser occipital nerve (C2–C3)

Infiltrate posterior to the ear, from the upper pole of the auricle to the level of the superior nuchal line (the bony ridge extending laterally from the occipital protuberance).

The greater occipital nerve (C2)

Insert a 25 or 27 G needle just medial to the occipital artery, at the level of the superior nuchal line. Care should be taken to avoid the occipital artery. Following injection of local anaesthetic, apply pressure to encourage spread.

The nasal cavity

The nasal cavity extends from the nares anteriorly through the vestibule, the atrium, and the conchae to the posterior pharyngeal wall.[15] It is lined with highly vascular mucous membrane (apart from the vestibule, which is lined with hairy skin) and has a large surface area, allowing it to warm and humidify inhaled air, and providing the sense of smell. The nasal cavity is formed by:

- Floor—hard palate (maxilla and palatine bones).
- Roof—sphenoid bone posteriorly, cribriform plate of the ethmoid bone (through which pass olfactory nerve fibres). Anteriorly, the frontal bone, then the nasal bone and the nasal cartilage.
- Medial wall—nasal septum. The upper part is the vertical plate of the ethmoid bone, the posterior part is formed by the vomer bone, the anterior part from septal cartilage.
- Lateral wall—three folds called conchae, each with an opening below it, called a meatus.

The conchae increase surface area and make air flow turbulent, slowing its passage, allowing it to be warmed and humidified. The air sinuses open onto the lateral wall of the nasal cavity:[15]

- The sphenoid sinus opens into the sphenoethmoidal recess.
- The posterior ethmoidal sinus opens into the superior meatus.
- The middle ethmoidal sinus opens into the middle meatus.

- The anterior ethmoidal sinus opens into the infundibulum of the middle meatus.
- The frontal sinus opens into the infundibulum of the middle meatus.
- The maxillary sinus opens into the hiatus semilunaris, a ridge that lies within the middle meatus.

The nasal cavity has a rich blood supply. The anterior ethmoidal artery, posterior ethmoidal artery, and sphenopalatine artery meet the superior labral artery in the part of the septum known as Little's area. It is therefore important to target the septum when administering vasoconstrictors to the nose in preparation for nasal procedures.

Sensory innervation of the nasal cavity

The nasal cavity has a dual sensory supply. Olfaction is supplied by the olfactory nerve (CN I). Olfactory nerves embedded in the olfactory mucosa perforate the cribriform plate to form the olfactory bulb intracranially.

Of more relevance to anaesthesia, however, is the provision of general sensation. The nasociliary nerve (a branch of the ophthalmic division of the trigeminal nerve) supplies sensation to the anterior and superior parts of the nasal cavity, directly and via the internal nasal branches of the anterior ethmoidal nerve (one of the divisions of the nasociliary nerve).[3] The nasociliary nerve also supplies sensation to the sphenoidal, ethmoidal, and frontal sinuses. The posterior parts of the nasal cavity are supplied by the maxillary division of the trigeminal nerve. The nasopalatine nerve is a terminal branch of the zygomatic nerve, which arises from the maxillary division of the trigeminal nerve. It supplies the posterior septum, while the anterior septum and the lateral vestibule are supplied by nasal branches of the infraorbital nerve, a major branch of the maxillary division of the trigeminal nerve (Fig. 4.3).

Anaesthetizing the nasal cavity

Indications for nasal anaesthesia generally comprise ear, nose, and throat procedures such as functional endoscopic sinus surgery, septoplasty, rhinoplasty, septorhinoplasty, sphenopalatine artery ligation, or biopsy in the affected area. Other surgical specialties may also require nasal anaesthesia, such as in neurosurgery for an endoscopic approach to trans-sphenoidal hypophyseal resection, or for skull base resection. Usually this is as an adjunct to general anaesthesia, designed to augment intra- and postoperative analgesia, but there are reports of patients undergoing septoplasty under local anaesthesia alone.[16] For biopsies, local anaesthesia alone will frequently be sufficient. Passage of flexible fibreoptic scopes and nasotracheal tubes may also require anaesthesia of the nasal cavity (discussed below).

Topical anaesthesia

Most of the local anaesthesia applied to the nasal cavity will be topical. This is almost always combined with a vasoconstrictor to reduce the volume of the mucosa and reduce bleeding. This improves surgical access and visibility.

Moffett's solution

In 1947, Moffett described a solution of 2 mL of 8% cocaine, 2 mL of 1% sodium bicarbonate, and 1 mL of adrenaline 1:1000, to be instilled in a patient's nose.[17] Cocaine is an ester local anaesthetic which, unlike most amide local anaesthetics in use currently, is also a potent vasoconstrictor. Adrenaline further adds to the vasoconstriction, while the bicarbonate raises the pH and therefore increases the unionized proportion of the local anaesthetic (a weak base), and so speeds up the onset of action. Systemic absorption of the cocaine and adrenaline contained in Moffett's solution has been associated with hypertension, coronary artery vasospasm, exacerbation of ischaemic heart disease, arrhythmias, and postoperative cognitive dysfunction.[18] The maximum recommended dose for cocaine is 1.5 mg/kg[19] so the described recipe represents an overdose for most patients. For that reason, many practitioners choose to dilute the solution and there are many variations on this mixture in practice. Typically, the solution is sprayed into the nares, coating the mucosa. Alternatively, the solution can be instilled after insertion of a throat pack, such that it fills the nasal cavity and can be removed by suction after a few minutes (discussed in Chapter 9).

Co-phenylcaine

A preparation of local anaesthetic and vasoconstrictor that can be used in place of Moffett's solution. It contains lidocaine 5% and phenylephrine 0.5%, and typically comes in a bottle containing 2.5 mL of solution, to be used as a spray. The pump spray delivers the mixture in a directed fashion.

Field blocks

Submucosal infiltration of local anaesthetic solution (usually containing dilute adrenaline for its vasoconstrictor action) can be performed. While this technique may be useful for small procedures such as excision biopsies of intranasal lesions, it is unlikely to provide the widespread anaesthesia required for sinus surgery.

Nerve blocks

Although not commonly practised, various nerve block techniques have been described to provide anaesthesia to the nasal cavity. Note that these often need to be performed in combination, and bilaterally.

Nasociliary nerve block

Using a 27 G needle, 1–2 mL of local anaesthetic is injected 1–1.5 cm above the medial canthus, with the needle directed medially onto bone. No adrenaline may be used with this block as there is a risk of retinal artery vasoconstriction.[3]

External nasal nerve block

Using a 27 G needle, 1–2 mL of local anaesthetic is injected 0.5–1 cm from the midline at the osseocartilaginous junction of the nose.[3]

Infraorbital nerve block

As described in the section on nerve blocks of the face.

Maxillary nerve block

As described in the section on nerve blocks of the face.

Pterygopalatine ganglion block

This is essentially an intraoral approach to the maxillary nerve and is described in the dental nerve blocks section of this chapter.

The mouth

The mouth extends from the lips anteriorly to the oropharynx posteriorly, and comprises the vestibule (between the lips and teeth) and the main oral cavity, within the alveolar arches. It is lined with mucous membrane (in which the opening of the parotid duct can be identified at the level of the second upper molar). It contains the teeth, gums, tongue, hard palate, soft palate, and uvula.

Sensory innervation of the mouth

The buccal cavity

The roof is supplied by the greater palatine nerve and, anteriorly, by the nasopalatine nerve. Both are branches of the maxillary division of the trigeminal nerve. The floor is supplied by the lingual nerve, a branch of the mandibular division of the trigeminal nerve. The cheeks are supplied by the buccal nerves, branches of the mandibular division of the trigeminal nerve.[15]

The teeth

Humans have 20 deciduous teeth in childhood, replaced in adulthood by 32 permanent teeth. The maxillary arch and mandibular arch each contain four incisors, two canines, four premolars, and six molars (including the third molars, known as 'wisdom teeth').

The pulp, investing structures, and gingiva are supplied by branches of the trigeminal nerve. The upper jaw is supplied by the maxillary division and the lower jaw by the mandibular division, as shown in Fig. 4.4. There is also some periosteal supply to the upper jaw from the greater palatine nerve and nasopalatine nerve (branches of the maxillary division of the trigeminal nerve). Some periosteal sensation to the lower jaw is supplied by the long buccal

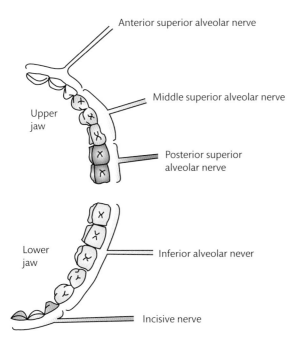

Fig. 4.4 Sensory innervation of the teeth. The upper jaw derives innervation from branches of the maxillary division of the trigeminal nerve. The lower jaw derives innervation from branches of the mandibular division of the trigeminal nerve.

nerve and the lingual nerve, which are both branches from the mandibular division of the trigeminal nerve.[15,20]

The tongue

The tongue is a structure of striated muscle, divided along the midline by the median fibrous septum. It is lined with mucous membrane, which form papillae on the superior surface. The underside contains lymphoid tissue. The anterior two-thirds reside in the mouth, while the posterior third sits in the pharynx and derives a different innervation. They are demarcated by the sulcus terminalis. At the pharyngeal level, the tongue can be thought of as congruent with the pharyngeal musculature.[15]

The intrinsic muscles

These have no bony attachment, consisting of longitudinal, transverse, and vertical fibres, and are supplied by the hypoglossal nerve (CN XII).

The extrinsic muscles

All the extrinsic muscles are supplied by the hypoglossal nerve, except palatoglossus which is supplied by the pharyngeal plexus (CN X, described later).

* Genioglossus—inserts on the genial body of mandible.
* Hypoglossus—inserts on the body and greater cornu of the hyoid bone.
* Styloglossus—inserts on the styloid process of the temporal bone.
* Palatoglossus—inserts on the palatine aponeurosis, and constricts the pharynx.

The sensory supply to the posterior third of the tongue (including the vallate papillae) is from the glossopharyngeal nerve (CN IX) (Fig. 4.5). In the anterior two-thirds, general sensation is supplied by the lingual nerve, a branch of the mandibular division of the trigeminal nerve. Taste is supplied by the chorda tympani, a branch of the facial nerve (CN VII).

Anaesthetizing the mouth

Topical anaesthesia

Topical application of local anaesthesia gel, for instance, benzocaine 10% or lidocaine 2%, is commonly used to provide anaesthesia for intraoral lesions and as preparation for intraoral injection of local anaesthesia.

Field block

This is the most common method of providing anaesthesia to the buccal mucosa and gingiva, and for excision of small tongue lesions. Since the nerves enter individual teeth via the root, local anaesthetic solution injected towards the apex of the tooth will adequately anaesthetize the tooth and periodontium (although the molars may require an additional nerve block). A narrow (27 G) needle is used, often with prefilled dental anaesthetic cartridges. These typically contain 2 mL of lidocaine 2% with adrenaline, up to 1:80,000 for vasoconstriction (a higher concentration than typically used in other surgical specialties).

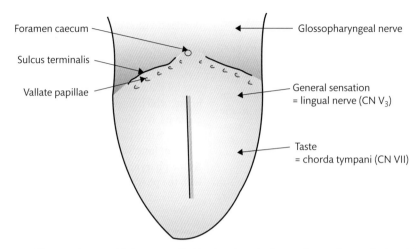

Fig. 4.5 Innervation of the tongue. The anterior two-thirds are supplied by the trigeminal nerve (general sensation) and the facial nerve (taste). The posterior third is supplied by the glossopharyngeal nerve.

Nerve blocks

There are many nerve blocks described in dental practice. For anaesthetists, an exhaustive knowledge of these is rarely required; however, they should be aware of common nerve blocks.

Inferior alveolar nerve block

This will anaesthetize the mandibular teeth on the ipsilateral side (incisors have some crossed innervation). Using a long 25 G needle, 2 mL of local anaesthetic solution can be injected through topicalized oral mucosa. The needle is inserted between the coronoid notch of the mandible and the pterygomandibular raphae (lateral to the mandible). Once bone is contacted, the needle is redirected posteriorly and most of the local anaesthetic injected. The lingual nerve can then be blocked by injecting the remainder of the local anaesthetic as the needle is withdrawn.[20] There are various alternative approaches to blocking this nerve, such as the Gow-Gates approach or the Akinosi–Vazirani approach.[21]

Maxillary nerve block

This can be used to anaesthetize ipsilateral maxillary teeth, when local infiltration is contraindicated. It is described earlier in this chapter in the section on nerve blocks of the face. Alternatively, the needle can be passed up the greater palatine foramen after topicalization of the hard palate. The foramen is just anterior to the border between the hard palate and the soft palate. A fine needle is passed approximately 30 mm up the foramen where 2 mL of local anaesthetic can be deposited.[20]

Infraorbital nerve block

As described in the section on nerve blocks of the face.

The pharynx

The pharynx is part of the aerodigestive tract, extending from the skull base to the larynx and oesophagus.

The pharyngeal wall

The pharyngeal wall consists of a two-layered muscular tube. The outer, mainly circular, layer of muscle consists of three overlapping constrictor muscles. The pharyngeal constrictors arise anteriorly and come together posteriorly to form the pharyngeal raphe.[5] There are gaps between the pharyngeal constrictor muscles that allow entry of a number of structures, including blood vessels and nerves. The constrictor muscles are responsible for swallowing. The inner, mainly longitudinal, layer of muscle consists of the palatopharyngeus, stylopharyngeus, and salpingopharyngeus. These muscles are responsible for lifting the larynx and pharynx during eating and speaking.

The inner pharynx

The inner part of the pharynx can be split into three anatomical areas:

- Nasopharynx.
- Oropharynx.
- Laryngopharynx.

The nasopharynx

The nasopharynx is the upper part of the pharynx, and communicates with the nasal cavity. The main features of the nasopharynx are the entry of the Eustachian tube in the lateral wall, and the presence of lymphoid tissue known as the adenoids. The nasopharynx ends at the level of the soft palate.[2]

The oropharynx

The oropharynx is the middle part of the pharynx, and communicates with the oral cavity via the oropharyngeal isthmus. This is formed by the soft palate, the palatoglossal arches, and the posterior third of the tongue.[2] The main feature of the oropharynx are two folds of mucosa known as the tonsillar pillars or fauces. The anterior fold is the palatoglossal arch, running between the soft palate and the lateral part of the tongue. The posterior fold is the palatopharyngeal arch, running between the soft palate and the lateral part of the oropharynx. The triangular space created between the two arches is the tonsillar fossa, and contains an aggregation of lymphoid tissue, the palatine tonsil.[5] This common surgical target is separated from surrounding tissue by a capsule and covered in mucous membrane. The inferior border of the oropharynx is formed by the base of the tongue and epiglottis.

The laryngopharynx

The laryngopharynx is the inferior part of the pharynx. It communicates with the oesophagus, and with the larynx via the laryngeal inlet. The laryngopharynx is at its widest at the level of the epiglottis, and then narrows at the level of the cricoid cartilage.[1] The inferior border of the laryngopharynx is the piriform fossa, a recess on either side of the laryngeal inlet.[5]

Sensory innervation of the pharynx

The nerve supply to the pharynx comes mainly from the pharyngeal plexus. This plexus of nerves lies in the external fascia of the pharynx and is formed by branches of the glossopharyngeal and vagus nerves.[1] Some of the structures within the pharynx are innervated by branches of the trigeminal nerve.

Glossopharyngeal nerve (CN IX)

The pharyngeal branch is a small sensory nerve that runs between the sphenoid and palatine bones. It supplies much of the mucosa of the pharynx and Eustachian tube. The tonsillar branch provides sensory supply to the structures of the oropharyngeal isthmus. The stylopharyngeus muscle receives motor supply from the glossopharyngeal nerve (**Table 4.1**).

Trigeminal nerve (CN V)

The maxillary branch supplies much of the mucosa of the nasopharynx.

Vagus nerve (CN X)

Pharyngeal and superior laryngeal branches provide motor supply to the major muscles of the pharynx, except the stylopharyngeus (**Table 4.1**).

Anaesthetizing the pharynx

Topical anaesthesia

The pharynx is rarely a target of regional anaesthesia for surgery, but it is discussed later in the section on topicalization techniques utilized for awake tracheal intubation.

Table 4.1 Extrinsic muscles of the larynx and pharynx, and their nerve supply

Muscle	Nerve supply
Digastric	Mandibular division of trigeminal (CN V3)
Mylohyoid	Mandibular division of trigeminal (CN V3)
Stylohyoid	Facial (CN VII)
Geniohyoid	C1–C3 (ansa cervicalis)
Stylopharyngeus	Glossopharyngeal (CN IX)
Palatopharyngeus	Glossopharyngeal (CN IX)
Salpingopharyngeus	Branch of vagus (CN X)
Sternothyroid	C1–C3 (ansa cervicalis)
Sternohyoid	C1–C3 (ansa cervicalis)
Omohyoid	C1–C3 (ansa cervicalis)
Thyrohyoid	C1–C3 (ansa cervicalis)

Nerve blocks

Glossopharyngeal nerve block

Most pharyngeal sensation derives from the glossopharyngeal nerve. It can be blocked via an intraoral or percutaneous approach. The intraoral approach requires the patient to have sufficient mouth opening to allow access. This may limit the use of this approach for patients requiring awake tracheal intubation for trismus. A tongue depressor or laryngoscope may be used to facilitate this approach. The glossopharyngeal nerve has a relatively superficial course at the base of the tonsillar pillars. As such, it is possible to block the nerve by applying gauze soaked in local anaesthetic to this area.[22] Alternatively, the surgeon may inject 2–3 mL of lidocaine at the base of the tonsillar pillar, lateral to the tongue, bilaterally.[22,23]

An external approach has also been described. The styloid process of the mandible is palpated between the angle of the jaw and the mastoid process, and a 25 or 27 G needle advanced towards it. The needle is then advanced posteriorly, off the bone, and 5 mL of local anaesthetic can be injected. This process should be repeated on both sides.[22] The nerve lies in close proximity to the carotid artery at this point, and care must be taken to avoid intravascular injection. Ultrasound guidance can be a useful adjunct.[24]

The larynx

The larynx separates the pharynx from the trachea, and performs the dual functions of protecting the airway and phonation. It is formed of cartilage, namely the thyroid cartilage and the ring-shaped cricoid cartilage, and muscle, attached to the hyoid bone. It is lined by a mucous membrane, except on the vocal cords where the epithelium becomes stratified squamous. The extrinsic muscles that act upon the larynx derive their innervation from the CNs and upper cervical nerve roots (**Table 4.1**).[15]

The intrinsic muscles close the glottic opening and adjust the vocal cord position during speech. They are innervated by branches of the vagus nerve (CN X)[15]:

- Oblique arytenoid passes from the muscular process of one arytenoid cartilage to the apex of the contralateral arytenoid. It adducts and lifts the vocal cords.
- Aryepiglottic muscles are extensions of the oblique arytenoid and close the glottis against the epiglottis, acting together as a sphincter.
- Cricothyroid tenses the vocal cords.
- Thyroarytenoid (also known as vocalis muscle) relaxes the vocal cords.
- Lateral cricoarytenoid adducts the vocal cords.
- Transverse arytenoid closes the glottis.
- Posterior cricoarytenoid abducts the vocal cords.

All intrinsic muscles of the larynx are supplied by the recurrent laryngeal nerves, except cricothyroid. The recurrent laryngeal nerves are bilateral branches of the vagus nerve, which leave the main vagus nerve distal to the larynx. The left nerve loops under the arch of the aorta, the right loops under the right subclavian artery. They then travel cranially alongside the trachea to the larynx. The cricothyroid muscle is supplied by the external laryngeal nerve, another branch of the vagus nerve.

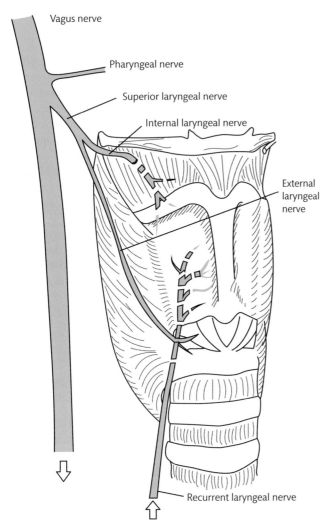

Fig. 4.6 Nerve supply to the larynx.

The sensory supply to the larynx is also derived from branches of the vagus nerve. The internal laryngeal nerve, a branch of the superior laryngeal nerve, supplies the mucosa above the vocal cords. The recurrent laryngeal nerve supplies sensation below the vocal cords (Fig. 4.6).

Anaesthetizing the larynx

Indications for anaesthetizing the larynx include awake fibreoptic tracheal intubation, awake videolaryngoscopic tracheal intubation, vocal cord surgery, flexible bronchoscopy, and occasionally as an adjunct to reduce coughing in other airway surgery.

Topical anaesthesia

Local anaesthetic solution can be applied topically to the larynx in several ways:

- In an anaesthetized patient, 5 mL of 2% or 2.5 mL of 4% lidocaine can be directly applied to the vocal cords during laryngoscopy. Mucosal atomization devices can be used to increase spread of the local anaesthetic.

- Lidocaine can be sprayed directly via an intubating bronchoscope ('spray-as-you-go' technique, discussed later in the section on awake tracheal intubation).
- An awake patient can gargle with 10 mL of 2% lidocaine.
- Nebulized local anaesthetic (e.g. 10 mL of 2% lidocaine or 5 mL of 4% lidocaine) can be inhaled through the upper airway, anaesthetizing the larynx and upper trachea. Although favoured by some anaesthetists for awake tracheal intubation, the nebulized route compares poorly with 'spray-as-you-go' or cricothyroid injection in patients undergoing bronchoscopy.[25]

Field block

Local anaesthetic, for example, 4 mL of 4% lidocaine, can be injected directly through the cricothyroid membrane. Studies in patients undergoing bronchoscopy suggest this achieves less coughing and better patient satisfaction.[26] The skin is cleaned with chlorhexidine and the cricothyroid membrane identified. A 27 G needle is passed perpendicular to the cricothyroid membrane, with gentle aspiration until air bubbles are observed. The lidocaine is then injected and the needle withdrawn rapidly. The patient will cough, spreading the local anaesthetic very effectively above and below the vocal cords. Ultrasound can be used to identify the cricothyroid membrane, especially in patients with large necks or altered anatomy, and this may improve the success of the technique.

Nerve blocks

The recurrent laryngeal nerve should never be blocked bilaterally as it can result in vocal cord abduction. The superior laryngeal nerve may be blocked with 2 mL of local anaesthetic injected below the superior cornu of the hyoid bone.[22] An alternative landmark is above the superior cornu of the thyroid cartilage. In both approaches, ultrasound can be used to identify the landmarks with greater accuracy. Superior laryngeal nerve block should be performed bilaterally as there is some cross-innervation.

Awake tracheal intubation

Various techniques exist for anaesthetizing the airway for awake tracheal intubation. Many practitioners combine airway topicalization techniques with 'light' sedation, in the form of a propofol target-controlled infusion (effect site concentration of 0.5–1.5 mcg/mL) or analgesia with a remifentanil target-controlled infusion (effect site concentration of 1–2 ng/mL). Both agents are easily and rapidly titratable, as well as having antitussive qualities. A second sedative agent, most commonly a benzodiazepine such as midazolam, can also be employed as an anxiolytic, but caution must be taken when using multiple agents due to the risk of inducing apnoea. The amnesic effects of midazolam are seldom required if effective local anaesthetic topicalization has been undertaken, and sedation should never be considered a substitute for poor topicalization.

A range of local anaesthetic topicalization techniques are available to facilitate awake tracheal intubation, depending upon the nature of the clinical situation, urgency, patient pathology, and intended route of tracheal intubation (oral/nasal)[22,27]:

- Mucosal atomization spray of local anaesthetic can be used to topicalize the nasal cavity or oropharynx. A vasoconstrictor can be added to the local anaesthetic when a nasal intubation is planned (e.g. co-phenylcaine).

- Cotton buds or ribbon gauze soaked in local anaesthetic can be applied to the nasal passages to topicalize the nasal cavity.
- Local anaesthetic ointment can be applied by the patient to their own nasal mucosa.
- Local anaesthetic gargle (e.g. 10 mL of 2% lidocaine) can be used to anaesthetize the pharynx and larynx.
- Nebulized local anaesthetic (e.g. 10 mL of 2% lidocaine or 5 mL of 4% lidocaine) can be used to anaesthetize the upper airway, larynx, and upper trachea. The patient should inhale the nebulized local anaesthetic for 10–20 minutes prior to the procedure. The British Thoracic Society does not recommend the nebulized route for bronchoscopy.[25,27]
- 'Spray-as-you-go' delivery of local anaesthetic solution (e.g. 2% or 4% lidocaine) can be achieved via the suction port of the bronchoscope, directing local anaesthetic at the vocal cords in particular. An epidural catheter can be passed down the suction port to facilitate this method of local anaesthetic administration.
- Trans-cricothyroid puncture and injection of local anaesthesia (as described earlier) can be employed in compliant patients. A cannula, rather than needle, can also be utilized for this purpose, and be left *in situ* after injection of the local anaesthetic. This cannula can then be used for oxygenation, end-tidal carbon dioxide monitoring, or to facilitate subsequent retrograde intubation.

The Difficult Airway Society, UK, has produced awake tracheal intubation guidelines, and these provide a useful resource to those unfamiliar with awake fibreoptic and awake videolaryngoscopic techniques.[28] Patients should be fully monitored at all times in accordance with local guidelines, have reliable intravenous access sited, and suitably trained personnel should be present. The awake tracheal intubation guidelines emphasize the importance of oxygenation (in particular, high-flow humidified nasal oxygenation), having the appropriate number of staff available, optimizing the ergonomics of the environment, and standardization of equipment set-up.

The maximum dose of local anaesthetic should be calculated prior to undertaking the topicalization procedure and resuscitation equipment (including Intralipid) should be immediately available. Traditionally, the maximum dose of lidocaine was considered to be 3 mg/kg. However, a significant proportion of nebulized local anaesthetic will not be absorbed, and similarly, topically applied anaesthetic may be swallowed. Patients have safely received 7–9 mg/kg lidocaine via the airway with no adverse effects, although case reports of toxicity have also occurred in much lower doses.[29]

Complications of regional anaesthesia

Although useful as either a stand-alone anaesthetic technique, or as part of a multimodal approach to anaesthesia and analgesia, the administration of local anaesthetic agents is not without risk. Strategies to minimize these risks are summarized in **Table 4.2**.

Complications of regional anaesthesia can be broadly divided into localized and generalized complications.

Table 4.2 Strategies to minimize the risk of complications from regional anaesthesia

Local anaesthetic agent	Utilize lowest mass of agent to achieve desired result
	Utilize lowest concentration of agent to achieve desired result
Local anaesthetic administration	Careful selection of appropriate needle size
	Careful selection of appropriate needle type
Ancillary equipment	Full anaesthetic monitoring and intravenous access
	Sterile equipment including gloves and needles
	Immediately available resuscitation equipment, Intralipid, and emergency algorithms
	Use of ultrasound to increase accuracy and minimize volume injected
	Use of nerve stimulator to increase accuracy

Localized complications

Any structure in the vicinity of the infiltrating/block needle has the potential to be damaged.

Nerve injury

Nerve injury may present with sensory or motor symptoms, and may be transient or permanent. The main mechanisms of nerve injury are:

- Direct damage to the nerve from the needle.
- Nerve ischaemia from local anaesthetic agents, or compressive haematoma.
- Cytotoxic axonal damage from the local anaesthetic agent.

Vascular injury

Vascular complications may be more likely in the head and neck due to the rich blood supply in this area. Inadvertent vessel puncture may present with localized bleeding and resultant haematoma formation. An expanding haematoma, dependent on its location, can have its own complications (e.g. airway compromise). Vascular injury from the infiltrating needle may also present with symptoms of systemic absorption of the drug, as described below.

Soft tissue damage

The local anaesthetic itself, or other components of the solution can cause localized soft tissue reactions in the area of infiltration. This may present with signs of a localized irritation such as oedema, erythema, and itch. Localized soft tissue infection can also occur as a complication of local anaesthetic infiltration. If local anaesthetic has been injected in the vicinity of the muscles of mastication, trismus can occur. This is more likely if there has been direct injection into the muscle, or if a high volume of local anaesthetic has been used.[30]

Generalized complications

Systemic absorption of adrenaline

Given the highly vascular nature of the tissues of the head and neck, the likelihood of systemic effects from adrenaline are increased when compared to other anatomical areas. This is likely to present as a short-lived tachycardia, with or without an associated rise in systemic blood pressure, although there is the risk of precipitating arrhythmias and ischaemia.

Local anaesthetic toxicity

Local anaesthetic toxicity can occur following injection of local anaesthesia. Care should be taken not to exceed the maximum advised dose, particularly when staged infiltration occurs. Toxic doses may be lower than those classically recognized due to increased vascularity and uptake from the tissues of the head and neck.[31] Toxicity classically presents with cardiovascular and/or neurological symptoms. If suspected, both cardiovascular and neurological status must be assessed and an appropriate management algorithm, such as that produced by the Association of Anaesthetists should be followed.[32] Intravenous lipid emulsion (Intralipid) is a specific treatment for local anaesthetic toxicity, thought to bind the local anaesthetic molecules and stabilize neuronal cell membranes. It is typically given as a 1.5 mL/kg bolus of 20% lipid emulsion, followed by an infusion at 15–30 mL/kg/hr, with a maximum dose of 12 mL/kg.[33]

Local anaesthetic allergy

An allergic reaction can occur in response to injection of local anaesthetic agents (Table 4.3).[33] This can be precipitated by either the local anaesthetic compound itself, or any of its preservatives. An attempt should be made to differentiate a true allergic reaction from the side effects of intravascular absorption of either the agent or accompanying vasoconstrictor. Symptoms and signs of hypersensitivity (rash, generalized oedema, or cardiorespiratory compromise) should be managed using an anaphylaxis guideline such as that produced by the Association of Anaesthetists.[34] The patient should be referred to an allergy clinic for follow-up and to definitively identify the responsible agent.

Other adverse drug reactions

A rare complication of local anaesthetic administration is the development of methaemoglobinaemia. This is most likely with prilocaine.

Table 4.3 Commonly used local anaesthetic preparations in oromaxillofacial surgery

Lidocaine	Amide local anaesthetic Presented with or without adrenaline (1 in 80,000–200,000) With adrenaline: 5, 10, 20 mg/mL solutions Without adrenaline: 5, 10, 20, 40 mg/mL solutions Available in prefilled dental cartridges
Bupivacaine	Amide local anaesthetic Presented with or without adrenaline (1 in 200,000) With adrenaline: 2.5, 5 mg/mL solutions Without adrenaline: 2.5, 5 mg/mL solutions
Articaine	Amide local anaesthetic Presented with adrenaline (1 in 100,000) With adrenaline: 40 mg/mL solution Available in prefilled 2.2 mL dental cartridges
Mepivacaine	Amide local anaesthetic Presented with or without adrenaline (1 in 100,000) With adrenaline: 20 mg/mL solution Without adrenaline: 30 mg/mL solutions Both available in prefilled 2.2 mL dental cartridges

Conclusion

Regional anaesthesia is a key component of oromaxillofacial surgery. Although anaesthetists rarely perform head and neck nerve blocks to facilitate surgery, they should be aware of the relevant anatomy, and the potential benefits of the regional anaesthetic techniques employed by their surgical colleagues. For the anaesthetist undertaking awake tracheal intubation, an understanding of the anatomy of the upper airway, and how this can be anaesthetized, is fundamental. It is crucial to also be aware of the potential complications of local anaesthetic administration, and how to manage and avoid them.

REFERENCES

1. Moore K, Agur A. *Essential Clinical Anatomy*. Baltimore, MD: Lippincott, Williams and Wilkins; 1995.
2. McMinn R, Hutchings R, Pegington J, Abrahams P. *A Colour Atlas of Human Anatomy*, 3rd ed. London: Wolfe; 1993.
3. New York School of Regional Anesthesia. Nerve blocks of the face. n.d. https://www.nysora.com/nerve-blocks-face
4. Hartstein ME, Holds JB, Massry GG. *Pearls and Pitfalls in Cosmetic Oculoplastic Surgery*. New York: Springer; 2008.
5. Ellis H. *Clinical Anatomy*, 9th ed. London: Blackwell Science; 1997.
6. Dartt D, Besharse J, Dana R. *Encyclopaedia of the Eye*. Cambridge: Academic Press; 2010.
7. Somerville N, Fenlon S. Anaesthesia for cleft lip and palate surgery. *CEACCP.* 2005;**5**(3):76–79.
8. Kanakaraj M, Shanmugasundaram N, Chandramohan M, Kannan R, Perumal SM, Nagendran J. Regional anesthesia in faciomaxillary and oral surgery. *J Pharm Bioallied Sci.* 2012; **4**(2):S264–S269.
9. Schiedler V, Sires B. Regional nerve blocks in oculofacial surgery. In: Harstein M, Holds J, Massry G (eds) *Pearls and Pitfalls in Cosmetic Oculoplastic Surgery*, pp. 22–26. New York: Springer; 2008.
10. Agur A, Dalley A. *Grant's Atlas of Anatomy*, 11th ed. Baltimore, MD: Lippincott, Williams and Wilkins; 2006.
11. Burnard C, Sebastien J. Anaesthesia for awake craniotomy. *CEACCP.* 2014;**14**(1):6–11.
12. Osborn I, Sebeo J. 'Scalp block' during craniotomy: a classic technique revisited. *J Neurosurg Anaesthesiol.* 2010;**22**(3):187–194.
13. Costello TG, Cormack JR, Mather LE, LaFerlita B, Murphy MA, Harris K. Plasma levobupivicaine concentrations following scalp block in patients undergoing awake craniotomy. *Br J Anaesth.* 2005;**94**(6):848–851.
14. Audu P, Wilkerson C, Bartowski R, Gingrich K, Viscusi E, Andrews D. Plasma ropivicaine levels during awake intracranial surgery. *J Neurosurg Anaesthesiol.* 2005;**17**(3):153–155.
15. Snell R. *Clinical Anatomy for Medical Students*, 4th ed. Boston, MA: Little, Brown and Company; 1992.
16. Vives I, Mateo D, Botana C, Agreda G, Salgado I. Septoplasties with local anesthetic and sedation in ambulatory surgery; clinical outcomes. *Eur J Anaesthesiol.* 2008;**25**:19.
17. Moffett A. Nasal analgesia by postural instillation. *Anaesthesia.* 1947;**2**:31–34.

18. Dwyer C, Sowerby L, Rotenberg BW. Is cocaine a safe topical agent for use during endoscopic sinus surgery? *Laryngoscope.* 2016;**126**(8):1721–1723.

19. Electronic Medicines Compendium. Cocaine hydrochloride solution 10% w/v. 2020. https://www.medicines.org.uk/emc/product/3692#gref

20. New York School of Regional Anesthesia. Oral & maxillofacial regional anesthesia. n.d. https://www.nysora.com/regional-anesthesia-for-specific-surgical-procedures/head-and-neck/maxillofacial/oral-maxillofacial-regional-anesthesia/

21. Haas D. Alternative mandibular nerve block techniques: a review of the Gow-Gates and Akinosi-Vazirani closed-mouth mandibular nerve block techniques. *J Am Dent Assoc.* 2011;**142**(9):8–12.

22. New York School of Regional Anesthesia. Regional and topical anesthesia for awake endotracheal intubation. n.d. https://www.nysora.com/regional-and-topical-anesthesia-for-awake-endotracheal-intubation

23. Benumof J. Management of the difficult airway. *Anaesthesiology.* 1991;**75**(6):1087–1110.

24. Ažman J, Stopar Pintaric T, Cvetko E. Ultrasound-guided glossopharyngeal nerve block: a cadaver and a volunteer sonoanatomy study. *Reg Anesth Pain Med.* 2017;**42**(2):252–258.

25. Stolz D, Chhajed P, Leuppi J, Pflimlin E, Tamm M. Nebulized lidocaine for flexible bronchoscopy: a randomized, double-blind, placebo-controlled trial. *Chest.* 2005;**128**(3):1756–1760.

26. Madan K, Mittal S, Gupta N, Biswal SK, Tiwari P, Hadda V, et al. The cricothyroid versus spray-as-you-go method for topical anesthesia during flexible bronchoscopy: the CRISP randomized clinical trial. *Respiration.* 2019;**98**(5):440–446.

27. Du Rand IA, Blaikley J, Booton R, Chaudhuri N, Gupta V, Khalid S, et al. British Thoracic Society guideline for diagnostic flexible bronchoscopy in adults: accredited by NICE. *Thorax.* 2013; **68** Suppl 1: i1–i44.

28. Ahmad I, El-Boghdadly K, Bhagrath R, Hodzovic I, McNarry AF, Mir F, et al. Difficult Airway Society guidelines for awake tracheal intubation (ATI) in adults. *Anaesthesia.* 2020;**75**:509–528.

29. Williams K, Barker G, Harwood R, Woodall N. Plasma lidocaine levels during local anaesthesia of the airway. *Anaesthesia.* 2003;**58**(5):508–509.

30. Stone J, Kaban L. Trismus after injection of local anaesthetic. *Oral Surg Oral Med Oral Pathol.* 1979;**48**(1):29–32.

31. Christie L, Picard J, Weinberg G. Local anaesthetic systemic toxicity *BJA Educ.* 2015;**15**(3):136–142.

32. Association of Anaesthetists of Great Britain and Ireland. Management of severe local anaesthetic toxicity. 2010. https://anaesthetists.org/Home/Resources-publications/Guidelines/Management-of-severe-local-anaesthetic-toxicity

33. British National Formulary. Local anaesthesia. 2020. https://bnf.nice.org.uk/treatment-summary/anaesthesia-local.html

34. Association of Anaesthetists of Great Britain and Ireland. Quick reference handbook: guidelines for crises in anaesthesia. Section 3-1. Anaphylaxis. 2022. https://anaesthetists.org/Portals/0/PDFs/QRH/QRH_3-1_Anaphylaxis_v5.pdf?ver=2022-04-12-124225-493

5

Imaging

Indu Mitra

Introduction

The head and neck region incorporates structures from the skull base to the thoracic inlet, encompassing numerous complex anatomical entities in a confined and vital area. An understanding of the complex anatomy is important when faced with oral and/or maxillofacial pathologies that can result in anaesthetic dilemmas such as airway compromise and skeletal instability. This chapter describes how imaging can assist in foreseeing possible anaesthetic difficulties, exploring the different imaging modalities available, looking at the strengths and weaknesses of each, and how traditional radiological studies are still used to complement the use of more modern techniques. Using radiological examples, clinically applicable anatomy is reviewed and common pathologies relevant to anaesthetic intervention are discussed.

Imaging modalities

The four main types of imaging modality commonly used in oromaxillofacial specialities are X-ray, ultrasound, computed tomography (CT), and magnetic resonance imaging (MRI). Each imaging modality has its strength and weakness, such that occasionally different modalities are used in conjunction to define certain structures such as bone, soft tissue, and cartilage.

X-ray

X-ray is one of the oldest and most commonly used modalities in dental imaging. Radiation exposure is low (0.005 mSv, which is equivalent to 0.2% of the annual UK average radiation dose). The images are used to assess not only bone architecture and dentition, but certain soft tissue structures as well. Many current practices have moved away from traditional X-rays which were captured on plain film as these have been replaced by digital X-rays. Although the image generation by X-rays is largely unaltered, the digital acquisition confers slightly less radiation, faster image production, and improved image quality. Software can also be used to manipulate the images with regard to contrast and magnification, resulting in enhanced image interpretation.

Dental radiographs can be taken intra- or extraorally. For intraoral images, a sensor is placed inside the mouth and can be used to generate periapical, bitewing, or occlusal views. Extraoral radiographic views, such as lateral cephalometric views, are primarily used in orthodontics and orthognathic surgery.

Panoramic views are generated by rotating the X-ray source and sensor around a patient who is standing in the upright position. This technique gives a good overview of the maxilla and mandible. The orthopantomogram is one of the most commonly seen panoramic radiographs. In addition to dentition, other bony landmarks, soft tissue structures, and paranasal sinuses are also visible (Fig. 5.1), and hence other non-dental pathologies can be seen on these views.

Ultrasound

This imaging modality is radiation free as it uses sound waves to generate images and is best used to assess soft tissue structures of the neck. The benefit of this modality is that it uses real-time imaging and can be tailored to answer specific questions, such as demonstrating neck vessel patency/stenosis or vocal cord paralysis.

Computed tomography

CT uses a gantry which contains a rotating X-ray source and digital sensors, resulting in multiple image slices, ranging from <1 mm to 10 mm in thickness. The very fine cuts (0.65 mm thick) are often used to assess detailed skull base bone anatomy. The cross-sectional images are acquired in minutes and provide comprehensive anatomical detail of the soft tissues and bone architecture. Iodine-based intravenous contrast can be used to highlight soft tissue structures more clearly. Since the images acquired are digital, they can be manipulated using imaging information technology. By varying window width and the grey level, the digital images can be optimized for visualization of different structures such as bone, brain, lung, liver, and so on (Fig. 5.2). Three-dimensional (3D) reconstructions can be generated from the two-dimensional (2D) images obtained. This is useful for identifying subtle cranial fractures and helps in the clinical interpretation of complex facial fractures. Often CT is used to image preoperative implant resin moulds. The 3D reconstruction images generated can be used

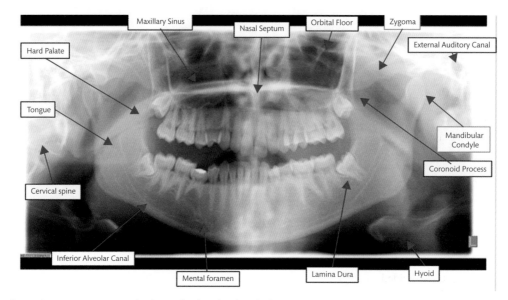

Fig. 5.1 Example of an orthopantomogram with relevant landmarks identified.

to assist in preoperative assessment prior to facial reconstructive surgery.

Magnetic resonance imaging

MRI does not use ionizing radiation, but utilizes a strong magnet to align protons within the body. Radiofrequency waves cause the protons to spin. When the radiofrequency pulse is removed, the protons return to a resting state and emit a signal which is detected by receptor coils around the patient. It is these signals which are used to generate an image, using complex software. By using different pulse sequences, varying signals can be generated dependent on the composition of the structures. The images generated enable structural and compositional assessment. Head and neck structures are separated anatomically into compartments with intervening fat planes. MRI can depict pathology that has resulted in distortion of these fat planes. Even when a pathology results in minimal structural change, MRI can demonstrate subtle signal changes, helping in the diagnosis of early pathologies.

Trauma imaging

X-ray and CT scanning are the most commonly used modalities in trauma imaging. A 2D image can be obtained quickly using X-rays, but the patient needs to be able to comply with positioning requirements. For example, for an orthopantomogram, the patient must be able to stand. When there are other synchronous injuries, this may not be possible, in which case a CT scan is often required. CT is often used to help assess more subtle injuries and better define soft tissue structures. The additional detail provided can help in pre-empting complications and assisting in management.[1]

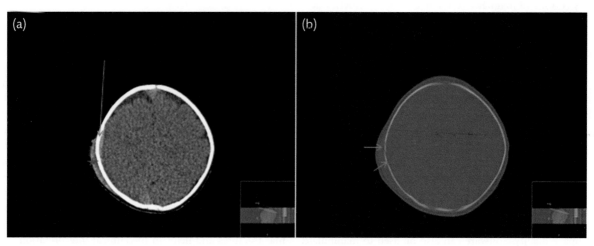

Fig. 5.2 Paediatric CT head axial images demonstrating how window width and greyscale level is used to assess different structures. For example, the soft tissue window level reconstructions (a) show a shallow right subdural haemorrhage (arrow) and a haematoma (star) overlying the right parietal bone. On the bone window levels (b), there are right parietal bone fractures evident.

Dentition

Within the field of medicine, it is crucial to standardize terminology to avoid confusion and facilitate reproducibility and communication between medical professionals. This is particularly pertinent to dental description, and relevant to all anaesthetists undertaking pre-operative dental assessment, not least since dental damage is one of the most common medicolegal claims against an anaesthetist.[2] As in medical imaging, dental description is based on the understanding that the patient's right-hand side corresponds to the left of the image.

Dental nomenclature

Dental nomenclature assists in standardizing dental description. Worldwide, there are several dental notation systems, with varying usage preference according to each country. The common basis of all these systems is to divide the mouth into four quadrants. The maxillary and mandibular components are divided into two at the midline between the front two incisors (Fig. 5.3).

The dental notation developed by the FDI World Dental Federation, often shortened to FDI (in French, *Fédération Dentaire Internationale*) is widely used, and the International Standards Organization Designation System (ISO 3950) defined by the World Health Organization is based on this. It uses two digits, where the first digit indicates the quadrant, and the second digit indicates the tooth within the quadrant. In addition to this, the first number also describes whether the tooth is primary (deciduous/baby) or permanent (adult). For example, 1–4 as the first digit indicates primary dentition, whereas 5–8 indicates permanent dentition.

Although the FDI system is easier for electronic documentation, the older Zsigmondy Palmer notation system from 1861 is still favoured in the UK. This system describes the quadrants as right upper, right lower, left upper, and left lower and gives each a symbol (⌐, ⌐, ⌐, and ⌐, respectively). Permanent teeth are numbered from 1 to 9, and primary teeth are numbered alphabetically from A to E.

The Universal notation system was devised in 1968 and is most commonly used in the US. For permanent dentition, each tooth is given a number from 1 to 32 in a clockwise manner starting with the right maxillary third molar and finishing at the right mandibular third molar. Primary teeth are numbered in a similar clockwise pattern, but the suffix 'd' is placed after the number.

Radiographic assessment of dentition

Dental disease can be assessed by a clinical history of predisposing factors such as smoking, xerostomia, diabetes, autoimmune conditions, immunocompromise, Down syndrome, and connective tissue disorders; by direct visualization of missing teeth, gingivitis, or abscess formation; and by radiological assessment, to identify potential problematic teeth.

The most commonly used modality is X-ray because the dental anatomy such as enamel, dentine, pulp, and alveolar bone can be demonstrated. The lamina dura (Fig. 5.1) is clearly demonstrated as a fine line of compact bone outlining the socket. This compacted bone margin, together with the periodontal ligaments, provides tooth stability. Loss of the lamina dura often occurs in periapical disease and can identify a potentially unstable tooth. Other causes of lamina dura loss include Paget's disease, leukaemia, multiple myeloma,

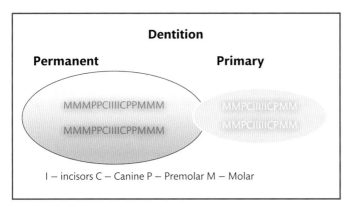

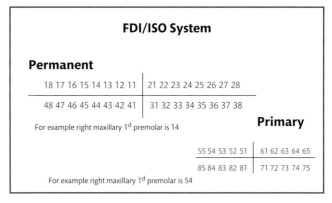

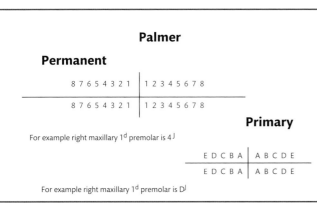

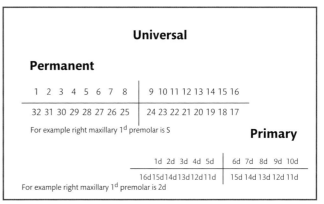

Fig. 5.3 Dental nomenclature.

osteomalacia, rickets, hypoparathyroidism, renal osteodystrophy, and histiocytosis.[2]

A variant of dental X-rays is cone-beam CT. This uses X-rays in the shape of a cone to generate multiple images which are reconstructed by the software to produce multiplanar (axial, coronal, sagittal) 2D and 3D images. Cone-beam CT differs from multidetector CT with regard to the temporal resolution of the detectors, resulting in slow acquisition, increased motion artefact, and increased image reconstruction time. However, when used for small field of view areas such as the mandible and maxilla, cone-beam CT can deliver diagnostic images at a lower radiation dose than conventional multidetector CT, which is useful in planning orthodontic surgery. The 3D images generated can be used in computer-assisted design or manufacturing to produce implants made from either titanium or resin to assist in complex facial reconstruction surgery.

Craniofacial anatomy

The skull (cranium) is composed of the vault and the skull base. The vault comprises several flat bones—frontal, parietal, occipital, temporal, and sphenoid bones. It is important to know conventional suture positions as fine, undisplaced skull fractures can occasionally be mistaken for sutures (Fig. 5.2). The skull base can be divided into the anterior (orbital plate of the frontal, lesser wing sphenoid, cribriform plate of the ethmoid bones), middle (greater wing sphenoid, temporal bones), and posterior (petrous temporal, occipital bones) cranial fossae. Throughout the skull base are foramina containing blood vessels and nerves.

The face is composed of the mandible, maxilla, pterygoid plates of the sphenoid, palatine, zygomatic, nasal, frontal, and lacrimal bones. When considering facial anatomy, the face can be divided into upper, middle, and lower thirds to aid in fracture description and planning

of surgical approach; or, it can be viewed as a buttress composed of four transverse and four paired vertical supports (Fig. 5.4)[4]:

- Upper transverse maxillary (nasofrontal suture, inferior orbital rim, zygoma, to temporozygomatic suture).
- Lower transverse maxillary (maxillary alveolar process and hard palate).
- Upper transverse mandibular (mandibular alveolar process, through mandibular ramus, to posterior cortical margin of the mandible).
- Lower transverse mandibular (inferior margin of the mandible).
- Medial maxillary (nasofrontal suture, medial orbital wall, medial wall maxillary sinus, to maxillary alveolar process).
- Lateral maxillary (frontozygomatic suture, lateral orbital wall, lateral maxillary sinus, body of zygoma, to maxillary alveolar process).
- Posterior maxillary (pterygoid plates).
- Posterior mandibular (mandibular rami).

These supports are characterized by increased bone thickness[5]; they connect to the skull base and calvarium, and provide structure for facial appearance, skeletal support for the orbits, assist in functioning of the facial soft tissues, and withstand the forces of mastication. Between these, there are areas of thin bone or bone containing foramina (e.g. infraorbital or mental nerve foramina), which in the context of trauma can act as 'crumple zones', dissipating energy to minimalize intracranial damage.

Craniofacial fractures

There are various classifications of craniofacial fractures.[6] The classifications can be anatomically based (e.g. skull base, midface, and lower face), based on skeletal support mechanisms,[7] or based on

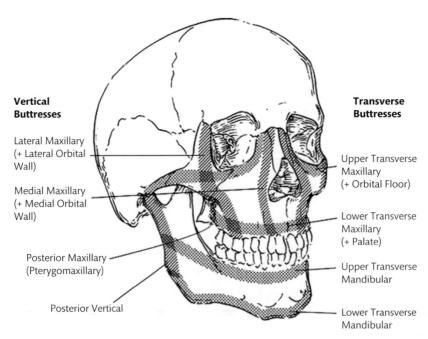

Vertical Buttresses

Lateral Maxillary (+ Lateral Orbital Wall)

Medial Maxillary (+ Medial Orbital Wall)

Posterior Maxillary (Pterygomaxillary)

Posterior Vertical

Transverse Buttresses

Upper Transverse Maxillary (+ Orbital Floor)

Lower Transverse Maxillary (+ Palate)

Upper Transverse Mandibular

Lower Transverse Mandibular

Fig. 5.4 Diagram of the horizontal and vertical buttresses and sites of potential complication following fractures at these positions.
Hopper, RA Salemy S, Sze RW. Diagnosis of midface fractures with CT: what the surgeon needs to know. *Radiographics*. 2006;26:783–793.

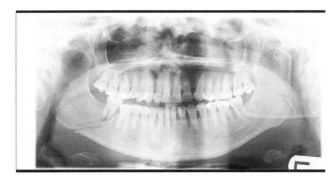

Fig. 5.5 Orthopantomogram showing a fracture through the angle of the right mandible, extending to the root of the lower mandibular molar tooth—a natural point of weakness. There is associated periapical lucency suggesting that this tooth may have become loose as a result of the fracture. Note that the temporomandibular condyles are appropriately enlocated and articulate with the articular eminence of the temporal bone bilaterally.

the severity of the injury and potential complications. The most common fracture trajectories and frequently used classifications are described below:

Lower facial fractures

These most commonly involve the mandible. The mandible should be thought of as forming a ring with the calvarium via the temporomandibular joints. This is because when it fractures, it often does so in more than one location. Occasionally, only a single fracture line is visible and this is most likely due to intermittent dislocation of a temporomandibular joint; hence, it is also important to check for temporomandibular joint continuity and exclude an 'empty temporomandibular joint socket'.

The natural lines of weakness in the mandible run through the roots of the teeth (Fig. 5.5); hence, teeth can become displaced, dislodged, or fragmented.

When the fracture line involves the anterior aspects of the mandible, there is the potential for a floating segment, which can lead to instability during positive pressure ventilation. Often mandibular fractures alone do not cause airway issues. However, the tongue is composed of the genioglossus muscles which attach into the genial tubercle on the lingual aspect of the mandibular symphysis, such that a bilateral anterior fracture can result in a floating bone segment and posterior tongue displacement in the supine position, causing airway compromise.

Midface fractures

The most popular midface fracture classification is the Le Fort classification which dates back to 1901 and is based upon experimental fracture patterns to identify the lines of weakness. It provides a system to describe three patterns of midface fractures, all of which involve the pterygoid plates. These fracture patterns can occur singularly or in combination. The Le Fort type I fracture pattern involves fractures through the lower transverse maxillary buttress, and is known as a 'floating palate' or Guérin fracture. This is best depicted on coronal views due to the transverse nature of the fracture. The Le Fort type II fracture involves the nasofrontal suture and extends along the medial orbital walls, orbital floor, and through the zygomaticomaxillary suture. This results in a pyramidal midface segment which may move independently from the rest of the upper midface and skull base. This fracture type is best seen on axial and coronal views due to the varying planes. The Le Fort type III fracture begins at the nasofrontal suture and extends through the medial and lateral orbital walls to involve the zygomatic arch. This fracture type involves complete craniofacial dissociation.

The Le Fort classification is based on cadavers and does not consider complex fractures which can often involve additional fronto-orbital or nasoethmoidal fractures.

Upper third craniofacial fractures

These fractures may include frontal bone, sphenoid, naso-orbital–ethmoidal complex, and paranasal sinuses. They are often associated with enophthalmos due to an increase in orbital volume, dural tears, or cerebrospinal fluid leak—with an increased risk of ascending infection. It is crucial for an anaesthetist to recognize these particular fractures as a nasotracheal tube, nasogastric tube, or nasopharyngeal temperature probe placed within the nasal passage may inadvertently pass into the cranial fossa.[8]

Zygomaticomaxillary complex fractures

These fractures are usually caused by direct trauma to the cheekbone, resulting in disruption of the zygomaticofrontal, zygomaticomaxillary, zygomaticotemporal, and zygomaticosphenoidal suture posteriorly. This complex fracture pattern is known as a tetrapod fracture—previously, tripod fracture, as only three of the fractures were visible on plain radiographs (Fig. 5.6). Potential complications include enophthalmos due to involvement of the lateral orbital wall, and fragment instability due to the forces applied by surrounding muscles (particularly the masseter muscle).

(a)   (b)   (c)

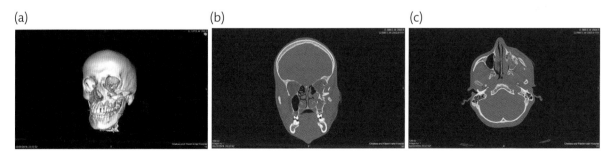

Fig. 5.6 Examples of a complex zygomaticomaxillary fracture: (a) 3D reconstruction demonstrating complex left zygomatic frontal and maxillary fractures; (b) coronal image demonstrating complex butterfly and displaced fractures of the left orbital lateral wall and floor, together with the left medial and lateral maxillary antral walls; (c) axial image, showing left anterior maxillary wall and zygomaticomaxillary fractures.

(a)   (b)

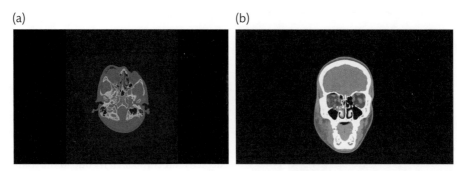

Fig. 5.7 CT images of the face and orbits of a patient who had been punched in the face. The axial bone reconstructions (a) demonstrate comminuted, depressed fractures of the right lamina papyracea, and surgical emphysema anterior to the right globe. The coronal soft tissue window levels image (b) shows a comminuted depressed fracture of the right orbital floor. Both the medial wall and floor of the right orbital fractures have associated herniation of the infraorbital fat, and the altered appearance of the medial and inferior recti muscles suggests that these may also be herniating or impinged.

Orbital fractures

A single buttress fracture of the orbital wall can occur following direct traumatic force to the globe—also known as a 'blowout' fracture because the resultant increase in orbital pressure causes fracture lines at the points of weakness, for example, fracture lines are common along the floor of the orbit (due to the natural weakness caused by the infraorbital foramen), or the medial orbital wall (which is formed by the thin lamina papyracea) (**Fig. 5.7**). When the orbital floor is involved, the fracture can be characterized as an 'open door' or 'trapdoor'. In an open-door fracture, there is a large

defect in the floor of the orbit, compared to a trapdoor fracture where the fracture is hinged and herniation of the orbital contents is followed by spontaneous reduction of the fracture fragment. The latter is also known as a 'white-eyed blowout' because of the few overt physical and radiological features.[9] Potential complications of blowout fractures include extraocular muscle herniation and entrapment, intraorbital haemorrhage, and globe or infraorbital nerve injury. CT is the modality of choice for this injury as 2D reconstructions can provide the necessary information to assess these potential complications, and because the thin slice thickness (0.75 mm) on the bone windows provides accurate fracture line analysis.

Cervical spine

When considering facial fractures, it is important to consider potential traumatic force to the cervical spine and likelihood of a cervical spine fracture. These can be easily missed when there is distracting pain from other injuries. Lateral view radiographs (**Fig. 5.8**) are often the most useful, with 90% of cervical spine fractures able to be diagnosed. The contour lines (anterior, posterior, and spinolaminar) should be aligned and there should be no prevertebral soft tissue thickening. In an adult, the prevertebral soft tissue should measure <6 mm at C2 and <22 mm at C6. In paediatric patients, the prevertebral soft tissue should be between half to two-thirds of the anterior posterior width of the vertebral body.

The mechanism of injury can sometimes help to predict the likely injury incurred:

Cervical spine flexion injuries

Flexion injuries are the most common mechanism and can result in rupture of posterior ligaments with subsequent anterior subluxation of the vertebral body—because the anterior and posterior columns are intact, this fracture is stable. However, high-impact flexion injuries can result in wedge fractures, which can be unstable when there is involvement of the anterior column and posterior interspinous ligaments. Flexion and rotation can result in unilateral facet dislocation. Bilateral facet dislocation can occur when there has been extreme flexion, and this is an unstable injury with a high incidence of cord damage. Flexion teardrop fractures occur after extreme flexion and axial loading—again, these are unstable with a high incidence of cord damage.

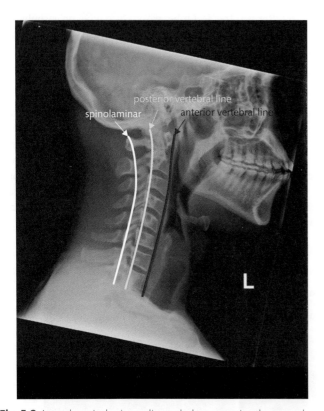

posterior vertebral line
spinolaminar   anterior vertebral line

Fig. 5.8 Lateral cervical spine radiograph demonstrating the normal contours such as the anterior vertebral, posterior vertebral, spinolaminar lines, and the normal prevertebral soft tissue thickness of an adult cervical spine.

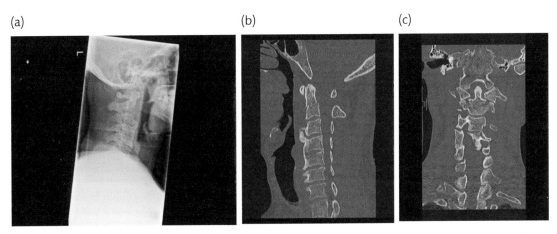

Fig. 5.9 Hangman's fracture. Lateral cervical spine radiograph (a) demonstrating disruption of the anterior and posterior contour lines with increase in prevertebral soft tissue thickness. Subsequent CT performed, with the sagittal (b) and coronal (c) bone reconstruction images demonstrating the displaced fracture involving the C2 vertebra.

Cervical spine extension injuries

Extension injuries, such as Hangman's fracture (**Fig. 5.9**), extension teardrop fracture, and axial compression, can result in a burst fracture. When this involves the C1 ring, it is known as a 'Jefferson fracture'. These are considered unstable fractures and require the utmost care during manipulation of the head and neck, especially during tracheal intubation.

Infection

Head and neck infections can present with life-threatening emergencies such as airway obstruction or mediastinal spread, both of which can hinder airway management (discussed in detail in Chapter 12). As previously mentioned, the head and neck region is composed of several virtual compartments separated by fascial layers and intervening fat planes (**Fig. 5.10**). The orofacial planes

permit odontogenic infection to spread from bone into the subperiosteal region, through to the fat planes superiorly and into the infratemporal fossa, posteriorly to the pharyngeal space, inferiorly into the submandibular fat planes, or in very severe cases into the mediastinal fat planes.

Tumours

Potential anaesthetic difficulties in oromaxillofacial patients may arise from the presence of head and neck masses, whether these are congenital, malignant, or benign. The best imaging modalities are cross-sectional modalities such as CT or MRI. Occasionally, both are required. For example, **Fig. 5.11** shows the imaging of a lung cancer patient who presented with neurological symptoms of headache, left trigeminal paraesthesia, diplopia, left ptosis, and left tongue deviation. The CT scan of the patient's brain did not depict the extent of skull base metastatic disease as comprehensively as the MRI scan.

Similarly, both CT and MRI were required in the diagnosis and in evaluating the extent of a large neuroplexiform mass (**Fig. 5.12**).

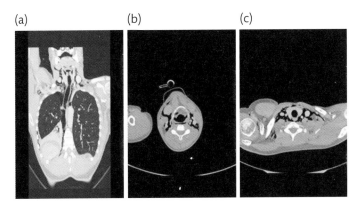

Fig. 5.10 CT images of a patient with spontaneous pneumomediastinum. The reconstructed CT coronal image (a) shows air tracking within the neck and chest, and demonstrates how the cervical and mediastinal fat planes communicate with one another. The reconstructed axial images (b) and (c) demonstrate how different structures in the neck region are divided by fascial planes, for example, the submandibular gland, carotid sheath, and thyroid are separated from each other by fascia.

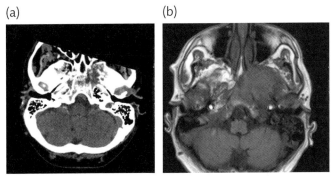

Fig. 5.11 Comparison of imaging modalities in the same patient. The CT axial slice (a) demonstrates architectural bone change within the left skull base. The MRI axial slice (b) shows the *extent* of the soft tissue mass central on the left skull base with infiltration of the clivus.

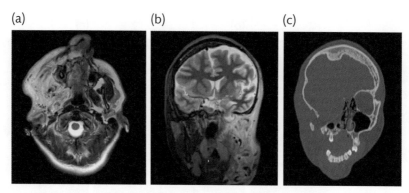

(a)   (b)   (c)

Fig. 5.12 Congenital neuroplexiform mass on (a) axial MRI and (b) coronal MRI, shown as a large soft tissue mass distorting the right facial structures. The mass involves the pterygoid muscles and extends into the right parapharyngeal fat space, potentially resulting in poor mouth opening and compromised airway calibre. The coronal CT image (c) shows right sphenoid wing absence and bone remodelling. These findings are in keeping with neurofibromatosis type 1.

There is a vast range of potential aetiologies relating to oromaxillofacial tumours.[10] With regard to anaesthesia, the difficulties faced may be primary, such that the mass itself results directly in airway compromise or difficult tracheal intubation; or secondary, where the mass involves other head and neck structures such as muscle or nerves, which may result in trismus. These issues are discussed in more detail in Chapter 15.

Conclusion

Although head and neck anatomy is complex, a basic understanding of the most common pathologies and fracture patterns can help when assessing oromaxillofacial patients for anaesthetic intervention. When the appropriate imaging investigation is used, it can aid patient assessment and help pre-empt potential anaesthetic problems that may arise as a result of the underlying pathology.

REFERENCES

1. Chesshire NJ, Knight DJW. The anaesthetic management of facial trauma and fractures. *BJA CEPD Rev.* 2001;**1**(4):108–112.

2. Abeysundara L, Creedon A, Soltanifar D. Dental knowledge for anaesthetists. *BJA Education.* 2016;**16**(11):362–368.

3. Mishra N, Shrivardhan K. Significance of lamina dura—a review. *Int J Contemp Med Surg Radiol.* 2017;**2**(1):1–4.

4. Hopper RA, Salemy S, Sze RW. Diagnosis of midface fractures with CT: what the surgeon needs to know. *Radiographics.* 2006;**26**(3):783–793.

5. Winegar BA, Murillo H, Tantiwongkosi B. Spectrum of critical imaging findings in complex facial skeletal trauma. *Radiographics.* 2013;**33**(1):3–19.

6. Hardt N, Kuttenberger J. Classification of craniofacial fractures. In: Hardt N, Kuttenberger J (eds), *Craniofacial Trauma*, pp. 31–54. Berlin: Springer; 2010.

7. Donat TL, Endress C, Mathog R. Facial fracture classification according to skeletal support mechanisms. *Arch Otolaryngol Head Neck Surg.* 1998;**124**(12):1306–1314.

8. Morosan M, Parbhoo A, Curry N. Anaesthesia and common oral and maxillo-facial emergencies. *Cont Educ Anaesth Crit Care Pain.* 2012;**12**(5):257–262.

9. Yew C, Shaar R, Rahman SA, Alam MK. White-eyed blowout fracture: diagnostic pitfalls and review of literature. *Injury.* 2015;**46**(9):1856–1859.

10. Harnsberger R. *Diagnostic Imaging: Head and Neck*, 3rd ed. Philadelphia, PA: Elsevier; 2016.

6

Sedation

James W. D. Mann and Vivian Yuen

Introduction

Sedation has a long and often fraught history in oromaxillofacial surgery and dentistry. When performed correctly, it improves patient comfort, reduces anxiety, and facilitates medical interventions and procedures to be performed without the need for general anaesthesia. Sedation, being a medical procedure in its own right, has its own associated risks, but is generally more straightforward, quicker, and cheaper than providing general anaesthesia. However, because sedation is deemed more straightforward, and can often be carried out by non-anaesthetists, the risks are not always fully appreciated by patients and medical professionals alike. The term sedation means different things to different people. Patients will often confuse sedation with meaning asleep or general anaesthesia; surgeons might sometimes suggest 'sedation' for a procedure, but still expect an unconscious and motionless patient, really alluding to a state of general anaesthesia. It is imperative that the intended level of sedation is clearly communicated to manage the expectations of the patient and the surgeon.

This chapter focuses on sedative agents and sedation techniques for maxillofacial, craniofacial, and dental procedures, though clearly some of these can be extrapolated to other settings. Whether or not the procedures are suitable to be performed under sedation will depend on the patient and the extent of the underlying pathology. Procedures that lend themselves well to sedation are those where concurrent local anaesthesia can attenuate most, if not all, of the pain. Sedation does not treat pain—analgesia is required for that purpose. Sedation treats procedure-related anxiety, and helps patients tolerate unpleasant procedures. Sedation may fail in some patients where they become disinhibited, confused, and non-compliant (so-called paradoxical effects). Very painful procedures are best carried out under general anaesthesia. Combining sedatives and opioids markedly increases the risk of patient complications, as seen in the American Society of Anesthesiologists (ASA) closed claims study, where poor technique led to significant harm (including cardiac arrest) during procedures under sedation in both adults and children. These cases also highlighted a lack of appropriate monitoring and the inability of staff to manage oversedation.

Logistically, there are not enough anaesthetists to meet the demand for provision of sedation for the number of procedures where it has been requested. This has led to an increasing number of non-anaesthetists providing a sedation service, often in settings away from the operating theatre. Doctors and allied health professionals of various grades and levels of training across many specialties have had to rise to meet the demand. Overall, demand has increased exponentially as new invasive diagnostic and therapeutic procedures have been developed and healthcare services have become more accessible. Patient expectations have risen, such that uncomfortable or painful procedures are, understandably, not tolerated without the relief provided by sedation. Fear and anxiety about dental work, or dental phobia, are common and place added demand on sedation services, when behavioural techniques do not suffice.

Aims of sedation

The principal objective of sedation is to reduce the anxiety and discomfort of patients undergoing procedures. Sedation is a drug-induced reduction in consciousness, the desired endpoints of which lie on a continuum between a state of wakefulness through to general anaesthesia. This altered state of consciousness can be achieved with a myriad of agents, in a number of different settings, to enable a wide range of procedures to be performed.

There are a number of recognized measures of depth of sedation, and the ASA has provided some clarity over the terminology used to describe these (Table 6.1).[1] Other validated measures of sedation include the Ramsay Sedation Scale, Observer's Assessment of Alertness/Sedation (OAA/S) scale, and the Richmond Agitation Sedation Score, though the latter is more applicable to sedation of patients in the intensive care unit (ICU).

- *Minimal sedation/anxiolysis*: this refers to a drug-induced state of calm, with a subtle reduction in cognition and coordination but no cardiorespiratory impairment. Patients should maintain a normal response to verbal stimulation.
- *Moderate sedation ('conscious sedation')*: this refers to a drug-induced depression of consciousness during which patients respond purposefully to verbal commands, either alone or accompanied by light tactile stimulation (reflex withdrawal from a painful stimulus is not considered a purposeful response). No

Table 6.1 The continuum of depth of sedation—definitions of general anaesthesia and levels of sedation

	Minimal sedation/anxiolysis	Moderate sedation/analgesia	Deep sedation/analgesia	General anaesthesia
Responsiveness	Normal response to verbal stimulation	Purposeful response to verbal or tactile stimulation	Purposeful response following repeated or painful stimulation	Unarousable, even with painful stimulation
Airway	Unaffected	No intervention required	Intervention may be required	Intervention often required
Spontaneous ventilation	Unaffected	Adequate	May be inadequate	Frequently inadequate
Cardiovascular function	Unaffected	Usually maintained	Usually maintained	May be impaired

Source: American Society of Anesthesiologists.[1]

interventions are required to maintain a patent airway, and spontaneous ventilation is adequate. Cardiovascular function is usually maintained.

- *Deep sedation*: this refers to a drug-induced depression of consciousness during which patients cannot easily be aroused but respond purposefully following repeated or painful stimulation. The ability to independently maintain ventilatory function may be impaired. Patients may require assistance in maintaining a patent airway.
- *General anaesthesia*: this refers to a drug-induced loss of consciousness, during which patients are not rousable, even by painful stimulation. The ability to independently maintain ventilatory function is often impaired. Patients often require assistance in maintaining a patent airway, and positive pressure ventilation may be required because of depressed spontaneous ventilation or drug-induced depression of neuromuscular function. Cardiovascular function may be impaired.[1]

'Conscious sedation' is an oxymoron[2]—a confusing and contradictory term, that unfortunately, is in common parlance. It is intended to mean sedation without the loss of consciousness—which is the definition of sedation! Deep sedation requires skills normally attributed to anaesthetists, in order to rescue the patient from unintended general anaesthesia.

It is important to differentiate between procedures that will require analgesia in addition to sedation, and those that just require anxiolysis or minimal sedation. The sedation technique is determined by a number of factors: the operative conditions required, the intended depth of sedation, the type of procedure, how painful the procedure is likely to be, and the comorbidities of the patient. The required procedural conditions then govern the level of training of the sedationist, level of monitoring, location, and level of support staff required. Analgesia can be achieved with a multimodal approach including local anaesthetic infiltration, nerve blocks, and analgesic medication, for example, paracetamol, non-steroidal anti-inflammatory drugs, and opioids. Oromaxillofacial surgical procedures are particularly amenable to infiltration of local anaesthesia or peripheral nerve blocks (discussed in Chapter 4). In dental procedures, general anaesthesia for the purposes of anxiolysis should be the last resort,[3] and only be employed when local anaesthesia and sedation techniques have either failed or are not suitable. Often, general anaesthesia is necessary for children requiring longer restorative and conservation dental treatments, and in those with learning difficulties.

For some procedures, good communication and rapport with the patient may be all that is needed. Using sedation does not negate the need to maintain a good rapport with the patient.

Advantages of sedation

- Avoids general anaesthesia.
- May be more acceptable to the patient.
- May be quicker.
- Less expensive than general anaesthesia.
- Fewer medications; lower doses than general anaesthesia.
- Less airway instrumentation/intervention.
- Less disruptive for patient; day case possible.

Potential complications of sedation

- Desaturation.
- Nausea and vomiting.
- Undersedation.
- Oversedation.
- Aspiration.
- Respiratory depression.
- Airway obstruction.
- Prolonged recovery.
- Failure of sedation/incomplete abandoned procedure.
- Fear; the potential for post-traumatic stress disorder.
- Cardiac arrest.

The Paediatric Sedation Research Consortium has published a retrospective report on the incidence and nature of adverse events during paediatric sedation/anaesthesia with propofol for procedures outside the operating room (Table 6.2).[4] The report involved almost 50,000 cases of propofol sedation. The consortium has

Table 6.2 A comparison of the incidence of adverse events during paediatric sedation/anaesthesia with propofol and dexmedetomidine

Adverse events	Number of events	
	Dexmedetomidine	Propofol
Cardiopulmonary resuscitation	0	2/49,836
Pulmonary aspiration	0	4/49,836
Oxygen desaturation <90%	57/13,072 (43.6/10,000)	154/10,000
Central apnoea /airway obstruction	35/13,072 (26.8/10,000)	575/10,000
Unexpected admission	5/13,072 (=3.8/10,000)	7.1/10,000

also published a similar report on dexmedetomidine sedation in >13,000 children.[5] Comparing propofol with dexmedetomidine sedation for paediatric sedation, the incidence of adverse respiratory events was higher when using propofol. Although these are only retrospective reports and it is difficult to make a direct comparison, large numbers of children were included. These reports reflect the relative safety margin of the two sedative agents on respiratory adverse events. Thus, the practitioner who uses propofol for sedation should be trained and proficient in airway management of the unconscious patient and they should be competent to rescue the patient from the deep sedation that can be produced with propofol.

The economic and morbidity burden of sedation-related adverse events is significant, but is also underreported. The online reporting tool (http://www.aesedationreporting.com) was set up in 2012 by the World Society of Intravenous Anaesthesia with the aim of collecting and evaluating sedation data and the incidence of adverse events.[6] The ASA also proposed a common language for describing and reporting adverse events. Additionally, the International Committee for the Advancement of Procedural Sedation (ICAPS) set up their own version of an online adverse event reporting tool (Tracking and Reporting Outcomes of Procedural Sedation: TROOPS) in 2018.[7] This anonymized tool aimed to track the adverse events, interventions, and outcomes for all types of sedation, delivered by all types of sedationists, for all procedures and patients. Continuous quality improvement relies on documenting these events and their outcomes, yet this is a voluntary online tool relying on individuals to self-report their experiences.

Complications of sedation can be minimized by good preoperative assessment and patient selection, appropriate technique, and safe conduct of sedation. However, the sedationist should be prepared for potentially life-threatening events, and be appropriately trained in their management. Oxygen desaturation is frequently the commonest adverse event in studies, and should be promptly detected by the mandatory use of pulse oximetry. It may be due to hypoventilation, apnoea, or upper airway obstruction. Patients with obstructive sleep apnoea (common in oromaxillofacial surgery) are particularly at risk, being highly sensitive to opioids. The sequence of partial airway obstruction, coughing, oversedation, complete airway obstruction, and then hypoxia should be avoided where possible, but promptly managed if it does occur.

The ideal sedative agent

The ideal sedative agent, like the ideal anaesthetic agent, does not yet exist (or remains elusive). Only one new sedative drug has been released and gained clinical utility in the last 20 years, namely dexmedetomidine. Other new drugs are in development, with trials of prodrugs of current agents and different formulations of inhalation agents (e.g. remimazolam is undergoing phase III clinical trials. Preliminary studies reveal a quicker onset time and much shorter duration of action compared to midazolam). The ideal sedative agent should have the following pharmacological properties:

Pharmacodynamics (effects):

- Anxiolytic.
- Analgesic.

- Amnesic.
- Maintain respiratory drive.
- Maintain laryngeal reflexes.
- Minimal haemodynamic changes.
- No side effects.
- Wide therapeutic window—increased margin of safety.

Pharmacokinetics (absorption, distribution, metabolism, elimination):

- Multi-route.
- Good parenteral bioavailability.
- Quick onset and offset (conferring a wider margin of safety).
- Easily titratable.
- Inactive metabolites.
- Predictable (short) duration of action.
- Context-insensitive half-life.
- Dose-dependent effects.
- Specific antagonist available.

A comparison of commonly used agents with the ideal agent is presented in **Table 6.3**.

Pharmacology of sedative agents

Midazolam

Midazolam has been a World Health Organization essential drug since the 1970s. In common with other drugs from the large benzodiazepine family, midazolam potentiates the effects of gamma-aminobutyric acid (GABA) on $GABA_A$ receptors by binding to closely located benzodiazepine binding sites throughout the brain and spinal cord. This results in increasing neural inhibition, thus reducing the number of neural impulses reaching higher centres of the brain. Its effects include anxiolysis, sedation, anterograde amnesia, muscle relaxation, and anticonvulsant properties. It is shorter acting than lorazepam or diazepam, with an elimination half-life of 1.5–2.5 hours, which makes it more suitable for procedural sedation. Its availability in three different concentrations (1 mg/mL, 2 mg/mL, and 5 mg/mL) has prompted the National Patient Safety Agency to issue an alert on the use of midazolam—it advises that in the settings where procedural sedation is performed, only the 5 mg in 5 mL ampoules should be made available, to help avoid accidental overdose.

Midazolam has been regarded as the gold standard for premedication in paediatric anaesthesia and it is the most commonly used preoperative sedative.[8] It is associated with significant anterograde amnesia[9] and this is frequently put forward as a specific advantage. Although midazolam causes explicit memory loss, it has been shown in both adults[10] and children[11] that implicit memory is unaffected. Although implicit memories are not intentionally or consciously retrievable, these memories may have an effect on patients' subsequent emotion and behaviour on similar future encounters.[12] Midazolam sedation may be associated with learning without awareness, or having experience of the event without recall.

Midazolam is painless when injected intravenously. It is water soluble in its ampoule, and more lipid soluble at physiological pH, contributing to uptake at its effect site. Onset of action is 2 minutes and peak effect is reached in about 5–10 minutes. The intravenous injection of midazolam should be given slowly at a rate of

Table 6.3 A comparison of the properties of commonly used sedative agents compared with the ideal sedative agent

Ideal agent	Midazolam	Propofol	Dexmedetomidine	Ketamine	Nitrous oxide	Fentanyl
Anxiolytic	Y	Y	Y	Y	Y	N
Analgesic	N	N	(Y)	Y	Y	Y
Amnesic	Y	Y	Y	Y	Y	N
Maintains respiratory drive	N	N	Y	Y	Y	N
Maintains laryngeal reflexes	N	N	Y	(Y)	Y	N
Cardiovascular effects	Cardiostable	Decreased	Biphasic	Increased	Cardiostable	Cardiostable
Wide therapeutic window	N	N	Y	Y	Y	N
Side effects	Y	Y	Y	Y	Y	Y
Contraindications			Digoxin			
Multi-route	Y	N	Y	Y	N	N
Quick onset	N	Y	N	Y	Y	Y
Quick offset	N	Y	N	N	Y	Y
Inactive metabolites	Y	Y	Y	Y	Y	N
Predictable duration of action	Mins/hrs	Mins	Mins/hrs	Mins	Secs	Mins
Dose-dependent effects	Y	Y	Y	Y	Y	Y
Antagonist	Y	N	N	N	N	Y
Elderly	Reduce	Reduce	Reduce	Reduce		Reduce
Liver disease			Reduce			
Renal disease			Normal			Caution

N, no; Y, yes.

approximately 1 mg over 30 seconds. This misconception of onset time and injection rate has led to many problems with midazolam in inexperienced hands.[13]

It can usefully be given via several routes: nasal, buccal, oral, intravenous, and intramuscular. Oral bioavailability is 50%, so relatively higher doses are required for this route (e.g. 0.5 mg/kg, maximum dose is 20 mg in children). Different flavoured syrups have been formulated for children to aid compliance. Active metabolites are generated by liver metabolism, but are not clinically significant. Midazolam only produces modest cardiovascular effects. Allergies are rare. It is used throughout the hospital by anaesthetist and non-anaesthetist alike, especially in endoscopy. Midazolam is inexpensive in its intravenous formulation, unlike the flavoured oral solutions.

Disadvantages

The disadvantages of midazolam should warrant particular care when used in certain situations, most notably the elderly and those with significant comorbidities where even small doses (0.5–1 mg) can have an exaggerated effect. Midazolam affords no appreciable analgesia, and therefore is likely to be co-administered with an opioid for a painful procedure. This combination greatly increases the likelihood of respiratory depression. Respiratory depression and airway obstruction is possible even in healthy adults after quick intravenous injection or a large dose. Unpredictable paradoxical effects or disinhibited behaviours are a feature (more often seen in children), and can clearly be counterproductive to the procedure.

Antagonism

A benzodiazepine overdose (either relative or absolute) can be reversed by the antagonist flumazenil, which should be reserved for emergencies. The patient must undergo continued monitoring and observation, because this reversal agent has a shorter duration of action than midazolam, and it is possible for the patient to become re-sedated once the effects wear off. Incremental dosing is recommended to reduce the total dose needed as flumazenil has a number of undesirable side effects, so routine use should be avoided. Dry mouth, diplopia, headache, hypotension, arrhythmias, and seizures have all been reported.

Propofol

Propofol, 2,6-diisopropylphenol, is a synthetic phenol derivative that is commonly used for the intravenous induction and maintenance of anaesthesia. It was introduced in the 1980s, and has since largely replaced the use of barbiturates. Propofol is administered with a predetermined mg/kg bolus dose, titrated to effect or by a target-controlled infusion (TCI). This hypnotic agent is thought to exert its effects through the potentiation of GABAergic inhibitory neurotransmission, though exactly how remains unclear. Its use can be modified to produce different levels of sedation without reaching a state of general anaesthesia. With smaller intravenous boluses or a lower TCI rate, any desired level of sedation can be achieved. The challenge is to keep the patient at the intended level of sedation for the duration of the procedure, and TCI is ideal for this. Other co-administered depressant drugs (opioids, benzodiazepines, ketamine) will have additive or even synergistic effects.

Propofol is ideally suited to achieving the desired level of sedation due to its favourable pharmacokinetic profile, with a quick onset (15–30 seconds) and rapid recovery (5–10 minutes), and short context-sensitive half-life. The short clinical effect is due to rapid redistribution from central compartments to peripheral tissue compartments, though its elimination half-life can exceed 24 hours. Propofol is versatile in that it can be used for very short procedures or prolonged periods, be given as a bolus, simple infusion, or TCI to produce sedation, or at higher levels general anaesthesia. With dose-dependent anxiolytic, amnesic, and sedative effects, propofol can be titrated carefully to produce the desired endpoint. Hence, it remains the most common sedative drug in current use by anaesthetists. It has potent antiemetic effects which also makes it particularly suitable for day case procedures (especially oromaxillofacial).

Disadvantages

The lipid emulsion in which propofol is formulated can produce pain on injection—although this can be attenuated by slower injection, using a larger vein, diluting with saline, or mixing with lidocaine. This seemingly minor side effect should not be dismissed, because it can make the patient unnecessarily agitated or uncooperative. It is seldom seen with the medium- or long-chain triglyceride formulations. Propofol has a particularly narrow therapeutic window and therefore a reduced margin of safety, so there is a very real risk of unintended general anaesthesia or at least a deeper-than-intended level of sedation. Dose-dependent respiratory depression, hypoventilation, hypoxia, upper airway obstruction, depressed protective airway reflexes, cardiovascular instability, hypotension, reduced systemic vascular resistance, reduced cardiac output, reduced contractility, and reduced myocardial blood flow are effects that warrant close monitoring and vigilance to allow prompt treatment that will prevent harm to the patient. Hence caution is required, especially in the elderly and patients with extensive comorbidities. High dosages in ICU sedation have been associated with propofol infusion syndrome that manifests as a collection of metabolic derangements and organ failure, and may cause death. Metabolic acidosis, rhabdomyolysis, renal failure, hyperlipidaemia, arrhythmias, and cardiac failure are all features of the syndrome.[13]

Opioids

Opioids are not particularly sedative and they should not be used as such. They can have a role as adjuncts to sedatives in providing analgesia for more painful procedures, where local anaesthesia will not suffice. The synthetic opioid, fentanyl is commonly used, as well as alfentanil, sufentanil (not licensed in the UK), and in some cases remifentanil as an infusion. These are very potent intravenous analgesics, notable for producing respiratory depression and airway obstruction.

Disadvantages

Potential undesirable effects of opioids include respiratory depression, suppression of airway reflexes, bradycardia and hypotension, nausea and vomiting, itching, constipation, and urinary retention.

Antagonism

Naloxone can be used to manage opioid overdose, as it is a nonselective and competitive opioid receptor antagonist. When given intravenously, naloxone works within 2 minutes, and within 5 minutes if given intramuscularly. It may also be sprayed into the nose. The effects of naloxone last about 30 minutes to an hour. Multiple doses may be required, as the duration of action of most opioids is greater than that of naloxone. Administration to opioid-dependent individuals may cause symptoms of opioid withdrawal, including restlessness, agitation, nausea, vomiting, tachycardia, and sweating.

Ketamine

Ketamine is a phencyclidine derivative presented in a variety of concentrations. It is manufactured in 10 mg/mL, 50 mg/mL, and 100 mg/mL solutions on account of its use in veterinary medicine as well as in humans. Used intravenously or intramuscularly, ketamine has analgesic, sedative, and anaesthetic effects (when used in increasing doses), exerted via N-methyl-D-aspartate (NMDA) receptors. These favourable properties mean it can theoretically be used as the sole sedative agent for a procedure—often the case in the developing world. It has quick onset and a moderate duration of action—a 2 mg/kg dose injected intravenously produces dissociative anaesthesia in about 30 seconds, with the effects lasting from 5 to 15 minutes. It is very popular in emergency anaesthesia, especially in prehospital care. Lower doses are required for analgesia and sedation, 0.5–1 mg/kg when given intravenously.

In contrast to other anaesthetic agents, ketamine causes stimulation of the sympathetic nervous system resulting in increased systolic blood pressure and heart rate, and should therefore be used with caution in the elderly and those with ischaemic heart disease. However, these undesirable sympathomimetic effects are not seen with subanaesthetic doses (up to 0.5 mg/kg), while the potent analgesic effects are, making it well suited to sedation for brief painful procedures.[14] Ketamine is therefore often used in combination with other sedatives, employed at lower subanaesthetic doses, exploiting its analgesic properties and avoiding its sympathetic stimulation.

Disadvantages

Emergence delirium and unpleasant hallucinations can be a feature (if not attenuated by a benzodiazepine). Nausea and vomiting can also complicate its use, and prophylactic antiemetics should be considered when ketamine is used for procedural sedation.[15] As such, it is not often the first-line agent for sedation for oromaxillofacial procedures, compared to propofol. Nevertheless, respiratory rate is often increased and airway reflexes are better preserved than with propofol. Increased salivation may preclude its use in dental surgery, potentially precipitating coughing and bronchospasm. No specific antagonist is available, though it is considered to have a good margin of safety.

Dexmedetomidine

Dexmedetomidine was first approved for use in 1999 in the US, and in 2001 in the UK for the sedation of patients in ICUs. Since then, its use has expanded, as an anaesthetic-sparing agent, a premedication, and an analgesia adjunct (though not yet licensed for procedural sedation). A potent α_2-adrenoreceptor agonist, it provides anxiolysis, sedation, and analgesia. It is eight times more selective for α_2 than clonidine, and about five times more potent.[16] Dexmedetomidine exerts its clinical effects via activation of central adrenoreceptors in the locus coeruleus in the brainstem resulting in dose-dependent inhibition of excitatory neurotransmission. The resulting sedation more closely resembles natural physiological sleep than the GABAergic-induced sedation with propofol or midazolam. Studies have demonstrated electroencephalograms (EEG) resembling normal phase II non-rapid eye movement sleep. In this state, it is possible to rouse the patient, while they still remain calm and able to follow simple commands. This quality of sedation is in contrast to that of midazolam or propofol, which is more likely to lead to disorientation and movement if the patient is disturbed from sleep.

Effects of dexmedetomidine include:

- Sedation and anxiolysis.
- Analgesia.
- Hypotension/hypertension.
- Bradycardia.
- Decongestant.
- Antisialagogue.
- Diuresis.

The cardiovascular effects are biphasic and the initial response following the loading dose is mediated by the α_{2B} receptors in the vascular smooth muscle, causing hypertension. This is followed by centrally mediated inhibition of sympathetic outflow, which leads to hypotension and bradycardia. Respiration and airway patency are preserved even at high (over)doses, but concomitant use with other sedatives or opioids may enhance their action causing a degree of respiratory depression and/or airway obstruction, due to reduction in muscle tone.

Dexmedetomidine is not sufficient to be the sole analgesic for painful procedures, but should be considered more analgesic or opioid sparing. Where additional analgesia will likely be required, a reduced starting dose may be considered. Dexmedetomidine is a viable alternative to midazolam for procedural sedation for unilateral third molar surgery in conjunction with local anaesthesia.[17]

In the ICU, a loading dose is not warranted, mitigating the unwanted haemodynamic effects in critically ill patients, who invariably have received other sedatives. An infusion can be started at a rate of 0.7 mcg/kg/hr, and then adjusted accordingly (in the range 0.2—1.4 mcg/kg/hr). A steady state may take an hour to achieve after dose alteration, and it is not recommended to be bolused, as can easily be done with propofol.[13]

A 200 mcg ampoule can be diluted with 0.9% sodium chloride solution to achieve a concentration of 4 mcg/mL in a volume of 50 mL. For procedural sedation, a loading dose of 1 mcg/kg can be given over at least 10 minutes, before starting at a rate of 0.6 mcg/kg/hr, then titrated to the desired effect (within the range of 0.2–1.0 mcg/kg/hr). Care must be taken not to confuse mcg/kg/hr and mcg/kg/min, which would result in an overdose 60 times the intended dose. For stimulating procedures, a rate of at least 0.7 mcg/kg/hr may be required. For the elderly and those who will not tolerate the haemodynamic changes, the loading dose can be reduced (e.g. 50%). This induction of sedation process can therefore take more time to achieve a clinically useful endpoint compared to propofol. Anecdotally, intermittent low-dose boluses have been given to speed up the process, but this is not recommended by the manufacturer.[13]

The nasal administration of dexmedetomidine is a particularly useful alternative to nasal midazolam. This has been used successfully in adults and children for dental surgery.[18] Non-intravenous routes of administration have the disadvantage of slower onset and limited ability to titrate to the desired effect. A bolus of 1–2 mcg/kg delivered onto the nasal mucosa can be used as a premedication or as part of procedural sedation.

Dexmedetomidine has a longer duration of action than propofol, such that patients often remain sleepy post procedure. They can be easily roused, but will fall back to sleep when left undisturbed. This could cause problems for day case procedures, with patients failing to meet discharge criteria. Dexmedetomidine is contraindicated in patients taking digoxin due to an increased risk of severe bradycardia and cardiac arrest. No specific reversal agent is available.

Nitrous oxide

Inhaled nitrous oxide (N_2O) has the longest history of use in the field of sedation, being first used in 1844. Its use remains widespread in dental practice today for anxiolysis, and for minimal sedation in children and adults.[19,20] It can be safely used in community dental practice as well as the pre-hospital and hospital environment.[21] Also referred to as relative analgesia, N_2O is generally delivered in concentrations of 20–50% (though up to 70% can be delivered) in a mixture with oxygen. The concentration of N_2O can be titrated to effect in increments of 5–10%, with the patient remaining responsive throughout. It requires cooperation with the patient to tolerate the nasal mask, mouthpiece, or face mask. For procedures in the oral cavity, a nasal mask is required. For single-agent use of N_2O in dentistry, an operator-sedationist technique can be used, in conjunction with a trained assistant to help monitor the patient. Nausea and vomiting is a common side effect,[19,22] especially when used in combination with fentanyl.[23] Consideration of gas scavenging is important—N_2O is an environmental hazard as it depletes the ozone layer. SEDARA* (Linde Gas, North America, LLC) is a relatively new portable inhalation device for delivering a fixed 50% N_2O and 50% oxygen mixture, adding to the more historical MDM (Matrx Medical Inc., Orchard Park, NY, USA) and McKesson relative analgesia machines (both of which allow titration of the inspired concentration of N_2O).

Sevoflurane

Sevoflurane is included here for completeness, as subanaesthetic doses can produce sedation, which can be titrated with the inspired concentration. Compared to the other volatile agents, it is the most pleasant smelling and non-irritant. An agent-specific vaporizer, breathing circuit, and scavenging are required. Routine use is limited by the equipment required, cost, and its emetogenic effects.

Synergy of agents

Some combinations of agents produce profound synergism that can be both beneficial and problematic. Opioids and propofol work synergistically to produce desirable conditions for both surgeon/operator and patient. However, opioids in the presence of propofol or benzodiazepines are several times more likely to produce respiratory depression, increasing the risk of adverse events.

If fentanyl is to be given with midazolam, it should be given first, and its relatively slow onset of action observed for 2–4 minutes prior to titration of midazolam. Further dosing with fentanyl should be restricted to those who are trained and experienced in dealing with deeper-than-intended sedation.

Table 6.4 Properties of dexmedetomidine and ketamine

Dexmedetomidine	Ketamine
Sedative	Mild sedation
Weak analgesic	Strong analgesic
Bradycardia	Tachycardia
Hypotension	Hypertension
Antisialagogue	Salivation
Reduce emergence agitation	Emergence phenomena

Remifentanil and propofol are ideal partners for total intravenous anaesthesia, but at lower effect site target concentrations of both agents, sedation can be achieved (minimal, moderate, and deep depths). The plasma concentration of remifentanil rises at different rates according to its use as a fixed-rate infusion (mcg/kg/min) or TCI, with the effects evident sooner with TCI and delayed with fixed rate infusion.

Ketofol is a 50:50 mixture of 1% propofol and 1% ketamine that is sometimes used in emergency departments for painful procedures that require both sedation and analgesia. It is combined to take advantage of their complementary effects, with the undesirable effects of one drug compensated by the beneficial effects of the other. Generally, lower doses equate to fewer side effects, and given that both drugs cause sedation, this effect will still be achieved at lower doses. In practice, only those experienced with the pharmacology of these drugs should be administering such a combination. Studies have yet to determine the most efficacious ratio of propofol to ketamine, and in which setting it is most beneficial.

Though not currently available, it is logical to combine ketamine with dexmedetomidine as the advantages and disadvantages of both drugs complement each other (**Table 6.4**).[24] While dexmedetomidine is a sedative with minimal analgesic properties, the addition of ketamine would allow brief painful procedures to be performed. Dexmedetomidine may decrease the tachycardia, hypertension, salivation, and emergence phenomena from ketamine, while ketamine may prevent the bradycardia and hypotension from dexmedetomidine. The disadvantage of this combination would be a slightly prolonged recovery after the procedure.

Conduct of sedation

Depth of sedation may change during the course of the procedure because of the methods of delivery, pharmacogenetic and interpatient variability, anxiety state, level of surgical stimulation, and the patient's concurrent medication. Achieving a steady state can be difficult.

Risk of oversedation is more likely with bolus drug delivery, due to potentially higher peak plasma concentrations than with TCI. The effect of each bolus should be observed within the appropriate time frame, before delivering the next dose. Otherwise, dose stacking can occur, where further boluses are delivered before the peak effect of the previous dose, leading to a higher-than-necessary plasma concentration and potential for oversedation. Titration of doses is advocated by the dental faculties of both the Royal College of Surgeons and the Royal College of Anaesthetists,[25] especially in light of the National Patient Safety Agency report of adverse events with midazolam. Extremes of age and weight, and genetic polymorphism, are some of the factors responsible for interpatient variability, and careful titration of sedation and analgesia helps to mitigate some of the risk. Titration is paramount for providing effective and safe sedation for each patient, whatever the technique or combination of agents. Whether using a bolus technique or TCI, one must also be very patient when sedating elderly patients, allowing more time for slow circulation and the time to reach equilibrium.

TCI techniques free up the anaesthetist to monitor the depth of sedation and maintain communication with the patient and surgeon. Adjusting the target concentration is easy, and there is often a display to demonstrate how quickly the new steady state will take to achieve (albeit an estimate). TCI pumps improve titration of the drug's plasma concentration and effect, according to the pharmacokinetic and pharmacodynamic properties of the agents (propofol or remifentanil). The Minto model, used in effect site mode, is the preferred remifentanil TCI model, which can be started at an effect site target concentration of 1 ng/mL and titrated in increments of 0.5 ng/mL. The rate of remifentanil should be titrated to the respiratory rate and effort, to avoid significant hypoventilation and apnoea. Since remifentanil is a very potent opioid with a high risk of respiratory depression, monitoring of ventilation should include continuous waveform capnography. The onset of respiratory depression occurs after the onset of sedation,[26] therefore it is necessary to wait and observe the effects on ventilation before increasing the infusion rate.[27] The Marsh model, in effect site mode, is the preferred propofol TCI model in adults, which can be started at an effect site target concentration of 0.5 mcg/mL and titrated in 0.2 mcg/mL increments according to clinical effect. TCIs tend to perform better than manual infusions, and benefit from fewer episodes of apnoea, better cardiovascular stability, better patient and surgeon satisfaction, and quicker patient recovery.[28]

For procedures where fentanyl is used for analgesia, the fentanyl can be diluted to enable administration of smaller aliquots (e.g. 10–25 mcg). Fentanyl is better suited to short procedures, which do not require continued repeated boluses (therefore avoiding a higher cumulative dose and the associated risks).

Patient-controlled sedation, analogous to patient-controlled analgesia, provides a bolus of sedation on demand at the push of a button, with a set lockout time before a further dose is permitted. Propofol, midazolam, and remifentanil have all been trialled, but propofol has the better pharmacokinetic profile for this method. Patient-controlled sedation gives autonomy back to the patient and some studies demonstrate better patient satisfaction and quicker recovery.[29] Lower-technology alternatives, such as when a patient signals to the sedationist that they require more sedation by squeezing a squeaky toy or pressing a buzzer can easily be introduced into routine practice. A TCI version of patient-controlled sedation, as opposed to bolus delivery, is currently being developed. In this case, the sedationist sets a target concentration, which the patient can then titrate themselves to their desired level of sedation. The TCI device relies upon inputs from the patient to continue at the higher target concentration, otherwise it will revert to a lower infusion rate until the patient is alert enough to press the button to demand more. Closed-loop delivery systems that use inputs from monitors (e.g. BIS™, Medtronic Limited, Watford, UK) to help determine infusion rates for individual patients have been studied. These devices will have to prove their benefit and superiority over established techniques, before they are accepted into routine clinical practice. SEDASYS® (Ethicon Endo-Surgery, Inc.) was one such device, but was discontinued in 2016 due to poor uptake. The CONCERT-CL® closed-loop infusion system (VERYARK™, Nanning, China) is currently marketed for clinical use,[30] but the system is not readily available.

Conduct of surgery

During oromaxillofacial procedures, direct access to the patient's head and airway is limited, and therefore it is important that communication is maintained with the surgeon so they may report any deteriorating situation to the sedationist before it even becomes apparent on the monitors. Infusions can then be titrated accordingly or airway interventions performed in a timely manner.

Injecting local anaesthetic can be particularly painful, especially if injected quickly. Some dentists use topical benzocaine (or other topically applied local anaesthetics) to numb the injection site prior to insertion of the needle. A slow injection of local anaesthetic is also much more comfortable for the patient.

Oral surgical techniques often require irrigation, and along with any blood, debris, or even dental prostheses, these have the potential to cause aspiration in a sedated patient.[31] Under general anaesthesia, a throat pack can be used to prevent soiling of the airway, but this practice is not directly transferable to procedures performed under sedation. Methods that can be employed include high-volume suction, restricted irrigation, and bite blocks with integrated light source, suction, and fluid capture. Fluid capture using absorbent sponges or barriers such as a rubber dental dam can help limit the fluid and debris reaching the oropharynx (**Fig. 6.1**).

During oromaxillofacial procedures performed under sedation, airway obstruction can easily be caused by poor positioning, the dentist leaning on the jaw, or applying force when working on the mandible. Good knowledge of the surgical procedures can help the sedationist to anticipate changes in sedation and analgesia requirements and to titrate appropriately, and pre-emptively (**Fig. 6.2**).

Safety and guidelines

There have been numerous new guidelines and updates in the last decade, issued from national and specialist societies in the UK, the US, and Europe, that cover procedural sedation across many different specialties. In the recent past, there have been conflicting recommendations from leading anaesthetic societies and non-anaesthetic societies regarding the use of propofol by non-anaesthetists. The latest guidelines from the ASA represent a collaboration with dental anaesthesiologists, oral and maxillofacial surgeons, and radiologists, and state that the use of sedatives (propofol and ketamine) for moderate sedation must be provided with the care consistent with that required for general anaesthesia (including the requirement that practitioners are competent at identifying and rescuing patients from deep sedation or general anaesthesia). There is also now good consensus from the various European societies of anaesthesia

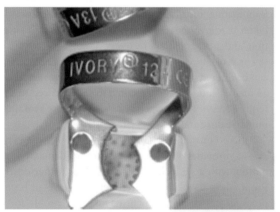
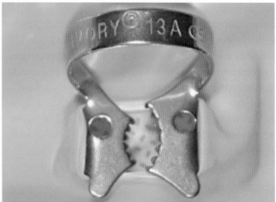
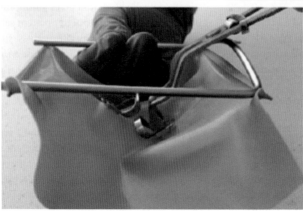
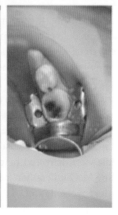

Fig. 6.1 Rubber dam used by dentists to contain and stop water/blood draining into the airway.

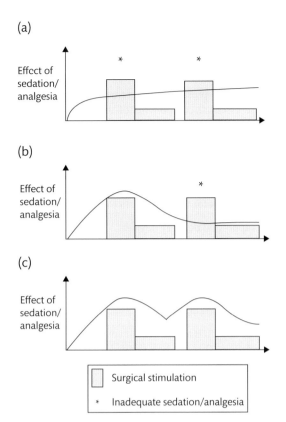

(a)

Effect of sedation/ analgesia

(b)

Effect of sedation/ analgesia

(c)

Effect of sedation/ analgesia

☐ Surgical stimulation

* Inadequate sedation/analgesia

Fig. 6.2 The importance of timing the peak effects of sedation/analgesia to coincide with peaks in surgical stimulation. (a) Insufficient sedation/ analgesia delivered for two episodes (*) of peak surgical stimulus, with the rest of the procedure adequately covered. (b) Sufficient titration of sedation/analgesia delivered for the start of the procedure, but not sufficient for the following peak (*) of surgical stimulation. (c) Sufficient titration of sedation/analgesia throughout the procedure.

that practitioners delivering the sedation should be appropriately trained, meet an accepted standard, and be objectively assessed. Anaesthesia-led training courses have now been developed for non-anaesthetists.

In the past, anaesthesia societies discouraged the non-anaesthetist use of sedative agents that have the potential to produce general anaesthesia, potentially denying patients a safe and effective drug when used appropriately. However, this has not stopped other specialties building up vast experience with propofol—for example, US gastroenterologists conduct >14,000,000 endoscopies annually, many of which require sedation.[32] An Australian study of 28,000 cases reported the incidence of adverse events during procedural sedation for endoscopy delivered by non-anaesthetists to be similar to the rate when sedation was delivered by anaesthetists.[33] It remains the interest, duty, and skillset of anaesthetists to help develop and set standards for all practitioners of sedation, in order to meet the increasing demand, and to ensure patient safety. In the UK, oromaxillofacial surgery procedures that do not require a general anaesthetic, but necessitate sedation, are attended by an anaesthetist. Conversely, in the US, surgeons and dentists are more often involved in the sedation and anaesthesia of their patients. In the UK, dental chair anaesthesia (delivered by a dentist) has not been permitted since 2001, following a series of fatal incidents. Dental chair sedation in community dental practice is, however, delivered by dentists in the UK—usually with N_2O or midazolam. A survey across six acute

National Health Service hospitals demonstrated the heterogeneity of sedation practice in the UK, with ten different agents in use (including opioids). The survey revealed 360 episodes of procedural sedation across all specialties over 2 days, with 71% being conducted by non-anaesthetists (only three episodes involved oromaxillofacial procedures). The total number of procedures performed under sedation in the UK remains unknown, and the incidence of adverse events is also unknown. This study was a proof-of-concept study that will hopefully lead on to a nationwide collaborative to help determine the total number of sedation episodes and the incidence of adverse events in order to help promote safety.[34]

Preoperative assessment and preparation

Preoperative assessment for sedation should be as thorough as it would be for a general anaesthetic, irrespective of the type of sedation and procedure that is being scheduled. Only by gaining vital information from the patient can one propose a safe and appropriate plan for sedation. A systemic enquiry with the main focus on cardiorespiratory and airway assessment informs the clinician, and helps determine the patient's physiological/cardiorespiratory reserve and their ASA classification. Other medical specialists should be consulted for advice on patient optimization, as indicated.

The airway assessment is crucial, given that oromaxillofacial procedures inevitably require a shared approach to airway management. The shared airway limits access and there is a risk of soiling with debris and irrigation fluid. The clinician must consider the following: will they be able to ventilate the patient? How will the procedure restrict them from performing airway rescue manoeuvres? And, what airway equipment might be needed in an emergency?

Discussion with the patient should include information on the procedure, the type and depth of intended sedation, the risks and benefits, and the alternative options. Only then can informed consent be obtained. Patients' concerns and expectations should be sought and addressed, indicating whether any psychological preparation or behavioural techniques can be employed to smooth each patient's journey. Total lack of awareness under sedation should not be guaranteed, as patients may well be aware of things going on around them at certain points during the procedure. Some drugs cause amnesia (particularly midazolam), which should be communicated to the patient. Amnesia may or may not be desirable for some patients. Some will find memory loss disconcerting and disorientating, whereas others will be glad to have no recollection of a potentially unpleasant experience.

Fasting prior to sedation remains relatively contentious, but in view of the potential risk of life-threatening pulmonary aspiration, it is generally safer to err on the side of caution. The risk of aspiration during sedation may well be lower than for general anaesthesia—there is less exposure to emetogenic drugs (especially volatile agents), and the target sedation level is usually moderate, such that airway reflexes are largely preserved. For simplicity and safety, adopting the same fasting regimen as for general anaesthesia is recommended for all elective procedures requiring sedation.[25,35–37] Exceptions might be made in the emergency department for very minor procedures, and when only minimal sedation is intended.[3] Those decisions should be justifiable, and determined on an individual patient basis.

Monitoring

The Association of Anaesthetists established recommendations for standards of monitoring during anaesthesia and recovery (updated in 2021), and these monitoring modalities (non-invasive blood pressure, electrocardiography, pulse oximetry, and capnography) can be considered the same minimal monitoring standards that should be employed for procedural sedation—in addition to assessing the level of sedation. Monitors are not surrogates for vigilance or situational awareness, and their output must be observed and acted upon. Monitor alarms should be set to appropriate ranges and should be easily audible.

Level of sedation

Although the ASA's continuum of sedation helps define the level of sedation,[1] it does not necessarily help the clinician assess the patient's level of sedation during a procedure. Evoking a response with verbal or tactile stimulation may interrupt the procedure as the patient rouses. Obviously, to prevent or manage adverse events it may be necessary to halt surgery from time to time, and this will no doubt be reflected in the surgeon's satisfaction with the sedation technique. The OAA/S scale, Ramsay Sedation Scale, and their modified derivatives can also be used to clinically assess the patient periodically throughout the procedure. Alternative options include the use of processed EEG (pEEG) monitoring, such as BIS™ or SedLine® (Masimo Corporation, Irvine, CA, USA), though in practice these devices are not routinely used for procedural sedation. The index values lack discrimination, and studies have shown poor correlation between sedation states based on pEEG values and clinical scoring systems.[38] The Anesthesia Responsiveness Monitor (ARM; Scott Laboratories Inc., Lubbock, TX, USA) is a device that can be used to objectively measure the patient's level of sedation, based on the reaction times of the patient to instruction (to push a button on a handset). Failure to respond correlates with a sedation level deeper than moderate. Integration into a closed-loop sedation delivery device has been achieved with the ARM.

Adequacy of respiration

The monitoring modalities of pulse oximetry and capnography are invaluable tools, but respiratory pattern and rate, sound of breathing, magnitude of chest excursion, and skin colour are all vital clinical signs that should also be observed—though clinical observation without monitors is insufficient and unreliable.

There are a number of devices on the market specifically designed to measure expired carbon dioxide during sedation, and some that can be adapted from common equipment supplies. The capnogram trace or graphic display must be interpreted carefully, as it will not exactly resemble that of a patient whose trachea has been intubated. It is also sensitive to the flow rate of oxygen being administered and whether the patient is breathing through their nose or their mouth. Nevertheless, despite a poor trace, capnography has been shown to detect many more episodes of apnoea than pulse oximetry alone. The recently developed Rainbow Acoustic Monitor® (Masimo Corporation, Irvine, CA, USA) uses a non-invasive skin transducer applied to the neck which measures turbulent airflow in the larynx in order to detect respiratory rate and apnoea—though the studies to prove its effect remain in their infancy.

Adequacy of circulation

Haemodynamic changes can be expected with deeper levels of sedation, especially in the elderly, and in patients with multiple comorbidities or dehydration. Continuous electrocardiography and non-invasive blood pressure measurement (set to cycle regularly) are therefore essential components of the minimum standards of monitoring for sedation.

Equipment availability

Essential equipment for the safe practice of sedation includes:

- Oxygen supply and delivery devices.
- Emergency drugs (including appropriate antagonists).
- Emergency rescue equipment (airway equipment, means of delivering positive pressure ventilation).
- Emergency alarm (or established means of getting help in an emergency).

Supplemental oxygen is advocated for any sedation depth exceeding minimal sedation. This can be provided by simple nasal cannulae, with a comfortable flow rate of 2–4 L/min (rates higher than this tend to be poorly tolerated by patients due to the drying effect of the gas). The use of Optiflow™ (Fisher & Paykel Healthcare, Auckland, New Zealand) could be considered in moderate or deep sedation, particularly if there are concerns about ventilatory insufficiency due to unfavourable body habitus or extensive comorbidities. This device provides high-flow humidified nasal oxygen (HFNO) at flow rates up to 70 L/min. The high flows produce continuous positive airway pressure that helps splint the airways open, and also aids ventilation by gaseous exchange through flow-dependent dead space flushing during spontaneous breathing or apnoea.[39] In practice, HFNO is not always compatible with oromaxillofacial procedures, but it has been used successfully in dental surgery. Newer models (AIRVO™ 2, Fisher & Paykel Healthcare, Auckland, New Zealand) allow the user to set the flow rate (10–60 L/min), temperature (31–37°C), and oxygen concentration (21–100%), whereas the earlier models only allow adjustment of the flow rate (0–70 L/min) with a fixed concentration (100%) of oxygen. On account of the high flow rates, consideration must be given to the availability and size of the oxygen cylinder (unless piped wall oxygen is used). Crucially, a patent airway must be maintained to benefit from HFNO, so if a jaw thrust or other airway manoeuvre is required to manage upper airway obstruction, the patient is probably over-sedated. It should also be noted that standard capnography is not feasible when HFNO is utilized, due to the high gas flows. In one study of apnoeic patients with flow rates of 70 L/min, the rate of rise of carbon dioxide was 0.15 kPa/min, and the mean $PaCO_2$ was 7.8 kPa after 14 minutes[39]—thus, in the spontaneously breathing moderately sedated patient, the rate of rise of carbon dioxide should therefore be considerably less than 0.15 kPa/min.

Training and personnel

The ability to provide safe procedural sedation need not be defined by specialty training alone, but rather by the practitioner having the requisite knowledge, skills, and competencies to manage sedation for individual patients and procedures. As discussed earlier, this must include being able to rescue the patient from a deeper-than-intended level of sedation. A minimum of two trained professionals must be present during any procedure performed under sedation, so that one person's sole responsibility is to monitor the condition of the patient at all times throughout the procedure, while the other performs the procedure itself.

Recovery and discharge

Close monitoring and observation of the patient post procedure must be continued for at least 1 hour afterwards, in an appropriately equipped recovery facility, staffed with trained recovery personnel. Vital signs should return to their normal baseline values. Importantly, the patient should return to their baseline level of consciousness, and there must be no risk of further reduction in consciousness. Any pain, or nausea and vomiting, must be adequately controlled. In the day case setting, the patient (and/or carer) should be given information on any potential problems to look out for, and how to contact help following discharge.

Conclusion

All sedative agents deserve respect, given their capacity to cause harm through misuse. Inadequate preoperative assessment or failure to monitor the patient's condition adequately can lead to serious harm. Knowledge of each drug's time to onset of action, peak effect, and duration of action is essential in delivering sedation safely. The simplest regimen is often the safest. The heterogeneity among international guidelines governing sedation and local hospital practices is a cause for major concern. Greater safety in sedation can be achieved with better training for all sedation providers, and by application of agreed guidelines. Future agents and devices will hopefully confer a safety advantage, but better application of existing knowledge and skills would confer an enormous safety benefit.

REFERENCES

1. American Society of Anesthesiologists. Continuum of depth of sedation: definition of general anesthesia and levels of sedation/analgesia. 13 October 1999. Last amended 23 October 2019. https://www.asahq.org/standards-and-guidelines/continuum-of-depth-of-sedation-definition-of-general-anesthesia-and-levels-of-sedationanalgesia
2. Cote CJ. 'Conscious sedation': time for this oxymoron to go away! *J Pediatr.* 2001;**139**(1):15–17.
3. Sury M, Bullock I, Rabar S, DeMott KJB. Sedation for diagnostic and therapeutic procedures in children and young people: summary of NICE guidance. *BMJ.* 2010;**341**:c6819.
4. Cravero JP, Beach ML, Blike GT, Gallagher SM, Hertzog JH. The incidence and nature of adverse events during pediatric sedation/anesthesia with propofol for procedures outside the operating room: a report from the Pediatric Sedation Research Consortium. *Anesth Anal.* 2009;**108**(3):795–804.
5. Sulton C, McCracken C, Simon HK, Hebbar K, Reynolds J, Cravero J, et al. Pediatric procedural sedation using dexmedetomidine: a report from the Pediatric Sedation Research Consortium. *Hosp Pediatr.* 2016;**6**(9):536–544.
6. Mason K, Green SM, Piacevoli Q; International Sedation Task Force. Adverse event reporting tool to standardize the reporting and tracking of adverse events during procedural sedation: a consensus document from the World SIVA International Sedation Task Force. *Br J Anaesth.* 2012;**108**(1):13–20.
7. Roback MG, Green SM, Andolfatto G, Leroy PL, Mason KP. Tracking and Reporting Outcomes Of Procedural Sedation (TROOPS): standardized quality improvement and research tools from the International Committee for the Advancement of Procedural Sedation. *Br J Anaesth.* 2018;**120**(1):164–172.
8. Kain ZN, Caldwell-Andrews AA, Krivutza DM, Weinberg ME, Wang SM, Gaal D. Trends in the practice of parental presence during induction of anesthesia and the use of preoperative sedative premedication in the United States, 1995–2002: results of a follow-up national survey. *Anesth Anal.* 2004;**98**(5):1252–1259.
9. Kain ZN, Hofstadter MB, Mayes LC, Krivutza DM, Alexander G, Wang SM, et al. Midazolam: effects on amnesia and anxiety in children. *Anesthesiology.* 2000;**93**(3):676–684.
10. Polster MR, McCarthy RA, O'Sullivan G, Gray PA, Park GR. Midazolam-induced amnesia: implications for the implicit/explicit memory distinction. *Brain Cogn.* 1993;**22**(2):244–265.
11. Stewart SH, Buffett-Jerrott SE, Finley GA, Wright KD, Valois Gomez T. Effects of midazolam on explicit vs implicit memory in a pediatric surgery setting. *Psychopharmacol (Berl).* 2006;**188**(4):489–497.
12. Chen E, Zeltzer LK, Craske MG, Katz ER. Children's memories for painful cancer treatment procedures: implications for distress. *Child Dev.* 2000;**71**(1):933–947.
13. Electronic Medicines Compendium. Midazolam. 2019. https://www.medicines.org.uk/
14. Agarwal A, Sinha PK, Pandey CM, Gaur A, Pandey CK, Kaushik S. Effect of a subanesthetic dose of intravenous ketamine and/or local anesthetic infiltration on hemodynamic responses to skull-pin placement: a prospective, placebo-controlled, randomized, double-blind study. *J Neurosurg Anesthesiol.* 2001;**13**(3):189–194.
15. Langston WT, Wathen JE, Roback MG, Bajaj L. Effect of ondansetron on the incidence of vomiting associated with ketamine sedation in children: a double-blind, randomized, placebo-controlled trial. *Ann Emerg Med.* 2008;**52**(1):30–34.
16. Cheung CW, Ng KF, Liu J, Yuen MY, Ho MH, Irwin MG. Analgesic and sedative effects of intranasal dexmedetomidine in third molar surgery under local anaesthesia. *Br J Anaesth.* 2011;**107**(3):430–437.
17. Cheung CW, Ying CL, Chiu WK, Wong GT, Ng KF, Irwin MG. A comparison of dexmedetomidine and midazolam for sedation in third molar surgery. *Anaesthesia.* 2007;**62**(11):1132–1138.
18. Yuen VM, Hui TW, Irwin MG, Yuen MK. A comparison of intranasal dexmedetomidine and oral midazolam for premedication in pediatric anesthesia: a double-blinded randomized controlled trial. *Anesth Anal.* 2008;**106**(6):1715–1721.
19. Hallonsten AL, Koch G, Schröder U. Nitrous oxide-oxygen sedation in dental care. *Community Dent Oral Epidemiol.* 1983;**11**(6):347–355.
20. Faulks D, Hennequin M, Albecker-Grappe S, Manière MC, Tardieu C, Berthet A, et al. Sedation with 50% nitrous oxide/oxygen for outpatient dental treatment in individuals with intellectual disability. *Dev Med Child Neurol.* 2007;**49**(8):621–625.

21. Zier JL, Liu M. Safety of high-concentration nitrous oxide by nasal mask for pediatric procedural sedation: experience with 7802 cases. *Pediatr Emerg Care*. 2011;**27**(12):1107–1112.

22. Burnweit C, Diana-Zerpa JA, Nahmad MH, Lankau CA, Weinberger M, Malvezzi L, et al. Nitrous oxide analgesia for minor pediatric surgical procedures: an effective alternative to conscious sedation? *J Pediatr Surg*. 2004;**39**(3):495–499.

23. Seith RW, Theophilos T, Babl FE. Intranasal fentanyl and high-concentration inhaled nitrous oxide for procedural sedation: a prospective observational pilot study of adverse events and depth of sedation. *Acad Emerg Med*. 2012;**19**(1):31–36.

24. Tobias JD. Dexmedetomidine and ketamine: an effective alternative for procedural sedation? *Pediatr Crit Care Med*. 2012;**13**(4):423–427.

25. Dental Faculties of the Royal Colleges of Surgeons and the Royal College of Anaesthetists. Standards for conscious sedation in the provision of dental care: report of the Intercollegiate Advisory Committee for Sedation in Dentistry. 2015. https://www.rcseng.ac.uk/dental-faculties/fds/publications-guidelines/standards-for-conscious-sedation-in-the-provision-of-dental-care-and-accreditation/

26. Babenco HD, Conard PF, Gross JB. The pharmacodynamic effect of a remifentanil bolus on ventilatory control. *Anesthesiology*. 2000;**92**(2):393–398.

27. Barker N, Lim J, Amari E, Malherbe S, Ansermino JM. Relationship between age and spontaneous ventilation during intravenous anesthesia in children. *Pediatr Anesth*. 2007;**17**(10):948–955.

28. Hinkelbein J, Lamperti M, Akeson J, Santos J, Costa J, De Robertis E, et al. European Society of Anaesthesiology and European Board of Anaesthesiology guidelines for procedural sedation and analgesia in adults. *Eur J Anaesthesiol*. 2018;**35**(1):6–24.

29. Ng J-M, Kong C-F, Nyam D. Patient-controlled sedation with propofol for colonoscopy. *Gastrointest Endosc*. 2001;**54**(1):8–13.

30. Liu Y, Li M, Yang D, Zhang X, Wu A, Yao S, et al. Closed-loop control better than open-loop control of profofol TCI guided by BIS: a randomized, controlled, multicenter clinical trial to evaluate the CONCERT-CL closed-loop system. *PLoS One*. 2015;**10**(4):e0123862.

31. Adewumi A, Kays DW. Stainless steel crown aspiration during sedation in pediatric dentistry. *J Pediatr Dent*. 2008;**30**(1):59–62.

32. Seeff LC, Richards TB, Shapiro JA, Nadel MR, Manninen DL, Given LS, et al. How many endoscopies are performed for colorectal cancer screening? Results from CDC's survey of endoscopic capacity. *Gastroenterology*. 2004;**127**(6):1670–1677.

33. Clarke AC, Chiragakis L, Hillman LC, Kaye GL. Sedation for endoscopy: the safe use of propofol by general practitioner sedationists. *Med J Aust*. 2002;**176**(4):159–161.

34. South West Anaesthetic Research Matrix (SWARM). Sedation practice in six acute hospitals—a snapshot survey. *Anaesthesia*. 2015;**70**(4):407–415.

35. Sury M, Bullock I, Rabar S, DeMott KJB. Sedation for diagnostic and therapeutic procedures in children and young people: summary of NICE guidance. *BMJ*. 2010;**341**:c6819.

36. Disma N, Thomas M, Afshari A, Veyckemans F, De Hert S. Clear fluids fasting for elective paediatric anaesthesia: the European Society of Anaesthesiology consensus statement. *Eur J Anaesthesiol*. 2019;**36**(3):173–174.

37. Practice guidelines for moderate procedural sedation and analgesia 2018: a report by the American Society of Anesthesiologists Task Force on Moderate Procedural Sedation and Analgesia, the American Association of Oral and Maxillofacial Surgeons, American College of Radiology, American Dental Association, American Society of Dentist Anesthesiologists, and Society of Interventional Radiology. *Anesthesiology*. 2018;**128**(3):437–479.

38. Sheahan C, Mathews D. Monitoring and delivery of sedation. *Br J Anaesth*. 2014;**113** Suppl 2:ii37–ii47.

39. Patel A, Nouraei S. Transnasal humidified rapid-insufflation ventilatory exchange (THRIVE): a physiological method of increasing apnoea time in patients with difficult airways. *Anaesthesia*. 2015;**70**(3):323–329.

7

Hypotensive anaesthesia

Kimberley Hodge, Patrick A. Ward, and Michael G. Irwin

Introduction

The intentional lowering of a patient's blood pressure under anaesthesia is a technique known as 'hypotensive anaesthesia', or controlled or deliberate hypotension. It can be utilized for:

- Improving visualization of the surgical field and surgical accuracy (better identification of pathological tissue, enabling greater precision of tumour or infective foci excision).
- Reducing blood loss and blood transfusion requirements.
- Decreasing surgical time (reducing the negative sequelae associated with prolonged procedures).
- Reducing reactionary bleeding, postoperative bleeding and haematoma formation.

Lowering the systemic blood pressure may cause organ ischaemia if there is inadequate blood flow, therefore deliberate hypotension should only be employed when absolutely necessary, for the minimum duration possible, and appropriate patient selection is crucial.

Background

Despite the concept of deliberate hypotension for surgery being proposed by Cushing in 1917,[1] the first documented use of the technique was in the 1940s. Benign olfactory groove meningiomas were noted to be difficult to resect due to the tumours' relative inaccessibility and high vascularity, with blood vessels located within the base of the skull, inferior to the tumour. It was observed by Gardner that during the first hour or so of the procedure, resection was painstakingly tedious and taxing. Once the patient had lost a substantial amount of blood and became hypotensive, the surgery became much easier, and faster to complete. He hypothesized that preoperative bloodletting via arteriotomy may be of use, optimizing surgical conditions at the onset of the operation, rather than waiting for haemorrhage to result in hypotension.[2] As the physiological response to bloodletting involves profound vasoconstriction, a brachial plexus block was performed first to prevent radial artery constriction, and the blood was then returned to the patient postoperatively.[3] Bloodletting was abandoned shortly afterwards when the patients were

noted to suffer from complications such as hypoxaemia, acidosis, irreversible shock, and excessive heparinization.[1]

During a similar epoch, total spinal anaesthesia, with resultant peripheral vasodilatation (and redistribution of blood volume), was also utilized to reduce blood loss in the operative field.[3] This technique was abandoned after a brief period, with the introduction of newer pharmacological agents (halothane, nitrous oxide, and vasodilatory drugs). The profound hypotensive effects of halothane were difficult to reverse quickly and so safer, more titratable alternatives were sought. Sodium nitroprusside and glyceryl trinitrate were found to be effective and remained the most popular pharmacological choices for many years.

Physiology

Autoregulation

Blood pressure varies naturally throughout the day and it is essential that flow to an organ is maintained despite these pressure fluctuations. The intrinsic ability of an organ (independent of neuronal or humoral control) to maintain flow despite changes in perfusion pressure is known as autoregulation. There is a window within which autoregulatory mechanisms operate effectively, thought to exist within a mean arterial pressure (MAP) range of 50–150 mmHg, but there is a huge degree of individual variability (affected by age, sex, and pre-existing disease such as hypertension, wherein the MAP will be higher). The efficacy of autoregulation depends upon the specific organ—the heart, brain, spinal cord, and kidneys are particularly proficient autoregulators, whereas skeletal muscle circulations are moderately effective, and cutaneous and splanchnic circulations have barely any autoregulatory capacity.[4] There are two main intrinsic autoregulatory mechanisms:

- *Myogenic autoregulation*: as arteriolar pressure increases, it causes more stretch within the vascular wall. A compensatory contraction occurs, which increases vascular resistance and produces a localized reduction in blood flow.
- *Metabolic autoregulation*: increased metabolic activity leads to an increased release of vasodilatory mediators such as adenosine,

nitric oxide, and hydrogen ions. This causes local arteriolar vaso-dilatation and therefore increased flow.[5]

Blood pressure regulation is complex and depends upon factors such as cardiac output, peripheral resistance, renal function, venous return, and blood volume.[6] Autoregulatory mechanisms are ineffective at low blood pressures (such as those that may be obtained under hypotensive anaesthesia) which may result in myocardial and cerebral ischaemia, renal injury, or death. When operating at blood pressures outside of those controlled by autoregulatory mechanisms, flow is dependent solely upon the perfusion pressure. If a patient is undergoing hypotensive anaesthesia, with the MAP outside the autoregulatory range, then flow may be insufficient for adequate organ perfusion. Currently, it is not possible to predict an individual patient's unique autoregulatory range, so it is better to err on the side of caution.

It is known that organ injury severity depends upon both the magnitude of perioperative hypotension and its duration.[7] While there is no conclusive evidence of an absolute systolic blood pressure value below which the risks become unacceptably high, there is evidence that <80 mmHg for >10 minutes puts the patient at increased risk of organ injury.[8] This threshold value will be higher in those with pre-existing cardiovascular disease. Recent observational studies suggest that MAP <55–65 mmHg for a prolonged period is particularly dangerous. The deeper and longer the patient's exposure to hypotension, the risk of myocardial injury after non-cardiac surgery and acute kidney injury increases exponentially.[9,10]

Indications

Potential benefits of hypotensive anaesthesia such as optimization of the surgical field, reduction in allogeneic transfusion requirements, and a possible reduction in operating time must be carefully weighed against the above-mentioned potentially devastating complications. Better knowledge of these adverse effects has made it harder to justify induction of significant hypotension in oromaxillofacial surgery, although bleeding in certain procedures can be challenging to control. This is not only related to high vascularity, but because bleeding points tend to be from intrabony capillaries which are more difficult to stop surgically than from more accessible bleeding sites.[11] The Le Fort I maxillary osteotomy, in particular, exemplifies these issues. Bleeding occurs when osteotomy cuts are made in the maxilla, and when the maxilla is down-fractured as this is especially stimulating. Bleeding cannot be controlled surgically until the down-fracture is completed. If systemic blood pressure is not reduced, significant bleeding can occur from branches of the maxillary artery, pterygoid, and greater palatine veins.

There is no consensus as to what degree of hypotension constitutes hypotensive anaesthesia. Definitions include reducing the systolic blood pressure to 80–90 mmHg, the MAP to 50–65 mmHg, or a 30% reduction in baseline MAP.[12]

Contraindications

Hypotensive anaesthesia, while providing potential benefit surgically, is most commonly a *non-essential* technique which does have the potential to cause serious harm to the patient. It is critical, therefore, that the patient undergoes a thorough preoperative physiological assessment to determine applicability and risk of complications. This is even more pertinent when faced with the older patient and those with comorbidities.

Relative contraindications include:

- Coronary and carotid atherosclerosis.
- Hypovolaemia.
- Renal impairment.
- Uncontrolled hypertension.
- Hepatic impairment.
- Severe anaemia and haemoglobinopathies (while there is little evidence for what constitutes a 'safe' haemoglobin to perform hypotensive anaesthesia, it would be prudent for the patient to have a haemoglobin concentration of at least 90 g/L, and higher than this if they have comorbidities).

Historically, it was felt that the risk of harm with hypotensive anaesthetic techniques, while possible, was slight. However, there is now a considerable body of research evidence which demonstrates more clearly that this is simply not the case. It is now apparent that hypotension during anaesthesia can detrimentally affect patients' postoperative outcome, so it follows that deliberate hypotensive anaesthesia must be used sparingly. Wesselink et al undertook a systematic review examining adverse postoperative outcomes after non-cardiac surgery in patients who had experienced unintended hypotension under anaesthesia—even if this was for a short duration (<1 minute).[8] As the authors themselves attested, there were several limitations in the review: the studies included disparate population groups, there was no consensus on how to determine the blood pressure value that constituted hypotension, and there were inconsistent definitions of what represented an adverse postoperative outcome. Nevertheless, they concluded that a MAP <80 mmHg for ≥10 minutes could result in organ injury. Potential organ dysfunction included acute kidney injury, myocardial injury or infarction, stroke, and delirium. The Perioperative Quality Initiative, in 2019, released a consensus statement about perioperative hypotension in adults. The key message when considering hypotensive anaesthesia was as follows: 'Intraoperative mean arterial blood pressures below 60–70 mmHg are associated with myocardial injury, acute kidney injury, and death. Systolic arterial pressures below 100 mmHg are associated with myocardial injury and death. Injury is a function of hypotension severity and duration.'[7] This statement has important clinical and medicolegal implications.

Deliberate or controlled hypotension implies that a lowering of the blood pressure is the only haemodynamic parameter being manipulated, with all other variables remaining constant. This, of course, is not the case. All the pharmacological agents and all the non-pharmacological methods, which will be discussed in detail later (controlled ventilation, positive end expiratory pressure, head-up tilt, etc.), have other physiological effects aside from lowering systemic blood pressure—many of which are difficult or impossible to directly measure. Systemic blood pressure is readily measurable (invasively or non-invasively), and, therefore, remains the principal monitoring tool (and target for adjustment), but it must be remembered that this does not fully reflect the myriad of other physiological changes and effects that may be occurring in various organ systems.

It is also worth noting that while the evidence supporting maintenance of 'normotension' in anaesthetic literature is ever increasing, there is relatively little published evidence supporting the technique of deliberate hypotension in the surgical literature (most publications advocating the technique are from anaesthetic journals). One might expect more vociferous support from surgeons for a technique specifically intended to improve *surgical* operating conditions and outcome. In many cases, surgeons may feel that there is not the necessity for deliberate hypotension. In other cases, rather than hypotensive anaesthesia, avoiding uncontrolled *hypertension* during critical phases of surgery may be more in accordance with their requirements.

Conduct of deliberate hypotensive anaesthesia

The practice of hypotensive anaesthesia should never be considered routine. The decision to employ such a technique must be discussed between the anaesthetist and surgeon preoperatively for every individual patient, and it must be their shared opinion that the patient will derive significant benefit to warrant the technique for that particular operation. The surgeon must be sufficiently experienced to take advantage of the improved operating conditions, the anaesthetist should be familiar with the technique, and all parties, including the patient, should be fully aware of the safety issues. The ultimate decision for the appropriateness of the technique lies with the anaesthetist, although mutual appreciation of each other's roles and priorities should engender collaborative decision-making. This cooperation and understanding is also necessary when the technique must be abandoned if there is evidence of compromised organ perfusion (e.g. electrocardiogram changes). In order to deliver hypotensive anaesthesia as safely and effectively as possible, there are several concepts to contemplate and some general principles that should be followed:

Firstly, the question of what constitutes a safe level of blood pressure must be considered. Aside from stating that the blood pressure must be sufficient to maintain organ perfusion (without being able to actually determine this), and understanding the pathophysiological changes that occur in different organ systems at low perfusion pressures (as described earlier), it is important to acknowledge that there is no fixed blood pressure value that can be considered safe for all patients—thus, every patient must be treated individually. The technique should only be considered for procedures where the potential benefits are most apparent—for example, maxillary osteotomy or temporomandibular joint replacement, where blood loss can be substantial and may significantly impair the operative field. Awareness of the patient's age, pre-existing comorbidities (especially coronary, renal, and cerebrovascular), and their preoperative 'normal' blood pressure is important. There remains considerable debate as to how this baseline blood pressure should be determined—whether this should occur in the community over a defined period of time, at the preoperative assessment clinic, preoperatively on the ward, or immediately prior to induction of anaesthesia, and how many measurements are necessary to determine a baseline value with any degree of reliability are contentious issues. Patients with ischaemic heart disease, cerebrovascular disease, hypertension, renal dysfunction, or diabetes are generally considered not suitable for hypotensive anaesthesia, although a modest reduction in blood pressure is likely to be safe.

Secondly, the question of what level of hypotension is necessary to control bleeding must be considered. Very commonly, an insignificant or ineffective reduction in systemic blood pressure is described as hypotensive anaesthesia, without causing any noticeable effects on capillary or arteriolar bleeding. The surgeon has an unrivalled view of the operative field, and can detect changes in blood pressure before it is reflected by the intermittent non-invasive reading, so they must provide constant feedback to assist the anaesthetist in achieving a clinically meaningful effect from blood pressure reduction (within predefined safe limits). Given the associated potential morbidity already discussed, only a *moderate* degree of *controlled* hypotension can be advocated, and this should be restricted to discreet periods of maximal blood loss and surgical stimulus only. Thus, the surgeon must also give sufficient warning prior to undertaking stages of the surgical procedure associated with high bleeding risk (e.g. maxillary down-fracture).

Careful patient monitoring is critical. Electrocardiography, with ST-segment analysis, is mandatory, and arterial blood pressure monitoring should be considered—this not only can facilitate immediate titration of blood pressure but can also enable arterial blood gas monitoring to track lactate and base excess levels, as surrogates of end-organ perfusion. Temperature monitoring is important as vasodilator hypotensive agents will facilitate greater intraoperative heat loss. Fluid balance and blood loss must be carefully monitored, as many of the drugs utilized for hypotensive anaesthesia will impair the normal physiological responses to bleeding. Meticulous care should be taken with patient positioning, as pressure areas are at particular risk during hypotensive anaesthesia. This includes the positioning of temperature probes, oxygen saturation probes and, in particular, the passive positioning of the nasotracheal tube at the nares (high risk for tissue necrosis).

It is crucial that hypotensive anaesthesia is discontinued well before completion of surgery, otherwise haemostasis cannot be reliably achieved. The surgeon must also be fastidious with coagulating any bleeding points prior to wound closure, as what may appear as just capillary ooze during a period of hypotensive anaesthesia may in fact represent bleeding from a larger blood vessel, that may bleed significantly on restoration of normotension.

Finally, when undertaking anaesthesia where deliberate hypotension is planned, anaesthetists should specifically inform patients preoperatively. Patients should be made aware of the indications, potential risks, benefits, and alternatives in accordance with the 2015 Montgomery Ruling, given that a reasonable patient is likely to attach material significance to the risks associated with the technique.

Pharmacological techniques for hypotensive anaesthesia

There are a number of drugs that can be utilized to induce hypotension. Historically, sodium nitroprusside, glyceryl trinitrate, and beta- and alpha-blockers were the preferred agents but newer agents may confer greater ease of delivery and a more favourable side effect profile.

Beta-blockers

Beta-adrenergic blocking agents lower blood pressure through negative inotropic and chronotropic actions. There are three beta receptors—β_1, β_2, and β_3. β_1 receptors are found in the heart and kidneys, β_2 in vascular smooth muscle, skeletal muscle, and the lungs, whereas β_3 are in adipose tissue. This is relevant when considering which beta-blocker to select to deliver hypotensive anaesthesia.

Labetalol is a non-selective beta-blocker, which also selectively antagonizes α_1-adrenergic receptors, with the beta-blocking effects being seven times more pronounced than the effects on α_1-adrenergic receptors. The α_1-adrenoreceptor antagonism leads to vasodilatation and decreased vascular resistance. It is inexpensive and can be administered as an intravenous bolus or infusion, up to approximately 160 mg/hr. Time of onset of activity varies between 5 and 30 minutes, effects can be unpredictable, and its mean duration of action of 50 minutes can make titration difficult. It has a slower onset and longer duration of action than other intravenous beta-blockers. Side effects include bronchoconstriction and heart failure in high doses.

Esmolol is reasonably cardioselective for β_1 receptors, has a quick onset of action (approximately 1 minute), and is metabolized by plasma esterases so has a short duration of action (approximately 10 minutes) making it easy to titrate. It is more expensive than labetalol and requires a syringe driver for administration (infusion rates between 50 and 200 mcg/kg/min). A risk of bronchoconstriction only occurs at high doses.

Dexmedetomidine

Dexmedetomidine is a potent centrally acting, highly selective α_2-adrenoceptor agonist which has sedative, analgesic, and anxiolytic properties. While not commonly used in the UK (due to its expense and lack of availability), it has been widely adopted throughout the rest of Europe, Asia, and the US, particularly in the critical care setting as a second-line sedative agent. It is typically administered with a 1 mcg/kg loading dose, and then infused at a rate of 0.2–0.7 mcg/kg/hr. The reduction in sympathetic activity may confer improved surgical field conditions when compared with agents such as sodium nitroprusside.[13] Its sedative and analgesic properties allow a reduction in co-administered anaesthetic agents (by 20–50%) and opioids, and it can facilitate a smooth tracheal extubation and emergence without respiratory depression—of particular benefit in the oromaxillofacial surgical patient. There is, however, the potential for patients to also be unduly sedated at emergence and the infusion should be stopped 30–60 minutes before emergence when patients have a difficult airway.

Magnesium

Magnesium is an incredibly versatile ion, impacting many physiological systems. It has direct effects upon the myocardium and vascular smooth muscle, directly blocks catecholamine receptors, and inhibits catecholamine release from the adrenal medulla among many other effects.[14] When utilized for the purposes of hypotensive anaesthesia, a bolus of approximately 40 mg/kg is administered, followed by a continuous infusion of 15 mg/kg/hr.[15] Onset of action can be slow, and the effects can be difficult to titrate; however, it provides the additional benefits of being a reliable analgesic (N-methyl-D-aspartate (NMDA) antagonism), reducing anaesthetic requirements and reducing postoperative nausea and vomiting and shivering. While magnesium is generally safe, hypermagnesaemia can result in complications such as nausea and vomiting, but also potentially life-threatening effects, including cardiorespiratory arrest with very high serum concentrations. Rather more commonly, it potentiates non-depolarizing neuromuscular blocking agents, and quantitative neuromuscular monitoring is important.

Remifentanil

Analgesia for oromaxillofacial surgery presents a unique pharmacological challenge as it needs to be titrated according to rapidly changing surgical stimuli. Remifentanil specifically addresses this issue, being fast acting, potent, and with a short half-life. It is a mu opioid agonist that reaches peak effect within 1–3 minutes,[16] and has a context insensitive half-time of 3–5 minutes as it undergoes rapid ester hydrolysis by non-specific plasma and tissue esterases, making it easy to titrate irrespective of organ function. Remifentanil is generally administered as an intravenous infusion, usually at a rate of 0.1–0.35 mcg/kg/min or 3–7 ng/mL using target-controlled infusion, with a predictable onset and offset. Opioids are not negatively inotropic but can depress the vasomotor centre causing bradycardia and hypotension. High doses can induce chest wall rigidity, tolerance, and (rarely) hyperalgesia. Remifentanil is undoubtedly well suited to oromaxillofacial surgery as a rapidly titratable analgesic, conferring haemodynamic stability despite intense surgical stimulus.

Propofol

Propofol is an easily titrated intravenous anaesthetic agent. It is a phenol derivative metabolized in the liver which is extensively and rapidly redistributed making it suitable for infusion. Propofol can induce hypotension without a compensatory increase in heart rate, by causing vasodilatation and via a negative inotropic effect. However, it is not safe or appropriate to use excessive doses of an anaesthetic agent to induce hypotension.

Inhalational anaesthetic agents

All inhalational agents lower blood pressure in a dose-dependent manner by reducing the systemic vascular resistance (with some additional effects on myocardial contractility and cardiac output with some agents). However, as with propofol, it is not safe or appropriate to use excessive doses of an anaesthetic agent for the purposes of deliberate hypotension and, while commonly used in the past, this cannot be condoned nowadays.

Other pharmacological agents

While the above-discussed drugs are those commonly used in modern anaesthetic practice, there are other agents utilized to induce intraoperative hypotension (Table 7.1), particularly where resources may be scarce.

Other, very rarely used drugs include adenosine, and ganglion-blocking agents such as trimetaphan. Premedication with oral angiotensin-converting enzyme inhibitors has also been tried, but this is unconventional, impractical, and unpredictable.

Table 7.1 Properties of pharmacological agents less commonly used to induce intraoperative hypotension

Drug	Advantage	Disadvantage	Dose
Oral clonidine	Resource sparing Analgesic Opioid sparing	Not easily titratable Postoperative sedation	300 mcg 1.5 hr preoperatively (adults)
Intravenous clonidine	Resource sparing Analgesic Opioid sparing	Less titratable Rebound hypertension Postoperative sedation	3 mcg/kg 30 min preoperatively
Calcium channel antagonists	Titratable, with short half-life Bolus or infusion	Reflex tachycardia	IV nicardipine 1–4 mcg/kg/min
Glyceryl trinitrate infusion	Rapid onset	Not as effective at lowering blood pressure as sodium nitroprusside Tachyphylaxis	10–400 mcg/min
Sodium nitroprusside	Rapid onset Very potent Titratable	Rate-dependent cyanide toxicity Needs protection from sunlight Metabolic acidosis Tachyphylaxis Reflex tachycardia, often requires small dose of beta-blocker Rebound hypertension Requires arterial line and hourly blood gas measurement for cyanide toxicity (acidosis)	0.5–0.6 mcg/kg/min (with normal renal function)

Table 7.2 Non-pharmacological techniques to minimize blood loss

Method	Rationale	Disadvantages
Coagulation optimization	Ensure patient's intrinsic ability to clot is not impaired: • Avoid acidosis • Maintain normothermia • Ensure normocalcaemia • Judicious fluid administration to avoid dilutional coagulopathy	Nil
Haemostatic sealants	Varied modes of action—mechanical, flowable, fibrin/synthetic sealants, and thrombins[17] Useful for difficult-to-access areas	Availability, cost
Harmonic scalpel	Ultrasonic device that coagulates while cutting through tissues. Utilizes the principle of thermal generation	Only coagulates as it cuts
Head-up positioning (reverse Trendelenburg)	Decreases venous congestion by 2 mmHg for each 2.5 cm of vertical height above the heart	Risk of air embolus (especially if hypotensive)
Laser surgery	'Light Amplification by Stimulated Emission of Radiation.' Coagulates blood vessels, sterilizes the target area, and eliminates postoperative sutures	Potential for iatrogenic damage due to lack of tactile feedback
Regional nerve blocks, such as trigeminal	Decreases physiological stress response to surgery	Familiarity with technique is essential as regional blocks for oromaxillofacial surgery are challenging Risk of generic block complications—including local anaesthetic toxicity
Surgical draping	Loosely secure the drapes, to prevent venous congestion if applied too tightly	Nil
Tranexamic acid (intravenous and topical)	Antifibrinolytic agent Consider for all surgeries where blood loss >500 mL	Use intravenously with caution in thromboembolic disease
Transoral robotic surgery	Causes reduction in tissue trauma, and increased surgical accuracy	Familiarity with the equipment is essential; limited to specialist centres. Access to the airway in event of an emergency is severely compromised
Vasoconstrictors (local application)	Dilute adrenaline applied topically or in combination with local anaesthetics	Caution must be taken not to exceed the maximum dose of adrenaline Systemic absorption of adrenaline can precipitate unwanted cardiovascular sequelae in patients with pre-existing cardiac disease, or the associated rise in blood pressure and heart rate can be misinterpreted as a light plane of anaesthesia
Ventilatory strategies	Controlled positive pressure ventilation, maintain normocapnia	If long inspiratory times are used, or excessive positive end-expiratory pressure, intrathoracic pressure may rise impeding venous return

Non-pharmacological techniques to minimize blood loss

While hypotensive anaesthesia is one way to minimize blood loss for oromaxillofacial surgery, there are extremely important techniques that should be used first or in conjunction with these (Table 7.2).

Conclusion

The role of hypotensive anaesthesia in oromaxillofacial surgery is controversial. While effectively delivered hypotension may help improve operative field conditions, minimize blood loss (and transfusion requirements), and reduce operating time, in doing so, perfusion may be compromised to important organ systems, resulting in significant morbidity. The anaesthetist, surgeon, and patient must fully understand the implications. Patient selection is key, along with adequate monitoring and constant vigilance. Hypotensive anaesthesia should never be considered or conducted as routine practice, and the potential risks and benefits specific to each individual patient should be fully contemplated and discussed before employing this technique.

REFERENCES

1. Corber Z, Salem R, Crystal G, Fahmy R. Deliberate hypotension: a historical perspective. In: Proceedings of the 2010 Annual Meeting of the American Society Anesthesiologists, San Diego, 2010. Abstract A568.
2. Gardner WJ. The control of bleeding during operation by induced hypotension. *J Am Med Assoc.* 1946;**132**(10):572–574.
3. Adams AP. Techniques of vascular control for deliberate hypotension during anaesthesia. *Br J Anaesth.* 1975;**47**(7):777–792.
4. Meng L, Wang Y, Zhang L, McDonagh DL. Heterogeneity and variability in pressure autoregulation of organ blood flow: lessons learned over 100+ years. *Crit Care Med.* 2019;**47**(3):436–448.
5. Barrett K, Barman S, Boitano S, Heddwen B. Cardiovascular regulatory mechanisms. In: *Ganong's Review of Medical Physiology*, 23rd ed., p 563. New York: McGraw-Hill; 2010.
6. El-Ghazali SK, Pandit JJ. Pre-incision hypotension and the association with postoperative acute kidney injury—an opportunity to improve peri-operative outcomes? *Anaesthesia.* 2019;**74**(12):1611–1614.
7. Sessler DI, Bloomstone JA, Aronson S, Berry C, Gan TJ, Kellum JA, et al. Perioperative Quality Initiative consensus statement on intraoperative blood pressure, risk and outcomes for elective surgery. *Br J Anaesth.* 2019;**122**(5):563–574.
8. Wesselink EM, Kappen TH, Torn HM, Slooter AJC, van Klei WA. Intraoperative hypotension and the risk of postoperative adverse outcomes: a systematic review. *Br J Anaesth.* 2018;**121**(4):706–721.
9. Salmasi V, Maheshwari K, Yang D, Mascha EJ, Singh A, Sessler DI, et al. Relationship between intraoperative hypotension, defined by either reduction from baseline or absolute thresholds, and acute kidney and myocardial injury after noncardiac surgery. *Anesthesiology.* 2017;**126**(1):47–62.
10. Monk TG, Bronsert MR, Henderson WG, Mangione MP, Sum-Ping ST, Bentt DR, et al. Association between intraoperative hypotension and hypertension and 30-day postoperative mortality in noncardiac surgery. *Anesthesiology.* 2015;**123**(2):307–319.
11. Praveen K, Narayanan V, Muthusekhar MR, Baig MF. Hypotensive anaesthesia and blood loss in orthognathic surgery: a clinical study. *Br J Oral Maxillofac Surg.* 2001;**39**(2):138–140.
12. Degoute C-S. Controlled hypotension. *Drugs.* 2007;**67**(7):1053–1076.
13. El-Kalla RS, El Mourad MB. Deliberate hypotensive anesthesia during maxillofacial surgery: a comparative study between dexmedetomidine and sodium nitroprusside. *Ain-Shams J Anaesthesiol.* 2016;**9**(2):201.
14. Watson VF, Vaughan RS. Magnesium and the anaesthetist. *Cont Educ Anaesth Crit Care Pain.* 2001;**1**(1):16–20.
15. Elsharnouby N, Elsharnouby M. Magnesium sulphate as a technique of hypotensive anaesthesia. *Br J Anaesth.* 2006;**96**(6):727–731.
16. Scarth E, Smith S. Remifentanil. In: *Drugs in Anaesthesia and Intensive Care*, 5th ed., pp. 338–341 Oxford: Oxford University Press; 2016.
17. Forcillo J, Perrault LP. Armentarium of topical hemostatic products in cardiovascular surgery: an update. *Transfus Apher Sci.* 2014;**50**(1):26–31.

8

Dental anaesthesia

Jennifer Gosling and John Myatt

Introduction

Dental anaesthesia is a challenging area of anaesthetic practice. The majority of dental surgery is carried out under local anaesthesia, with or without sedation. Patients who require general anaesthesia to facilitate their dental surgery often have additional requirements, including paediatric or adult patients presenting with learning difficulties, medical comorbidities, or severe anxiety. Operations involve a 'shared airway', and are predominantly day case procedures, with a high turnover of cases. Dental anaesthesia continues to evolve as a subspecialty, with several key developments in recent years.

Background and history

Once delivered mainly in the community, dental anaesthesia is now carried out exclusively in the hospital environment in the UK. These restrictions are intended to improve patient safety.

Dentistry and anaesthesia are inextricably linked, with the first recorded inhalational general anaesthetic using nitrous oxide being undertaken for a dental extraction.[1] After an initial early reliance upon nitrous oxide, different combinations of hypnotics and sedatives were gradually introduced. By the late twentieth century, dental anaesthesia was provided in both community dental surgeries and hospitals. The skills and experience of those providing anaesthesia varied widely and many dentists acted as both operator and anaesthetist. Provision of monitoring and resuscitation equipment was similarly variable, particularly in the community setting. During the 1970s, 1980s, and 1990s, a number of deaths occurred as a result of unsafe anaesthesia or excessive sedation, leading to a series of recommendations for the conduct of dental anaesthesia.[2–4] Since 2002, it has been illegal in England for general anaesthesia to be carried out for dental surgery, unless in a hospital setting, administered by an appropriately trained anaesthetist.[5] Nevertheless, sedation is still permitted in dental surgeries, including inhalational sedation with nitrous oxide, as well as intravenous sedation with benzodiazepines, opioids, and, increasingly, propofol. Multidisciplinary standards inform the administration of sedation for dentistry, as well as the resources and training that underpin its practice.[6,7] Concepts and the practice of sedation are discussed in detail in Chapter 6.

Current activity

Substantial numbers of anaesthetics are given for dental procedures, for a variety of indications, with many patients having repeat attendances. Poor oral health remains a significant public health issue, even in well-developed countries. In 2015–2016, 40% of children in England had no dental check-up despite being entitled to free treatment,[8] and in 2017–2018, dental caries was the most common reason for hospital admission in children aged 5–9 years.[9] Dental decay is associated with significant complications, including periodontitis, abscess formation, and uncommonly systemic sepsis, as well as contributing to poor feeding and weight gain. Data from the Royal College of Anaesthetists fifth National Audit Project reported an annual anaesthetic caseload of 110,600 dental cases[10]; of these, 60% were children (<16 years), 38.5% adults (16–65 years), and 1.5% the elderly (>65 years) with the overwhelming majority of patients undergoing general anaesthesia as a day case procedure.[10] In Wales, 1 in 86 children undergo general anaesthesia for dental work.[11] Of those children presenting for general anaesthesia, approximately 3% will have repeated anaesthetics, a third of whom have learning difficulties or physical comorbidities.[12]

Indications for general anaesthesia for dental surgery include:

- Children.
- Patients with learning difficulties.
- Patients with needle phobia.
- Complex reconstructive procedures.
- Dental extractions to facilitate surgical access for complex oromaxillofacial procedures.

The contribution of anaesthetists in facilitating dental procedures in these patients is now reflected by the specific references to dental anaesthesia in competency-based anaesthetic curricula, with considerable overlap in the training competencies required for sedation, paediatrics, and day surgery.[13,14]

The future

There is a projected decline in the numbers of registered dental practitioners specializing in 'special care dentistry',[15] which may result in increased referrals to secondary care for adult patients with additional needs. There may also be increasing numbers of older patients with cognitive impairment requiring anaesthetic input for dentistry in the future. While some of the patients presenting for dental surgery may have complex needs, syndromes, or difficult airways, by far the majority of dental surgery requiring general anaesthesia will be undertaken electively, such that thorough preoperative assessment, optimization of any medical conditions, and patient consent should all be undertaken during the lead time. Personalized and patient-centred care is paramount in managing these patient groups, particularly given the high number of re-attendances.[11,16]

Preoperative assessment

Patients requiring anaesthesia for dental surgery should receive the same standard of preoperative assessment as other patients, recognizing that the reasons they require general anaesthesia may also make preoperative assessment challenging.[29]

History

Patients may find it difficult to give a comprehensive history, either because of cognitive problems or communication difficulties. Collateral history can be obtained from parents or carers, patient notes, general practitioners (GPs), or community paediatricians. Electronic record-keeping may assist with this, and any previous anaesthetic charts should be reviewed. The reason for referral should be determined, together with the source of the referral. A full anaesthetic history should be taken, including details of comorbidities, previous anaesthetics, allergies, and current medication.

Rare unifying syndromes may be encountered and, if necessary, specific review of the possible complications should be carried out. Many syndromes are well recognized for their association with potentially difficult airway management, including Down syndrome, the Pierre Robin sequence, and Treacher Collins syndrome.

Screening questions should determine the presence and severity of obstructive sleep apnoea syndrome, any cardiac disease, or epilepsy. Timings of any regular medication should be noted, with the plan to maintain the normal regimen as far as possible.

Patients with learning difficulties or mental health issues may be taking psychotropic medications that have the potential to interact with anaesthetic drugs. Noradrenaline selective reuptake inhibitors and monoamine oxidase inhibitors limit the use of indirect sympathomimetics, and anticonvulsant medications which interact with cytochrome P450 enzymes.

If necessary, a medication switch or washout may be appropriate. This should be a joint decision in conjunction with the patient, dental surgeon, GP, and psychiatrist.

Examination and investigations

Extensive examination may not be possible if patients are uncooperative, but as far as possible should include examination of the airway and assessment for signs of uncontrolled cardiorespiratory disease. There is a relatively high incidence of undiagnosed cardiac disease in paediatric dental patients, which may be revealed by examination.[17]

The patient's weight should be noted, as with any paediatric case. Dental caries is associated with a diet rich in sugary foods and drinks, which also predisposes to obesity[18,19] and type 2 diabetes, with all of the attendant risks. Diabetics also have an increased risk of developing caries.[20]

Preoperative investigations depend upon the presence of comorbidities and also upon the likelihood of the particular tests being feasible in that particular patient—simple exodontia in an otherwise well child should not require investigation.

Information provided

The preoperative assessment visit should be used as an opportunity to provide patients and carers with appropriate information about their child's dental anaesthetic. The Royal College of Anaesthetists publishes a range of information leaflets targeted at different age groups (available from their website).[21] Patients with additional needs, including autism, may benefit from a multidisciplinary approach, involving play therapists, use of social stories, and specific visual aids (Fig. 8.1) to prepare them for the experience of surgery and anaesthesia.[22] Patients with generalized or specific anxieties (e.g. needle phobia) may benefit from cognitive behavioural therapy preoperatively.[23] Psychological interventions are increasingly available in self-guided computerized formats, even if face-to-face services are not readily accessible.[24]

Fasting guidance

Detailed fasting guidelines are produced locally by institutions. Most are based upon the principles of the European Society of Anaesthetists guidelines,[25] allowing solid food up to 6 hours before the time of surgery. Clear, non-carbonated fluids are encouraged up until 2 hours before surgery, as this is associated with increased gastric emptying and less acidity of the remaining gastric contents. More recently, several institutions have trialled permitting clear fluids right up until surgery, with no evidence of an increase in aspiration rates. Furthermore, dental patients may have additional needs that make it difficult for them to adhere to fasting guidelines and it is good practice to consider in advance how to proceed if faced with an unfasted patient on the day of surgery. Rapid sequence induction provides a technique for rapid control of the airway, minimizing the risk of aspiration, but is not feasible unless intravenous access is possible, and may be undesirable in the setting of anticipated difficult airway management. Cancelling or delaying a case because the patient is inadequately fasted is an option. One factor influencing the decision to postpone surgery is whether or not better adherence to fasting guidelines is likely in the future. If it is not, it may be more appropriate to proceed with surgery, accepting the additional risks.

Consent

Consent for treatment should be obtained from the patient where they have capacity. If the patient is not competent to give consent, a decision may be made by the parents (in the case of children) or in the patient's best interests (for adults).

General considerations

It is important to recognize that the law relating to consent differs between legal systems and differs even within the UK. Most systems have some provision for those unable to give informed consent themselves. Detailed information on consent is available from the General Medical Council.[25] In England, a person over the age of 18 can consent for themselves, if they have capacity to do so. Under the

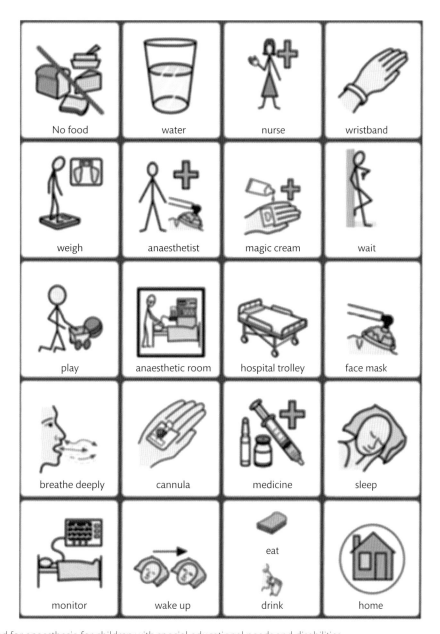

Fig. 8.1 Visual aids utilized for anaesthesia for children with special educational needs and disabilities.
Short J, Calder A. Anaesthesia for children with special needs, including autistic spectrum disorder. *Contin Educ Anaesth Crit Care Pain.* 2013;13(4):107–112.

Mental Capacity Act 2005,[26] capacity is specific to the decision being made. It requires the ability to:

- Understand information.
- Retain information.
- Use information for decision-making.
- Communicate the decision made.

It is recognized that capacity may fluctuate.[26] Every attempt possible should be made to enable people with capacity to make decisions for themselves. This might require the use of communication aids, different formats for information provision, and allowing sufficient time to be set aside, in an environment that facilitates decision-making. Independent mental capacity advocates should be appointed to petition on behalf of the patient and assist with decision-making when a patient lacks capacity. Advance directives

refusing particular treatments are legally binding even if the patient subsequently lacks capacity. In practice, most advance directives relate to end of life care and dental work is not within their scope. If an adult does not have capacity to make a decision about their healthcare needs, a decision can be made for them to proceed with treatment if it is deemed in his or her 'best interests' by the professionals involved. This decision must be carefully documented, and an appropriate consent form completed by the appropriate personnel if applicable. Note that one adult cannot give consent on behalf of another, even if the patient lacks capacity to consent. If this is the case, the path of 'best interests' should be followed. Legal systems contain provisions for consent in minors. Parents may consent on behalf of a child but cannot refuse treatment to which a competent young person has consented. From 16 years of age, a young person is presumed competent to make decisions to accept treatment. Younger children may also be competent, and this should be assessed on a case-by-case basis.

Specific considerations for dental anaesthesia

While consent is normally specific to procedures, in this context, preoperative examination may not be feasible, and the exact nature and extent of the treatment required might not be apparent until the patient is anaesthetized. The consent must include all possible procedures, including dental X-rays to inform future procedures. In patients with multiple medical problems, liaison with lead clinicians (e.g. GP or community paediatrician) should occur to enable coordination of investigations and procedures. It may be possible, for example, to take blood tests while under anaesthesia. This should also be included in the consent. In addition to the risks associated with surgery, relatively common anaesthetic risks should be discussed, including dental damage, sore throat, pain, drowsiness, and postoperative nausea and vomiting. Consent for analgesic suppositories should be specifically obtained.

It may be difficult to communicate risks appropriately and effectively in the setting of anxiety, particularly the rare but serious risks of anaesthesia (e.g. hypoxia, anaphylaxis, and death). Non-medical examples may help to give context, for example, the Association of Paediatric Anaesthetists, UK, states that in an otherwise well child for a minor procedure, 'the risk of a life-threatening problem is about 1 in 400,000. This risk is considerably less than that of your child being seriously injured in a road accident'.[27] Patients should also be given advice about return to work or normal activity, or school in the case of children.[22]

Anaesthesia

There are many considerations regarding the conduct of anaesthesia for dental surgery[28] and consensus guidelines exist to promote consistently high standards (e.g. the Royal College of Anaesthetists consensus guidelines for the management of children referred for dental extractions under general anaesthesia, published in 2011).[29] Dental surgery has a high rate of repeat attendance, and this should be remembered with each anaesthetic plan. The first experience of anaesthesia may 'set the tone' for subsequent attendances.

Premedication

Non-pharmacological methods

Distraction by parents or anaesthetic assistants can be invaluable in facilitating induction of anaesthesia. Most centres keep a range of appropriate distraction aids in anaesthetic rooms (e.g. 'hide and seek' books, bubbles, and sensory toys). Formal play therapy techniques may be helpful in calming patients, particularly children in the immediate preoperative period.

Hypnosis has not been shown to be of benefit in managing children's behaviour for dental interventions without general anaesthesia[30]—it is unclear if these findings can be extrapolated to the induction phase of anaesthesia. Interactive technologies (e.g. RELAX Anaesthetics™; Fig. 8.2) can be used to reduce anxiety[31] and potentially facilitate induction of anaesthesia, and these methods are likely to develop in the future with increased understanding of the nuances of digital distraction techniques.

Topical premedication

The Royal College of Anaesthetists advise that intravenous access 'should be considered for all children undergoing dental anaesthesia'.[30] Intravenous access should also be considered for all adult patients, where possible. Topically applied local anaesthetics can be used to facilitate intravenous access and therefore induction. EMLA™ (Eutectic Mixture of Local Anaesthetic, containing lidocaine and prilocaine) and Ametop™ (containing tetracaine) are the most commonly used. Topical local anaesthetic creams should be applied far enough in advance of intravenous cannulation attempts for them to reach full efficacy—approximately 40 minutes for Ametop™ and 1 hour for EMLA™. Ametop™ has the theoretical advantage of causing vasodilatation of underlying blood vessels, improving the target for cannulation.[32,33] While topical anaesthesia may be associated with

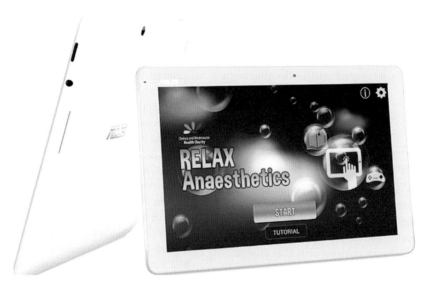

Fig. 8.2 RELAX Anaesthetics™, an NHS Innovation Challenge Acorn award-winning tablet-based app, which helps distract and calm children down before an operation.

reduced pain on venous cannulation, it has not consistently translated to improved success in paediatric practice.[34] Unlike EMLA™, Ametop™ is free of prilocaine and safe to use in patients susceptible to methaemoglobinaemia. Ethyl chloride spray provides immediate short-lived localized anaesthesia and may be an alternative to facilitate cannulation in nervous but cooperative and motivated patients.

Systemic premedication

Oral midazolam (0.25–0.75 mg/kg) may improve cooperation in children undergoing dental treatments,[35] although the patient must be able to comply with swallowing the medication, and it can sometimes result in paradoxical disinhibition.[36] The amnesic effect of midazolam may be beneficial in patients likely to undergo frequent procedures. Ketamine may be given orally (5–10 mg/kg), intranasally (3–5 mg/kg), or intramuscularly (5 mg/kg) and can be used to provide sedation in otherwise uncooperative patients. Side effects include excessive salivation, which may complicate the dental procedure, and sympathetic stimulation. There is no clear boundary between the sedation and the dissociative anaesthesia produced by higher doses of ketamine, such that its effects in an individual may be relatively unpredictable for a given dose. Full anaesthetic monitoring should be applied as soon as possible after administration.[37] Clonidine (oral) and dexmedetomidine (oral or intranasal) can also be used for premedication for dental procedures.

Induction of anaesthesia

Full anaesthetic monitoring is desirable prior to induction of anaesthesia, but often a pragmatic approach is necessary. If little monitoring is tolerated, pulse oximetry is probably the most desirable as this provides information about oxygenation and pulse rate, and the waveform can act as a surrogate for tissue perfusion. Intravenous induction is preferable, with propofol now the most frequently used agent. Total intravenous anaesthesia, utilizing target-controlled infusions of propofol and remifentanil, is becoming more commonplace due to reduced postoperative nausea and vomiting, faster emergence and recovery, and reduced incidence of postoperative delirium. Inhalational induction is an alternative, using oxygen, nitrous oxide, and up to 8% sevoflurane. Induction of anaesthesia with ketamine is possible via the intramuscular route (5–10 mg/kg), providing an alternative technique in particularly uncooperative patients.

Airway management

The choice of airway management technique and equipment depends upon surgical factors and patient factors (Table 8.1). Children are more likely to be undergoing primary exodontia procedures, which are usually quicker and less invasive than the complex reconstructive procedures potentially required in other patient groups.

Nasal masks (Fig. 8.3) are still used by some practitioners, although they are rapidly becoming obsolete. In their place, supraglottic airway devices (laryngeal mask airways) have become the mainstay for the majority of simple dental extractions in patients without risk factors for aspiration, or who have no significant anatomical or respiratory conditions that would make insertion or ventilation difficult. Laryngeal mask airways are associated with shorter insertion and recovery times compared to nasal intubation for dental anaesthesia.[38]

Reinforced or 'flexible' laryngeal mask airways enable manipulation of the position of the stem of the airway device to maximize surgical access.

If tracheal intubation is required, the technique for achieving optimum intubating conditions must to be balanced against the likely length of the surgical procedure. A multidisciplinary discussion with the operating surgeon about preferred choice of tracheal tube is most helpful. For short procedures, options for facilitating tracheal intubation include utilizing short-acting neuromuscular blocking agents (e.g. suxamethonium, mivacurium, and low-dose atracurium), rocuronium with subsequent sugammadex reversal, short-acting potent opioids (e.g. alfentanil), propofol boluses, or a deep plane of inhalational anaesthesia. The most important determining factors are patient comorbidities and the experience of the anaesthetist with a given technique. Nasal north-facing Ring–Adair–Elwyn (RAE) tracheal tubes provide maximum surgical access but may be contraindicated in patients with bleeding tendencies or adenoidal hypertrophy. South-facing RAE tubes and reinforced tracheal tubes are alternatives.

Table 8.1 Factors influencing choice of airway

Surgical factors	Patient factors
Predicted surgical time	Known or predicted difficult airway management
Number of dental extractions	
Additional procedures	History of gastro-oesophageal reflux
Area of oral cavity requiring access	Respiratory disease
Surgeon experience/preference	Anatomical abnormalities
	Bleeding/coagulation disorders
	Starvation status

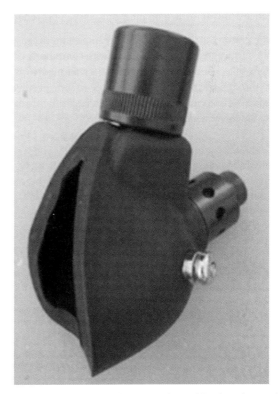

Fig. 8.3 Nasal anaesthetic mask, previously used for dental anaesthesia.
Reproduced with permission from Shaw et al, The Oxford textbook of anaesthesia for oral and maxillofacial surgery, First Edition, 2010, Oxford University Press, UK.

Throat packs

Historically, anaesthesia for dental surgery has routinely involved the anaesthetist inserting a throat pack, with the aim of limiting airway soiling from blood, excessive saliva, and surgical detritus. Debris in the airway may cause laryngospasm on emergence, while blood entering the stomach is potentially associated with increased postoperative nausea and vomiting. Throat packs may limit airway soiling but are potentially hazardous if accidentally retained. At least one visual and one documentary procedure should be undertaken to ensure safe removal[39] (Table 8.2).

Throat packs can be inserted using Magill's forceps or the anaesthetist's fingers. Care should be taken to avoid dental or soft tissue trauma from instruments, and that the final position of the tongue is not likely to cause swelling. While a throat pack may stabilize and improve the seal of an imperfectly fitting airway device, dental procedures involve a 'shared airway' and restricted access to the airway and any airway device once surgery is underway. Doubts about the integrity of the airway device are better resolved by changing the device before surgery is commenced, rather than by attempting to compensate with a throat pack. Following a number of incidents of potential or actual harm to patients as a result of retained throat packs, the National Patient Safety Agency, UK, issued guidance on reducing the risk of retained throat packs after surgery in 2009.[39] The key recommendations were:

- The decision to use a throat pack should be justified by the anaesthetist or surgeon for each patient as appropriate. This person should assume responsibility for ensuring the chosen safety procedures are undertaken.
- At least one visually based and one documentary-based procedure is applied whenever a throat pack is deemed necessary.
- All staff are fully informed on the locally chosen procedures.

The final recommendation is particularly important because members of the surgical team may be familiar with community dentistry, involving awake patients, and therefore less attuned to the risks posed by throat packs in anaesthetized patients. The prevailing evidence, controversies, and current guidance regarding throat packs are discussed in greater detail in Chapter 10.

Analgesia and antiemesis

Provision of adequate analgesia and prophylactic antiemetic administration is crucial in dental patients. The majority of these patients undergo day case procedures where unplanned admissions would have a significant impact upon their care needs. Assessment of pain in these patients can often be more challenging due to their young age or learning difficulties, which may also make requests for additional analgesia more difficult, if not impossible. Liberal use of simple analgesics is therefore advised. In adults, ibuprofen alone provides better pain relief than paracetamol alone after wisdom tooth extraction, and the combination is superior to either agent alone at 6 hours postoperatively.[40]

Paracetamol is given in a dose of 15 mg/kg intravenously (7.5 mg/kg if <10 kg) or 20 mg/kg orally. Intravenous paracetamol has been associated with deaths in underweight adults and guidelines for its use are available from the Association of Anaesthetists.[41] Ibuprofen doses are in the range of 5–10 mg/kg (maximum 30 mg/kg/day in three or four divided doses), but also depend upon age. Codeine is no longer permitted in the UK for children <12 years old, except in acute moderate pain uncontrollable by simple analgesics. It is contraindicated after tonsillectomy/adenoidectomy in patients with obstructive sleep apnoea or in any child at risk of respiratory depression.[42] Many dental patients will fall into this group as a result of their comorbidities and opioid analgesia should be used with caution. Local anaesthetics are frequently infiltrated by the dental surgeons. While, intuitively, this should reduce postoperative pain, heterogeneity in patient trials means that there is no conclusive evidence to this effect.[43] If local anaesthetic is used, it is important to inform patients and/or carers of their likely duration. In a minority of cases an insensate mouth, lips, or tongue may be problematic—for example, where repetitive behaviours like lip-smacking or tongue biting are a pre-existing issue—and in these situations, local anaesthetic may be best avoided, or at least used judiciously. Antiemetics such as ondansetron and cyclizine can be used for postoperative nausea and vomiting prophylaxis for the vast majority of patients. Dexamethasone has the dual benefit of antiemetic and anti-inflammatory activity.[44,45] However, it is associated with increased blood glucose levels in both diabetics and non-diabetics,[46] therefore patients requiring insulin or oral hypoglycaemic agents may require dose adjustment for a short time postoperatively.

Antibiotic prophylaxis

Historically, structural cardiac disease was considered a risk factor for infective endocarditis after dental procedures. This included patients with unrepaired septal defects (aside from an isolated atrial septal defect), hypertrophic obstructive cardiomyopathy, acquired valvular heart disease, prosthetic valves, and those with a previous history of infective endocarditis. Dental procedures were believed to result in significant translocation of oral commensal organisms into the blood, causing a bacteraemia and leading to vegetative bacterial growth on structurally abnormal cardiac tissue. Given the seriousness of infective endocarditis, the risk:benefit balance was thought to favour antibiotic prophylaxis.[47] In 2008, a review of the existing evidence suggested that dental procedures can result in a bacteraemia, but there is no causal link between dental procedures and infective endocarditis, even in high-risk patients.[48] Routine administration of antibiotics is not without risk, both on an individual basis (e.g. anaphylaxis) and on a wider population level, through the propagation of resistant organisms.[49] Consequently, current guidance from the National Institute for Health and Care Excellence (NICE), UK, highlights that patients with structural cardiac disease are at high

Table 8.2 Procedures undertaken to reduce accidental retention of throat packs

Procedures involving visual checks	Procedures involving documented evidence
Putting a label or mark on the patient. (The label is an adherent sticker that is put on either the patient's head or, exceptionally, on another visible part of the body. In either situation the label or mark must be removed at the same time as the pack is removed)	Formalized, recorded 'two-person' check of insertion and removal of a throat pack
Putting a label on the artificial airway device (e.g. tracheal tube or supraglottic airway device)	Recording insertion and removal of throat pack on swab count board
Leaving part of the throat pack protruding externally	

Source: NPSA 'Reducing the risks of retained throat packs' 2009.

risk for the development of infective endocarditis, but that antimicrobial prophylaxis (including chlorhexidine mouthwash) is not routinely recommended for dental procedures, even in high-risk patients. A 2014 analysis of infective endocarditis incidence before and after the changes in antibiotic prophylaxis guidance demonstrated an increased incidence in reported cases in parallel with the reduced use of antibiotics after the introduction of the NICE guidelines, but did not demonstrate causality.[50] NICE reviewed its guidance in 2015 taking into account these findings, and other evidence arising since 2008, but concluded that there was no case for reverting to routine antibiotic prophylaxis for dentistry at present.[50]

Maintenance of anaesthesia

Inhalational agents are most commonly used in the UK for maintenance of anaesthesia, with air or nitrous oxide supplementing oxygen as carrier gases. Sevoflurane has a faster onset and offset than isoflurane, but is associated with higher rates of emergence delirium in children.[51] As mentioned earlier, total intravenous anaesthesia may be of particular benefit in day case dental procedures, with reduced incidence of postoperative nausea and vomiting, faster emergence, and reduced cognitive deficits. Experience of target-controlled infusions in children is accumulating as models develop,[52] and its use is becoming more widespread.

Emergence from anaesthesia

Deep extubation of the trachea can be employed if there are no concerns about maintenance of the airway or the risk of pulmonary aspiration. A common technique for deep extubation is as follows:

- Position the patient in the left lateral position with slight head-down tilt.
- Reverse any residual neuromuscular blocking agents.
- Preoxygenate.
- Remove any throat pack, under direct vision.
- Suction the airway under direct vision, including behind the uvula (seeking the 'coroner's clot').
- Establish regular breathing pattern.
- Increase the depth of anaesthetic.
- Deflate the tracheal tube cuff slowly, ensuring no coughing or breath-holding.
- Extubate the trachea, removing the tracheal tube gently.

If there are concerns about potentially difficult airway management or the risk of aspiration, an awake tracheal extubation technique should be employed, as the safer option. Laryngeal mask airways can be removed as the patient wakes, having already established spontaneous ventilation.

Postoperative complications and follow-up

The most common postoperative complications are pain and nausea and vomiting, which should usually be avoided by prophylactic administration of adequate analgesia and antiemetic medications. Airway swelling, laryngospasm, bleeding, and pulmonary aspiration are also possible, and it is important that patients receive appropriate postanaesthetic care, even for simple cases. While dental surgery per se is unlikely to require high levels of postoperative care,

patients' pre-existing comorbidities may warrant admission to either a general ward or critical care unit postoperatively. Oral intake should be established early, particularly in patients who require regular medication for chronic conditions. Patients and/or parents/carers should be provided with emergency contact details on discharge, should any unexpected postoperative complications arise at home/at the care facility.

As patients will often undergo multiple anaesthetics for dental procedures, meticulous records should be kept on the anaesthetic chart and in-patient notes as these will often inform future anaesthetic plans. It can be very helpful to hold a debrief with patients and carers to determine which aspects of the anaesthetic and surgery were perceived to have gone well, as this may also be useful for repeat attendances. Communication with the patient's GP or community paediatrician is also imperative.

Sedation

Although general anaesthesia in the community setting is now prohibited, sedation is still permitted.[5–7] Both the Royal College of Anaesthetists and the General Dental Council are clear that general anaesthesia should be a last resort for patients who are unable to tolerate procedures with local anaesthesia and/or sedation. A staged transition from general anaesthesia to sedation is desirable for patients undergoing repeated dental surgery.

Anaesthetists may become involved in forward planning for transitions from general anaesthesia to sedation for individual patients, as well as developing protocols for non-anaesthetic delivered sedation services. Sedation is also discussed in detail in Chapter 6.

General considerations

Guidelines have been developed to improve the safety of sedation.[7,52,53] Sedation should take place in settings that have access to full anaesthetic monitoring and resuscitation equipment, and should only be administered by professionals competent in both sedation practice and life support. In 2015, the Society for the Advancement of Anaesthesia in Dentistry published a 'Safe Sedation Practice Scheme', covering all aspects of sedation specific to dentistry.[54] The Academy of Royal Medical Colleges define 'levels' of sedation and emphasize the need for practitioners to be able to 'rescue' a level of sedation deeper than that intended.[55] For dental surgery, 'conscious sedation' (according to the American Society of Anesthesiology depth of sedation continuum; Table 8.3) is the goal, although, as discussed in Chapter 6, this term is rather confusing.

Most recently, in 2020, a multidisciplinary consensus statement has been produced with guidance on fasting and prevention of aspiration before sedation in adults and children (on behalf of the International Committee for the Advancement of Procedural Sedation).[56]

Sedative and analgesic agents

Sedation has most commonly been provided using inhaled nitrous oxide, benzodiazepines, propofol, or ketamine. Potent short-acting opioids have also been used (in combination with sedatives, or as the sole agent) to provide adequate analgesic conditions for minor procedures. There is no conclusive evidence that one agent is significantly better or safer than another, such that the choice is largely

Table 8.3 Continuum of depth of sedation: definition of general anaesthesia and levels of sedation/analgesia

	Minimal sedation/anxiolysis	Moderate sedation/analgesia ('conscious sedation')	Deep sedation/analgesia
Responsiveness	Normal response to verbal stimulation	Purposeful[a] response to verbal tactile stimulation	Purposeful[a] response following repeated or painful stimulation
Airway	Unaffected	No intervention required	Intervention may be required
Spontaneous ventilation	Unaffected	Adequate	May be inadequate
Cardiovascular function	Unaffected	Usually maintained	Usually maintained
Escalation of required competencies			

[a] Reflex withdrawal from a painful stimulus is *not* considered a purposeful response.

Source: Excerpted from Continuum of Depth of Sedation. Definition of General Anesthesia and Levels of Sedation/Analgesia of the American Society of Anaesthesiology. October 2009.

dependent upon local protocols and the experience and preference of the sedation practitioner. General principles to increase the margin of safety include:

- Single-agent sedation.
- Incremental doses—'start low, go slow'.
- When an opioid–benzodiazepine combination is utilized (e.g. fentanyl and midazolam), the opioid should be given first and allowed to reach peak effect before the benzodiazepine is given.[52]

More recently, there has been particular interest in dexmedetomidine, a highly selective α_2-adrenergic receptor agonist, which can be given both intravenously and intranasally. In adults, intranasal dexmedetomidine with dental local anaesthetic has been shown to provide adequate sedation and superior postoperative analgesia for third molar extractions, when compared with local anaesthetic alone.[57] Several trials have also demonstrated its efficacy for paediatric dental sedation.[58,59] The relative preservation of cardio-respiratory stability and its additional analgesic action mean that dexmedetomidine is likely to gain popularity when it becomes more widely available.

Conclusion

Dental anaesthesia is a rewarding field, due to the demanding patient population, the additional consideration of the 'shared airway', and the high-turnover day case nature of the subspecialty. These challenges can be met by applying meticulous attention to detail and by providing genuinely individualized, patient-centred care. The anaesthetic workload for dental procedures is unlikely to reduce significantly in the near future, making it a key element of oromaxillofacial anaesthesia.

REFERENCES

1. Lyman HM. History of anaesthesia. In: *Artificial Anaesthesia and Anaesthetics*, p. 6. New York: William Wood and Company; 1881.
2. Poswillo D. *General Anaesthesia, Sedation and Resuscitation in Dentistry. Report of an Expert Working Party for the Standing Dental Advisory Committee*. London: Department of Health; 1990.
3. General Dental Council. *Maintaining Standards: Guidance to Dentists on Professional and Personal Conduct*. London: General Dental Council; 1998.
4. Royal College of Anaesthetists. *Standards and Guidelines for General Anaesthesia for Dentistry*. London: Royal College of Anaesthetists; 1999.
5. Department of Health. *A Conscious Decision: Report of an Expert Group Chaired by the Chief Medical and Dental Officer*. London: Department of Health; 2000.
6. Intercollegiate Advisory Committee for Sedation in Dentistry. *Standards for Conscious Sedation in the Provision of Dental Care*. London: Royal College of Anaesthetists; 2015.
7. Scottish Dental Clinical Effectiveness Programme. *Conscious Sedation in Dentistry: Dental Clinical Guidance*, 2nd ed. Dundee: Scottish Clinical Dental Effectiveness Programme; 2012.
8. NHS Digital. NHS dental statistics 2015–16. 2016. http://content. digital.nhs.uk/catalogue/PUB21701/nhs-dent-stat-eng-15-16-rep.pdf
9. NHS Digital. NHS dental statistics 2017–18. 2018. https://digital. nhs.uk/data-and-information/publications/staistical/nhs-dental-statistics/2017-18-annual -report
10. Sury MR, Palmer JH, Cook TM, Pandit JJ. The state of UK dental anaesthesia: results from the NAP5 activity survey. A national survey by the 5th National Audit Project of the Royal College of Anaesthetists and the Association of Anaesthetists of Great Britain and Ireland. *SAAD Dig.* 2016;**32**:34–36.
11. Dental Public Health Team. *Child Dental General Anaesthetics in Wales*. Cardiff: Public Health Wales; 2015.
12. Jogezai U, Ackuaku N, Dowson E, Nguyen E, Townsend D. Repeat paediatric dental general anaesthetics: a study of two regions. *J Dent Oral Health.* 2016;**3**:1–6.
13. Royal College of Anaesthetists. *Curriculum for a CCT in Anaesthetics*. London: Royal College of Anaesthetists; 2010.
14. Australia & New Zealand College of Anaesthesia. *Anaesthesia Training Program Curriculum*. Melbourne: Australia & New Zealand College of Anaesthesia; 2016.
15. NHS England. *Guides for Commissioning Dental Specialties—Special Care Dentistry*. London: NHS England; 2015.
16. Albadri SS, Jarad FD, Lee GT, Mackie IC. The frequency of repeat general anaesthesia for teeth extractions in children. *Int J Paediatr Dent.* 2006;**16**(1):45–48.
17. Rutherford J, Stevenson R. Careful physical examination is essential in the preoperative assessment of children for dental extractions under general anesthesia. *Pediatr Anesth.* 2004;**14**(11):920–923.
18. Gerdin EW, Angbratt M, Aronsson K, Eriksson E, Johansson I. Dental caries and body mass index by socio-economic status in Swedish children. *Community Dent Oral Epidemiol.* 2008;**36**(5):459–465.

19. Alm A, Fåhraeus C, Wendt LK, Koch G, Andersson-Gäre B, Birkhed D. Body adiposity status in teenagers and snacking habits in early childhood in relation to approximal caries at 15 years of age. *Int J Paediatr Dent*. 2008;**18**(3):189–196.

20. Johnston L, Vieira AR. Caries experience and overall health status. *Oral Health Prev Dent*. 2014;**12**(2):163–170.

21. Royal College of Anaesthetists. Information for Children and Parents. 2022. http://www.rcoa.ac.uk/childrensinfo

22. Short J, Calder A. Anaesthesia for children with special needs, including autistic spectrum disorder. *Contin Educ Anaesth Crit Care Pain*. 2013;**13**(4):107–112.

23. Jenkins K. Needle-phobia: a psychological perspective. *Br J Anaesth*. 2014;**113**(1):4–6.

24. NHS Self-help therapies. 2022. https://www.nhs.uk/mental-health/talking-therapies-medicine-treatments/talking-therpaies-and-counselling/self-help-therapies/

25. General Medical Council. *Consent: Patients and Doctors Making Decisions Together*. London: General Medical Council; 2008.

26. Legislation.gov.uk. Mental Capacity Act 2005. 2005. https://www.legislation.gov.uk/ukpga/2005/9/contents

27. Association of Paediatric Anaesthetists of Great Britain & Ireland. *Your Child's General Anaesthetic for Dental Treatment*. London: Association of Paediatric Anaesthetists of Great Britain & Ireland; 2009.

28. Cantlay K, Williamson S, Hawkings J. Anaesthesia for dental surgery. *Contin Educ Anaesth Crit Care Pain*. 2005;**5**(3):71–75.

29. Royal College of Anaesthetists. *Consensus Guidelines for the Management of Children Referred for Dental Extractions Under General Anaesthesia*. London: Royal College of Anaesthetists; 2011.

30. Al-Harasi S, Ashley PF, Moles DR, Parekh S, Walters V. Hypnosis for children undergoing dental treatment. *Cochrane Database Syst Rev*. 2010;**8**:CD007154.

31. Fancourt D, Lee C, Baltzer Nielsen S, Capps S, Brooks P. Abstract PR230. Relax anaesthetics: the effect of a bespoke distraction app on anxiety levels in children undergoing induction of anaesthesia. *Anesth Anal*. 2016;**123**(3S):298–299.

32. Browne J, Awad I, Plant R, McAdoo J, Shorten G. Topical amethocaine (Ametop) is superior to EMLA for intravenous cannulation. Eutectic mixture of local anesthetics. *Can J Anaesth*. 1999;**46**(11):1014–1018.

33. Arrowsmith J, Campbell C. A comparison of local anaesthetics for venepuncture. *Arch Dis Child*. 2000;**82**(4):309–310.

34. Newbury C, Herd DW. Amethocaine versus EMLA for successful intravenous cannulation in a children's emergency department: a randomised controlled study. *Emerg Med J*. 2009;**26**(7):487–491.

35. Lourenço-Matharu L, Ashley PF, Furness S. Sedation of children undergoing dental treatment. *Cochrane Database Syst Rev*. 2012;**3**:CD003877.

36. Allen Finley G, Stewart S, Buffett-Jerrott S, Wright K, Millington D. High levels of impulsivity may contraindicate midazolam premedication in children. *Can J Anesth*. 2006;**53**(1):73–78.

37. Association of Anaesthetists of Great Britain & Ireland. *Recommendations for Standards of Monitoring During Anaesthesia and Recovery*. London: Association of Anaesthetists of Great Britain & Ireland; 2016.

38. Zhao N, Deng F, Yu C. Anesthesia for pediatric day-case dental surgery: a study comparing the classic laryngeal mask airway with nasal trachea intubation. *J Craniofac Surg*. 2014;**25**(3):e245–e248.

39. National Patient Safety Agency. *Reducing the Risk of Retained Throat Packs: Supporting Information*. London: National Patient Safety Agency; 2009.

40. Bailey E, Worthington HV, van Wijk A, Yates JM, Coulthard P, Afzal Z. Ibuprofen and/or paracetamol (acetaminophen) for pain relief after surgical removal of lower wisdom teeth. *Cochrane Database Syst Rev*. 2013;**12**:CD004624.

41. Safe Anaesthesia Liaison Group. *Intravenous Paracetamol*. London: Royal College of Anaesthetists Safe Anaesthesia Liaison Group; 2013.

42. Medicines and Healthcare Regulatory Authority. *Codeine for Analgesia: Restricted Use in Children Because of Reports of Morphine Toxicity*. London: Medicines and Healthcare Regulatory Authority; 2013.

43. Parekh S, Gardener C, Ashley PF, Walsh T. Intraoperative local anaesthesia for reduction of postoperative pain following general anaesthesia for dental treatment in children and adolescents. *Cochrane Database Syst Rev*. 2014;**12**:CD009742.

44. Laureano Filho JR, Maurette PE, Allais M, Cotinho M, Fernandes C. Clinical comparative study of the effectiveness of two dosages of dexamethasone to control postoperative swelling, trismus and pain after the surgical extraction of mandibular impacted third molars. *Med Oral Patol Oral Cir Bucal*. 2008;**13**(2):129–132.

45. Markiewicz MR, Brady MF, Ding EL, Dodson TB. Corticosteroids reduce postoperative morbidity after third molar surgery: a systematic review and meta-analysis. *J Oral Maxillofac Surg*. 2008;**66**(9):1881–1894.

46. Tien M, Gan TJ, Dhakal I, White WD, Olufolabi AJ, Fink R, et al. The effect of anti-emetic doses of dexamethasone on postoperative blood glucose levels in non-diabetic and diabetic patients: a prospective randomised controlled study. *Anaesthesia*. 2016;**71**(9):1037–1043.

47. Gould IM, Buckingham JK. Cost effectiveness of prophylaxis in dental practice to prevent infective endocarditis. *Br Heart J*. 1993;**70**(1):79–83.

48. National Institute for Clinical Excellence. *Prophylaxis Against Infective Endocarditis. Clinical Guideline 64*. London: National Institute for Clinical Excellence; 2008.

49. National Institute for Clinical Excellence. *Prophylaxis Against Infective Endocarditis. Clinical Guideline 64.1*. London: National Institute for Clinical Excellence; 2015.

50. Dayer MJ, Jones S, Prendergast B, Baddour LM, Lockhart PB, Thornhill MH. Incidence of infective endocarditis in England, 2000–13: a secular trend, interrupted time-series analysis. *Lancet*. 2015;**385**(9974):1219–1228.

51. Costi D, Cyna AM, Ahmed S, Stephens K, Strickland P, Ellwood J, et al. Effects of sevoflurane versus other general anaesthesia on emergence agitation in children. *Cochrane Database Syst Rev*. 2014;**12**(9):CD007084.

52. Sepúlveda P, Cortínez LI, Sáez C, Penna A, Solari S, Guerra I, Absalom AR. Performance evaluation of paediatric propofol pharmacokinetic models in healthy young children. *Br J Anaesth*. 2011;**107**(4):593–600.

53. National Institute for Clinical Excellence. *Sedation in Children and Young People*. London: National Institute for Clinical Excellence; 2010.

54. Society for the Advancement of Anaesthesia in Dentistry. *A Quality Assurance Programme for Implementing National Standards in Conscious Sedation for Dentistry in the UK*.

London: Society for the Advancement of Anaesthesia in Dentistry; 2015.

55. Academy of Royal Medical Colleges. *Safe Sedation Practice for Healthcare Procedures.* London: Academy of Royal Medical Colleges; 2013.

56. Green SM, Leroy PL, Roback MG, Irwin MG, Andolfatto G, Babl FE, et al. An international multidisciplinary consensus statement on fasting before procedural sedation in adults and children. *Anaesthesia.* 2020;**75**(3):374–385.

57. Cheung CW, Ng KF, Liu J, Yuen MY, Ho MH, Irwin MG. Analgesic and sedative effects of intranasal dexmedetomidine in third molar surgery under local anaesthesia. *Br J Anaesth.* 2011;**107**(3):430–437.

58. Malhotra PU, Thakur S, Singhal P, Chauhan D, Jayam C, Sood R, et al. Comparative evaluation of dexmedetomidine and midazolam-ketamine combination as sedative agents in pediatric dentistry: a double-blinded randomized controlled trial *Contemp Clin Dent.* 2016;**7**(2):186–192.

59. Kim HS, Kim JW, Jang KT, Lee SH, Kim CC, Shin TJ. Initial experience with dexmedetomidine for dental sedation in children. *J Clin Pediatr Dent.* 2013;**38**(1): 79–81.

9

Aesthetic surgery

Corina Lee

Introduction

The title 'aesthetic surgery' can be ambiguous, with the terms 'aesthetic', 'cosmetic', 'plastic', and 'reconstructive' often being used interchangeably, such that the layperson may perceive plastic and reconstructive as meaning purely cosmetic or aesthetic surgery. Ultimately, an element of crossover exists—procedures that are primarily functional or reconstructive in nature may be performed with excellent aesthetic results. Indeed, almost all operations have an aesthetic component to a varying degree, and the terms 'aesthetic' and 'cosmetic' are widely accepted as transposable. The Royal College of Surgeons defines cosmetic surgery as 'the choice to undergo an operation, or invasive medical procedure, to alter one's physical appearance for aesthetic rather than medical reasons'.[1] Conversely, reconstructive surgery is that which is performed to improve the function of structures that are abnormal, due to congenital, trauma, or acquired causes, in an attempt to make them as near 'normal' as possible. Any aesthetic component is inextricably linked with the restoration of function in reconstructive surgery. This chapter focuses on purely aesthetic procedures for primary cosmetic gain.

Orofacial aesthetic surgery

Aesthetic surgery on the mouth and face may be broadly divided into two categories: firstly, where the shape or size of a feature is changed because the patient dislikes it; and, secondly, involving facial rejuvenation or anti-ageing surgery in patients who were previously content with their features but are now seeking a more youthful appearance. The procedures can be classified as surgical or non-surgical. Surgical options for those seeking a change in a disliked facial feature include rhinoplasty, otoplasty, insertion of facial implants, or genioplasty. Anti-ageing options including face lift, brow lift, and blepharoplasty. Non-surgical treatments include laser, botulinum toxin type A (commonly referred to as 'Botox'), or filler injections. Orthognathic surgery can be functional, or have a largely cosmetic component, and is discussed in Chapter 10. Genioplasty may be performed at the time of orthognathic surgery or independently. In adults, non-surgical procedures are often performed with local or topical anaesthesia; however, in children, general anaesthesia

(GA) or sedation may be required for laser or Botox (non-aesthetic) treatments. Surgical procedures vary from minor to major, such that local anaesthesia (LA) alone may suffice, or may be used in conjunction with sedation or GA.

Aesthetic surgery was, until recently, one of the fastest growing medical practices in the UK. However, following a 'peak' in 2015, a decline of 8% was seen in the total number of patients undergoing cosmetic surgery in the UK by 2017.[2] Potential explanations for this downturn include the widespread availability of less invasive treatments and, perhaps, an increased acceptance of 'real' bodies through the influence of social media, shifting from the previously desired 'model' image. A British Association of Aesthetic Plastic Surgery audit highlighted that gender differences may also exist, with men being more accepting of their bodies, tending to opt for brow lift and blepharoplasty surgery, with women more focused upon body rather than facial surgery.

Due to the nature of cosmetic surgery, there is a paucity of clinical trials, such that some of the anaesthesia techniques utilized are less evidence based and more centred upon what works well with a particular surgeon, complemented by practices translated from non-aesthetic surgeries. Many of the publications in aesthetic surgery are from the US, where this type of surgery is largely undertaken in an office-based setting, contrasting with the more hospital-based practice in the UK. It is the assumption that all procedures requiring GA or sedation in the UK take place in fully equipped hospital facilities, with monitoring, equipment, and trained staff complying with the Association of Anaesthetists standards of monitoring for anaesthesia and recovery.[3] These principles cannot necessarily be universally applied to international practice of aesthetic surgery, therefore this chapter describes the anaesthesia considerations and techniques based upon common collective practice, supported by research evidence where possible.

Preoperative assessment

Patient considerations

Preoperative assessment of patients for cosmetic surgery has some special considerations, precisely because they are a self-selecting group. Although this cohort of patients is usually physically well, a thorough preoperative assessment remains essential, particularly on account of specific surgical requirements. Patients' psychological status and expectations should also be addressed, given their willingness to undergo aesthetic surgery and its inherent risks. Indeed, it is the recommendation of the Royal College of Surgeons that patients' psychological status is assessed alongside medical fitness prior to surgery.[1]

Medical assessment

Patients undergoing cosmetic surgery are generally well. However, there is a subgroup of patients, particularly those undergoing anti-ageing procedures, who may have concomitant disease. It is prudent to keep in mind the elective nature of aesthetic surgery. Surgery is requested only because of the patient's desire to change their physical appearance or an aspect of their features, which may be functionally and structurally normal. The balance of risk versus benefit must be carefully considered. The patient's physiological status should ideally be classified as American Society of Anesthesiologists[4] (ASA) 1 or 2 (healthy or mild systemic disease) to justify proceeding, minimizing the risk of anaesthesia and surgery. Patients who are ASA 3 must be carefully assessed, with the risk:benefit ratio fully considered and discussed between the surgeon, anaesthetist, and patient.

A comprehensive medical history should be undertaken, focusing specifically on the presence of hypertension, ischaemic heart disease, obstructive sleep apnoea syndrome, cerebrovascular disease, smoking, asthma, and chronic obstructive pulmonary disease.

Adequate control of hypertension should be sought preoperatively. The Association of Anaesthetists guideline for the preoperative management of hypertension (2016) recommended that if 'in-hospital' systolic blood pressures are <180 mmHg and diastolic <110 mmHg (systolic <160 mmHg and diastolic <100 mmHg at time of referral from primary care), elective surgery may proceed.[5] However, there is evidence that patients with a preoperative systolic pressure >150 mmHg undergoing face lift surgery are at an increased risk of postoperative haematoma, therefore adequate assessment and tighter preoperative control of hypertension may be necessary.[6] For similar reasons, intraoperative locally infiltrated adrenaline may require greater dilution in select patients.[7,8]

Medication such as anticoagulants and antiplatelets should ideally be stopped prior to surgery to reduce the risk of intraoperative bleeding and haematoma formation. It is also important to consider antidepressants such as tricyclic agents and monoamine oxidase inhibitors due to the high doses of adrenaline used during LA infiltration (discussed in detail in Chapter 10).[8,9]

Psychological assessment

A review of complications of breast implant procedures in the UK (2014) identified certain psychosocial factors associated with poor patient outcome. Underlying reasons motivating patients to undergo surgery included dissatisfaction with body image, appearance-related self-consciousness, social anxiety, and life stressors. Changes in their physical appearance alone may fail to fulfil patients' needs and expectations, and may even lead to deterioration in their psychological status and significant distress.[10] Consequently, the Royal College of Surgeons 'Professional Standards for Cosmetic Surgery' (2016) recommended that surgeons should be prepared to defer or avoid surgery pending psychological health assessment in vulnerable patients. This includes patients with unrealistic expectations of surgery not resolved during the consultation process, a history of repeated cosmetic procedures (particularly in one anatomical area), and coexisting psychological disorders.[1]

Anaesthesia for orofacial aesthetic procedures

General principles

The overall aim of anaesthesia for these procedures is to provide a safe, dry operating surgical field, in a patient who is stationary during surgery, wakes up smoothly at emergence without coughing, and is ready to be discharged in a timely manner with well-controlled pain and the absence of nausea, vomiting, or drowsiness.[7] Many other aspects of general patient care are covered in more detail in previous chapters, therefore only those aspects pertinent to aesthetic surgery and the common types of surgery are discussed.

The specific anaesthetic challenges in orofacial aesthetic surgery include potentially prolonged surgery, achieving a dry surgical field, minimizing the risk of postoperative haematoma formation, ensuring safe airway management (with restricted access), and employing safe sedation techniques. The patient's experience of surgery and its outcome can be influenced by the anaesthetist, particularly in the first 72 hours when oedema and pain are at their maximal degree. Good intraoperative communication between surgeon and anaesthetist is key to achieving the optimal postoperative outcome.

Often the head of the patient is away from the anaesthetic machine, therefore particular consideration should be given to the length of breathing circuits, monitoring cables, and intravenous access lines. Patients should wear anti-venous thromboembolism stockings and sequential pneumatic inflatable calf compressors should be applied intraoperatively to prevent deep vein thrombosis. The use of prophylactic anticoagulants should be considered for patients undergoing prolonged surgery or where a significant period of postoperative immobility is expected; however, this must be specifically discussed with the operating surgeon, given the potential risk of haematoma formation. Generally, a single prophylactic dose of a broad-spectrum antibiotic is given intravenously at induction of anaesthesia in most aesthetic surgical procedures, followed by regular oral antibiotics for up to 1 week following surgery involving any implants or grafts (including cartilage)—although local policies should be followed. Normothermia should be maintained perioperatively using warmed intravenous fluids and active warming blankets as necessary, in order to avoid issues relating to hypothermia such as altered coagulation and wound healing. Large volume blood loss is rare in these procedures, and a relatively restrictive perioperative intravenous fluid regimen is advised, to avoid bladder distension (causing patient irritability and hypertension) and facial oedema in the early postoperative period.

Anaesthesia technique

Most of these surgical procedures require GA or sedation to augment LA infiltration, though there is some variation depending upon the specific procedure and the duration of surgery, further influenced by the preference of the patient, surgeon, and anaesthetist.

Sedation

Sedation is discussed in detail in Chapter 6; however, in the context of orofacial aesthetic surgery, it is best reserved for superficial procedures of short duration, in compliant patients. The potential advantages include avoidance of invasive airway management and emergence phenomena, reduced postoperative nausea and vomiting and sore throat, and expedited hospital discharge. Delivery of safe and appropriate sedation is a skill that requires practice, and most anaesthetists would agree that achieving the desired depth of sedation requires a great deal of skill. It can be challenging to achieve the fine balance required, in the face of fluctuating surgical stimuli, variable onset/offset of different pharmacological agents, additive and synergistic effects of combinations of agents, and the varied response of individual patients to them.[7]

The ASA defines the continuum of depth of sedation as follows[11]:

- Minimal sedation (anxiolysis): a drug-induced state during which patients respond normally to verbal commands. Although cognitive function and physical coordination may be impaired, airway reflexes, ventilatory functions, and cardiovascular functions are unaffected.
- Moderate sedation/analgesia ('conscious sedation'): a drug-induced depression of consciousness during which patients respond purposefully to verbal commands, either alone or accompanied by light tactile stimulation. No interventions are required to maintain a patent airway, and spontaneous ventilation is adequate. Cardiovascular function is usually maintained.
- Deep sedation/analgesia: a drug-induced depression of consciousness during which patients cannot be easily aroused but respond purposefully following repeated or painful stimulation. The ability to independently maintain ventilatory function may be impaired. Patients may require assistance in maintaining a patent airway, and spontaneous ventilation may be inadequate. Cardiovascular function is usually maintained.
- GA: a drug-induced loss of consciousness during which patients are not rousable, even by painful stimulation. The ability to independently maintain ventilatory function is often impaired. Patients often require assistance in maintaining a patent airway and positive pressure ventilation may be required because of depressed spontaneous ventilation or drug-induced depression of neuromuscular function. Cardiovascular function may be impaired.

The greatest risk of sedation is unintended airway obstruction, leading to hypoxia. This is particularly pertinent during facial surgery where the unsecured airway may be lost without immediate access or easy early detection. Inadequate sedation of the patient for a particular phase of surgery may lead to deepening of the level of sedation, which in turn may cause the patient to become restless and more uncooperative, leading to a further increase in the depth of sedation, such that the patient inadvertently drifts into GA and subsequent airway obstruction. Immediate detection of airway obstruction may be hindered by interference with monitoring systems following patient movement, surgical draping, or during surgery on the surrounding area.[7,12] Nasal cannulae and face masks with continuous end-tidal carbon dioxide monitoring are now widely available.

Patients often perceive that sedation may be less 'risky'[13] compared with GA, and in some cases this may have influenced their overall decision-making and justification to undergo cosmetic surgery. Patients should be fully counselled about the risks of sedation, and given no false reassurances. The desired depth of sedation must be agreed by the anaesthetist and surgeon, and the potential for GA must be prepared for—the patient must be appropriately starved, and the necessary facilities, equipment, and personnel must be available.[12–14]

Successful sedation should complement good-quality LA infiltration, and relies upon close communication between surgeon and anaesthetist. Patient selection is also important, and caution should be applied in patients with obstructive sleep apnoea syndrome. The ideal sedation technique facilitates rapid onset of sedation, provides additional analgesia, causes minimal respiratory or cardiovascular depression, and allows rapid recovery. The key is often to ensure provision of adequate analgesia at the time of LA injection, whose intense stimulation may provoke a response; thereafter sedation may be titrated to provide patient comfort without respiratory impairment. Many different combinations of propofol, opioids, benzodiazepines, and ketamine have been described and used successfully for sedation, and are discussed in greater detail in Chapter 6. Dexmedetomidine has gained popularity more recently, and can be used for short, minimally stimulating procedures, such as laser treatments. It can be administered as a premedication, orally or intranasally, or as a continuous infusion intraoperatively (after an initial loading dose of 0.5–1.0 mcg/kg bolus over 10 minutes). This centrally acting α_2-adrenoceptor agonist attenuates sympathetic activity[7,15] and its properties of sedation, anxiolysis, and mild analgesia, with minimal respiratory depression, make it an attractive agent for aesthetic facial surgery. In the UK, it is most commonly used as a sedative adjunct in critical care, and it is often used in combination with other agents due to its mild analgesic properties; however, this may potentiate the risk of hypoventilation and airway compromise. Intravenous dexmedetomidine has been used in patients undergoing facelift surgery under sedation, demonstrating a reduction in opioid and other anxiolytic medications, with fewer episodes of intraoperative hypoxaemia requiring supplemental oxygen. Side effects include hypotension and bradycardia, and intraoperative administration of vasopressors may be required more frequently.[15–17]

General anaesthesia

The choice of airway device should reflect the potential for head and neck movement intraoperatively, surgical access requirements, and the type of surgery. As there is a risk of displacement of the airway, particularly during application of surgical drapes and during head turning, the device must be safely secured. South-facing Ring–Adair–Elwyn (RAE) tubes, reinforced tracheal tubes, and nasotracheal tubes are commonly used as well as flexible laryngeal mask airways (recommended airway devices for specific surgical procedures are described later in the chapter). The advantage of the laryngeal mask airway is the ability to insert and remove it in a smooth manner, minimizing sympathetic and airway reflex stimulation. The obvious disadvantage is its easier dislodgement from head movement during surgery, therefore it is prudent to check the position and seal after insertion and before commencing surgery, and to secure it thoroughly. Tracheal tubes provide greater security, being less easily displaced during head movement, and they can be optimally positioned away from the surgical site; however, they are more likely to invoke coughing and a sympathetic response at tracheal extubation. The eyes should be protected during all facial surgery, as they are at particular risk of desiccation from the heat of the operating lights. Regular and liberal eye lubrication, eye taping, and corneal shields should be used where appropriate, and especially during prolonged surgery.[7,9,18] The use of throat packs is discussed in detail in Chapter 10, but should no longer be considered routine practice, and evidence is lacking for their efficacy.[19,20]

Propofol is used most commonly for induction of anaesthesia for orofacial aesthetic surgery, and maintenance of anaesthesia may be either inhalational or total intravenous anaesthesia (TIVA). Commonly used inhalational agents include desflurane (for its rapid emergence properties) and sevoflurane (for its smooth emergence properties). Intraoperative analgesia is most commonly provided by remifentanil, via a target-controlled infusion that allows titration to the level of surgical stimuli, supplemented with either fentanyl or morphine for postoperative analgesia. Recent guidelines have been published by the Association of Anaesthetists for the safe practice of TIVA.[21] Processed electroencephalography is recommended for patients at high risk of awareness (e.g. when neuromuscular blocking agents are required) and if surgical access permits its use. The intravenous cannula should be directly visible when using TIVA. Intraoperative monitoring standards should comply with Association of Anaesthetists guidance.[3]

Local anaesthesia

LA is often administered in the form of a regional anaesthetic block, or by tumescent anaesthesia. The former allows small targeted LA doses to be delivered, with minimal tissue distortion. The latter delivers large volumes of LA diluted in 0.9% sodium chloride solution (often with additives), and allows tissue hydrodissection, anaesthesia, and haemostasis. An initial dose of LA administered at the start of the procedure attenuates the stress response to surgery, and reduces intraoperative analgesic requirements. Various dilutions, additives, and LA agents can be used, therefore the surgeon and anaesthetist must agree the maximum safe dose to avoid LA toxicity. As there is a rich blood supply to the face, LA may be absorbed easily, so the risk should be minimized by using dilute concentrations of LA, adding adrenaline, and fractionating the dosing over prescribed time intervals.[8]

Adrenaline

The addition of this vasoconstrictor to LA is well established. Advantages include prolonging the effect of the LA by decreasing its systemic absorption, minimizing the risk of systemic toxicity, and providing haemostasis. The addition of 5 mcg of adrenaline to 1 mL of LA agent produces a 1:200,000 concentration[22] (preprepared vials also exist). Larger doses of LA are permitted if adrenaline is added. It requires several minutes following injection in order to take effect. Caution should be observed in patients susceptible to the haemodynamic effects of systemic absorption of adrenaline.[8]

Hyaluronidase

By catalysing the hydrolysis of hyaluronic acid, a major constituent of the interstitial barrier, hyaluronidase lowers the viscosity of hyaluronic acid, thereby enhancing permeation of the LA, and also potentially reducing tissue distortion. The dose is usually 1500 IU, added to the LA solution.

Sodium bicarbonate

Commonly used amide LA agents are poorly soluble in water.[22] They are prepared as hydrochloride salts with an acidic pH (in the range of 4–6) to improve water solubility and increase shelf life. The addition of sodium bicarbonate as a buffer will raise the pH to nearer physiological values, which can decrease pain on injection. This alkalinization can also increase the rate of onset by raising the proportion of lipid-soluble uncharged base, which readily penetrates neural tissue. The main limitation is the amount of sodium bicarbonate that may be added, before precipitation of the LA.

Steroids

As well as being given intravenously, dexamethasone may be added to LA agents to prolong their duration of action. There is limited evidence of its efficacy in LA infiltration and it is probably more effective as an adjunct in regional anaesthetic nerve blocks.[23] Alternatively, triamcinolone acetonide (Kenalog®) is sometimes used to minimize postoperative swelling.

Regional anaesthesia

Regional anaesthesia is the deposition of low doses of LA around or near a specific nerve or nerve bundle, aiming to block the nerve territory. This technique minimizes tissue distension at the surgical site and can cover a large area. It may be used as a sole technique depending on the type of surgery, or used in combination with sedation or GA. The sensory supply of the face is complex, and is discussed in detail in Chapter 4. The relevant nerve blocks for specific orofacial aesthetic surgical procedures are described later in this chapter.

Surgical requirements for orofacial aesthetic procedures

Dry surgical field

A dry surgical field provides optimal operating conditions for surgery, as well as reducing blood transfusion requirements. There are several methods of providing these conditions (discussed in greater detail in Chapters 7 and 10):

- Head-up tilt: 20–30° to improve venous drainage.[24]
- Tranexamic acid: the highly vascular orofacial region is at risk of bleeding, and a single intravenous dose of this antifibrinolytic agent may reduce intraoperative blood loss in orthognathic surgery.[25,26] A meta-analysis of 10,000 patients undergoing a range of surgical procedures found the probability of requiring blood transfusion reduced by approximately a third. The effects on thromboembolic events and mortality remain uncertain, however.[27] The translation to aesthetic facial surgery depends upon the specific procedure and associated risk of blood loss, and it should be considered on a case-by-case basis.
- Controlled hypotension: its use in reducing intraoperative blood loss in major orthognathic surgery is well documented[28–31];

however, there is a paucity of evidence for this technique in aesthetic facial surgery. Generally, a moderate degree of hypotension for major surgery where the bleeding risk is relatively high is accepted practice, with profound hypotension or prolonged periods avoided. There is no clear blood pressure target that will minimize blood loss and protect the patient from postoperative organ injury; however, prolonged duration at low blood pressures should be avoided.[32,33]

- Local vasoconstrictor: adrenaline, at varying concentrations, may be used locally to achieve haemostasis.

Identification of bleeding points

Identification of potential bleeding blood vessels is paramount in minimizing the risk of postoperative haematoma formation. Several strategies may be employed for this purpose. Firstly, 'normal' (or even supra-normal) blood pressure should be restored towards the end of surgery, to ensure that any bleeding points are found and haemostasis achieved. Secondly, surgeons may request head-down tilt or a Valsalva manoeuvre in order to raise venous pressure. Additionally, some surgeons advocate avoidance of a vasoconstrictor in the LA in order to avoid rebound vasodilatation. Crucially, surgeons must dissect accurately in the correct plane to avoid bleeding, rather than potentially masking bleeding by suboptimal dissection.

Emergence and tracheal extubation

Due to the nature of the surgery and inherent risk of bleeding, the aim is to perform a smooth wake-up with no coughing, laryngospasm, or airway obstruction. This can be achieved either with the patient awake or in a deep plane of anaesthesia. Each patient must be evaluated individually as to whether they represent a 'high' or 'low' risk for deep tracheal extubation and managed accordingly.[34] Deep tracheal extubation requires experience, skill, and often requires insertion of an oropharyngeal airway and/or jaw thrust—manoeuvres that may not always be feasible or desirable in patients undergoing facial surgery. Tracheal extubation in the awake patient minimizes the risk of airway obstruction and laryngospasm, but is associated with sympathetic stimulation and potential risk of coughing, causing bleeding at the operative site. These responses may be attenuated to some extent with opioids, and a continued infusion of remifentanil during this period can assist due to its antitussive properties. Achieving the desired level to suppress coughing without causing apnoea requires experience and attention to detail.[34] Alternatively, well-timed administration of an alternative opioid or propofol bolus just preceding tracheal extubation may be utilized.

Laryngeal mask airways tend to cause less adverse stimulation on removal. For this reason, the Bailey manoeuvre[35] may be employed in carefully selected patients, where the tracheal tube is exchanged for a laryngeal mask airway at the end of surgery. This is performed in a deep plane of anaesthesia, with 100% oxygen and follows meticulous oropharyngeal suctioning. The laryngeal mask airway is inserted and inflated behind the tracheal tube, which in turn is deflated and removed. The laryngeal mask may then be removed in recovery ensuring minimal interference or stimulation. This should be undertaken with the patient placed in an upright position, and a bite block may be inserted to minimize airway obstruction.[34]

The aim is to achieve an awake, comfortable patient who has a clear protected airway, is normotensive, and has no nausea or vomiting. This optimizes patient experience, and reduces haematoma formation. Where possible, the patient should be nursed in an upright position to promote venous drainage and minimize facial oedema.

Blood pressure management

Systemic blood pressure may elevate on emergence from anaesthesia, and may require active treatment to minimize haematoma formation, particularly following face lift or blepharoplasty surgery. Pain and postoperative nausea and vomiting should be treated promptly to avoid the associated sympathetic response. Hypertension may be addressed with increments of intravenous labetalol or hydralazine (if not contraindicated), depending on the patient's heart rate. Alternatives include sublingual nifedipine or intravenous clonidine, the latter having additional analgesic properties.

Nausea and vomiting

Prophylaxis should be the tenet of care for these patients. TIVA, avoidance of nitrous oxide, and administration of ondansetron 4–8 mg and cyclizine 50 mg contributes to minimizing the postoperative risk of nausea and vomiting. Dexamethasone 3.3–6.6 mg is also useful given its dual effect on reducing oedema as well as antiemesis.

Cooling masks

Hilotherapy delivers cooled, temperature-regulated water through a contoured, anatomically designed face mask. While there is no high-quality evidence for its use currently, systematic reviews suggest that it is well tolerated by patients and that it reduces oedema and pain in the immediate postoperative recovery period.[36,37]

Analgesia

Generally, orofacial aesthetic procedures are not particularly painful, being largely superficial surgery, where good-quality local or regional anaesthesia has also been used. Nevertheless, intravenous opioids may still be required in the immediate recovery period. At discharge, a balanced approach to analgesia should be employed, with regular paracetamol, supplemented by codeine, dihydrocodeine, or tramadol. Non-steroidal anti-inflammatories may also be utilized, reducing opioid requirements (and the associated risk of nausea and vomiting). Cyclooxygenase-2 (COX-2) inhibitors may be preferable due to the lesser effect on platelet function; however, the potential increased risk of cardiovascular complications must also be considered.

Common orofacial aesthetic procedures and the principal anaesthetic considerations are summarized in **Table 9.1** and discussed in more detail below.

Table 9.1 Common orofacial aesthetic procedures and considerations for anaesthesia

Site	Procedure	Duration	Pain	Anaesthetic modality	Airway management	Anaesthetic considerations	Other
Upper face	Blepharoplasty (upper)	60–90 minutes	Minimal, with appropriate local anaesthesia (LA) intraoperatively; use of longer-acting bupivacaine for post-procedure reduction in pain	LA +/− sedation, or general anaesthesia (GA)	If GA, usually supraglottic airway device (SAD) unless contraindicated	Requires stationary patient under sedation. Intense stimulation on LA infiltration, followed by minimal surgical stimulus. May require eye opening intraoperatively if ptosis surgery	Postoperative haematoma risk—ensure adequate analgesia, prevention of nausea and vomiting, and good blood pressure control. Ensure patient aware of eye padding on emergence
	Blepharoplasty (lower)	60–120 minutes	Moderate	LA +/− sedation, GA	SAD unless contraindicated	LA may not cover all areas	Good blood pressure control
	Brow lift	30–90 minutes	Minimal if direct or local approach; moderate if endoscopic approach	LA + sedation; GA if endoscopic approach or if combined with blepharoplasty	SAD or tracheal tube (SAD may dislodge with head movement)	Dry surgical field	May be combined with blepharoplasty
Middle face	Face lift (rhytidectomy)	2–5 hours	Mild–moderate	LA +/− sedation possible if superficial; GA if deeper dissection or if combined with other procedures	SAD or tracheal tube (SAD may dislodge with head movement. Tracheal tube best for longer cases). May be difficult to secure tracheal tube	Identify potential bleeding points intraoperatively. May require tranexamic acid	Postoperative haematoma risk—ensure adequate analgesia, prevention of nausea and vomiting, and good blood pressure control
	Rhinoplasty	1–4 hours	May be minimal; moderate if osteotomies or if rib graft used	GA	Flexible SAD or reinforced tracheal tube	Dry surgical field; nasal decongestant; avoid distortion of upper lip when securing airway device	May require tranexamic acid to minimize bleeding +/− dexamethasone to reduce oedema
	Otoplasty	60–90 minutes	Minimal	LA or GA (usually children)	If GA, SAD unless contraindicated	Head movement on changing sides	
Lower face	Genioplasty	30–90 minutes	Minimal if implant used; moderate if sliding genioplasty	LA +/− sedation or GA	SAD; nasotracheal tube if intermaxillary fixation	Avoid pressure on the chin postoperatively	
	Liposuction	30–90 minutes	Mild	LA +/− sedation if sole procedure	Nasal cannulae oxygen with end-tidal carbon dioxide monitoring	Large doses of LA—ensure care with maximum doses	
Other	Laser superficial lesions	Varies depending on site and size	Mild–moderate	Usually LA/regional; may require GA for children; oral sedation may suffice	SAD for GA unless contraindicated	Laser fire hazard—use lowest oxygen concentration and protective safety measures	Ensure laser safety protection for patient and staff
	Insertion of on-lay implants for augmentation	60–90 minutes	Mild	LA +/− sedation or GA (depends on surgical site)	SAD unless contraindicated	Commonly cheek, jaw, chin implants	
	Autologous fat transfer	60–120 minutes	Mild	LA +/− sedation, GA		Large doses tumescent LA—care with maximum doses	

Blepharoplasty

Blepharoplasty may be performed on the upper or lower eyelids and is the third most frequently undertaken aesthetic procedure in the UK.[2] Upper blepharoplasty, to correct hooding of the eyes, is the most common of the two, and may be performed for both functional and aesthetic reasons. It is sometimes also combined with a brow lift. Lower lid blepharoplasty may be performed either via transconjunctival or transcutaneous approaches, and aims to achieve a youthful appearance and a smooth continuum of the lower lid and midface, and it may be combined with midface surgery. Isolated blepharoplasty can be performed under LA with sedation or GA. Skin markings are performed in the sitting and lying position prior to anaesthesia. Proxymetacaine eye drops are first administered topically. Tetracaine drops, which are more potent, are also used but should be administered after the proxymetacaine as they cause considerable discomfort. A rubber corneal shield, generously

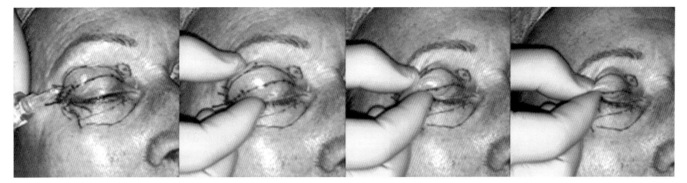

Fig. 9.1 Infiltration of the upper eyelid using the 'pinch and roll' technique.

covered with ocular surface lubricant, is used to protect the cornea during surgery. LA mixture is injected subcutaneously using a 30 G needle. The 'pinch and roll' technique separates the orbicularis from the skin, creating a subcutaneous, relatively avascular plane for injection[38,39] (Fig. 9.1). LA injection is the most stimulating phase of the surgery, with speed of injection proportional to patient discomfort, and maximal analgesia should pre-empt injection. The medial half of both eyelids (at the pretarsal zone, near the eyelashes) and the medial canthal region are the most sensitive areas.

Adequate LA renders the operative site insensate during the procedure. Once the LA has taken effect, there is very little surgical stimulation for the remainder of the procedure. Addition of bupivacaine together with the lidocaine and adrenaline mixture, prolongs the duration of the LA. Ocular/ophthalmic complications during blepharoplasty are extremely rare, but may be associated with inadvertent patient movement or hypertension. Effective LA administration improves patient cooperation, reduces perioperative hypertension, and minimizes unwanted patient movements during surgery in this delicate area. For GA, limiting coughing at tracheal extubation and treating postoperative nausea and vomiting promptly may also reduce any risk.[40]

Occasionally, patient participation may be required intraoperatively, to open and close their eyes, particularly in ptosis surgery—in order to gauge lid position. Sedation techniques, such as propofol target-controlled infusions, may facilitate this. A single prophylactic dose of intravenous antibiotics, meticulous skin preparation (with water-based iodine or chlorhexidine), and topical chloramphenicol are employed to reduce the risk of infection. Simple oral analgesia is generally sufficient postoperatively. The eyes are padded for several hours after the procedure, and the patient should be prewarned of this to reduce anxiety/disorientation in the recovery room.

Brow lift

Ageing of the brow may cause ptosis due to loss of volume, or can be positional relating to laxity of the frontalis muscle.[39] There are several treatment options:

- Botox injection may be used to correct brow ptosis in appropriately selected patients, performed as an outpatient, with minimal risks associated. Results are temporary and therefore repeated treatments are required, and it is not universally successful.
- Surgical brow lifts can be direct (in the supra-brow region), local (pre-trichial, at the forehead and near the lower hairline),[38] or distant (endoscopic or transcranial). A modification of the direct

lift is the 'crenated browlift', which involves a zigzag incision (to disguise the scar) just above the eyebrow, with resection of skin, subcutaneous tissue, and muscle. The direct and local approaches can be performed with regional anaesthesia, but the distant approaches often require sedation or GA. The post-trichial endoscopic approach allows access to the brow as well as the midfacial area.[41] GA is preferred since extensive deep dissection, within multiple tissue planes, may be required—including detachment of the firmly adherent periosteum from the underlying bone, which can be extremely uncomfortable. Continuous intraoperative infusion of remifentanil is particularly well suited, titrated to the varying magnitude of surgical stimulus. The airway is usually away from the site of surgery, and may be secured in the usual manner, although care should be taken during head turning, such that a tracheal tube may be preferred to a supraglottic airway device (SAD).

Surgical face lift (rhytidectomy)

Face lift surgery is only the seventh most common aesthetic surgical procedure in the UK.[2] Less invasive techniques that utilize limited incisions and fewer dissection planes (minimizing patient discomfort and complications) are more popular. Almost all modern face lift surgery is performed using the superficial muscular aponeurotic system (SMAS). Cutaneous facelifts are now only performed for select patients, such as those with skin disorders or the more elderly patient, as the skin is not a good vehicle for repositioning descended facial tissues. SMAS flaps and lateral SMAS-ectomy are the main techniques for facial rejuvenation. SMAS plication may be helpful in patients who have undergone multiple surgical procedures to decrease the risk to the facial nerve, but results are often short-lived. In line with patient demand for more minimally invasive procedures and faster recovery, non-surgical procedures such as thread lifts and minimal access cranial suspension lifts are becoming increasingly popular. These can be performed under LA, though, like SMAS plication, the results are often not long-lasting. Endoscopic brow lifts and SMAS facelifts can often be combined, and produce a more harmonious rejuvenation. Face lifts may also be combined with other rejuvenating surgery such as blepharoplasty, liposuction, or removal of submental/submandibular fat.

Face lift surgery is generally performed under GA. TIVA or inhalational anaesthetic techniques may be used, though TIVA is generally preferred. Surgery may be prolonged, sometimes taking up to 5 hours, therefore maintenance of normothermia, venous

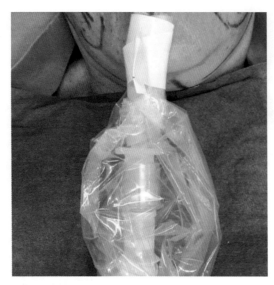

Fig. 9.2 Sterile draping of the breathing circuit within the sterile surgical field.

thromboembolic prophylaxis, protection of pressure areas and eyes, and close attention to optimizing fluid balance are essential. The greatest challenge is ensuring that any airway device is not interfering with the surgical field, and that it remains secure during head turning. Either a flexible laryngeal mask airway or a tracheal tube may be used; however, a RAE tube offers a degree of security while also enabling positioning away from the surgical field. The airway device may be held in place with either tape or ties if access to the lower jaw is permitted, or may be left un-taped, relying upon care from the surgeon to not dislodge it. The breathing circuit can be contained within a sterile clear drape such that it can pass through/over the sterile field and enable the surgeon to move the breathing circuit in concert with the head[13] (Fig. 9.2). Alternatively, a reinforced tracheal tube can be used, sutured to the mandibular dentition.[42]

Facial nerve monitoring may be used to minimize the risk of nerve damage during flap dissection. In such cases, neuromuscular blocking agents should be avoided at tracheal intubation. Where a judicious dose of neuromuscular blocking agent is necessary to facilitate challenging airway management, quantitative neuromuscular monitoring is advisable to ensure return of neuromuscular function before surgery commences—by the time the patient has been positioned, skin preparation performed, and surgical drapes applied, pharmacological reversal is rarely required.

Postoperative haematoma formation is the most common and serious complication,[43,44] with an incidence of 0.2–8% (depending on the definition of haematoma). One of the most important risk factors that has been identified is hypertension—either pre-existing uncontrolled hypertension, or rebound hypertension following surgery.[6,44] To minimize the risk of hypertension and haematoma formation, care and attention should be paid to the following: avoidance of coughing and straining at time of tracheal extubation; restoration of normotension prior to skin closure to identify bleeding points; control of postoperative blood pressure; nursing with head elevated in the recovery period; prevention and prompt treatment of postoperative nausea and vomiting; avoidance of excessive intravenous fluids, which may cause bladder distension, discomfort, and agitation; and, adequate analgesia. Intraoperative hypotensive

anaesthesia may contribute to postoperative haematoma formation if bleeding points are not identified before the end of surgery, in addition to the potential associated risk of 'rebound' hypertension.[44] Other risk factors include male sex, smoking, and preoperative non-steroidal anti-inflammatories.[6] There is little consensus on the optimal method for postoperative blood pressure control. The key is prompt management after excluding/treating pain. In patients without pre-existing hypertension, a systolic blood pressure of <140 mmHg is often targeted.[13,44,45]

Pain is generally mild to moderate following facelift procedures. LA infiltration at the time of surgery and simple analgesics such as paracetamol, codeine/dihydrocodeine, or tramadol normally suffice.

The surgeon and anaesthetist should ensure that they (or a nominated colleague) are immediately available during the postoperative recovery period in case urgent haematoma evacuation is required.

Rhinoplasty

Rhinoplasty surgery involves modifying the shape of the nose for aesthetic purposes, and is the fifth most popular cosmetic surgery in the UK.[2] Possible reasons for rhinoplasty include hump or saddle nose, nasal length too short or too long, previous nasal fracture/trauma, or bent/buckled nose structure. It may also be combined with a septoplasty to improve nasal breathing, in which case the procedure is termed functional septorhinoplasty. There are two main rhinoplasty approaches—closed and open—depending upon patient requirements and surgeon preference.

Closed rhinoplasty corrects the nasal structures via an incision inside the nose, and visible scars are avoided. Open rhinoplasty requires a transcolumellar incision in combination with an internal incision, allowing elevation of a nasal skin flap, and degloving of the lower alar cartilages for direct and wide exposure of the nasal frame. The skin of the nose tip is carefully lifted and the nasal cartilages and bones are surgically corrected. At the end of the surgery, the incisions are closed with fine suture material. The small incisions usually heal very well, and in most cases are barely noticeable after a few months. There is currently a trend towards more open surgery. Postoperative pain is similar whether an open or closed technique is used. Although the skin incision is tiny, the operative field is much bigger, with dissection from the nasolabial angle to the nasion, extending to the lateral nasal sidewall. If the Piezo technique is used to cut the bone for remodelling, there is even wider undermining, almost to the infraorbital nerve. When osteotomies are performed, there is increased surgical stimulus regardless of the technique used.

Lidocaine with adrenaline is delivered into the septum by injection into the columella and base of septum—which is covered by squamous epithelium, so will not absorb topically applied LA (Fig. 9.3a). The long sphenopalatine nerves (from the sphenopalatine ganglion) innervate the posterior two-thirds of the septum and lateral walls, and may be regionally blocked with lidocaine/adrenaline. The skin is innervated by the ophthalmic and maxillary division of the trigeminal nerve. The infraorbital nerve (a branch of the maxillary nerve) innervates the lateral aspect. The intertrochlear branches and the anterior ethmoidal branch of the nasociliary nerve (both from the ophthalmic division) supply the skin from the superior to inferior aspect respectively. The infraorbital nerve may be blocked with bupivacaine 0.5% and adrenaline 1:200,000 to aid postoperative analgesia (Fig. 9.3b).

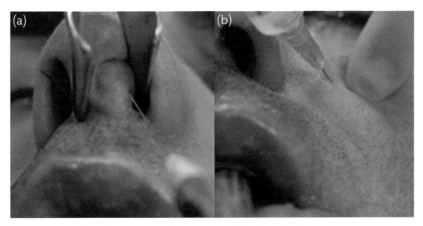

Fig. 9.3 Local anaesthetic injection sites for rhinoplasty surgery: (a) septum and (b) infraorbital nerve.

Nerve blocks with adrenaline also assist in decreasing bleeding at the site of surgery, optimizing the surgical field, so early administration ensures maximal efficacy during surgery.[46]

The nasal mucosa and nasopharynx are highly vascular zones, and a topical vasoconstrictor is often administered alongside the LA injected by the surgeon. Gauze soaked in cocaine (4–5%), a potent vasoconstrictor, can be used to pack the nasal cavities to provide a relatively avascular field. Similarly, Moffett's solution, containing cocaine, sodium bicarbonate, and adrenaline, may be used (constituent quantities tend to vary between institutions, and do not necessarily conform to the traditional description).[47] Care must be heeded in patients with cardiovascular disease, with particular vigilance for hypertension following surgical co-infiltration of adrenaline. Ideally, Moffett's solution is administered with the patient in the head-down position to facilitate pooling in the nasopharynx. Any excess volume can be absorbed by prior placement of an appropriately positioned throat pack (with the throat pack removed before commencing surgery) or by careful suctioning of the oropharynx, preventing postoperative mucosal injury/oropharyngeal discomfort from the residual solution. A safe approach to the use of throat packs (discussed in Chapter 10) must be employed. Alternatively, premixed co-phenylcaine spray (lidocaine 5% with phenylephrine 0.5%) can be used, which ensures a standardized concentration, and avoids some of the safety issues surrounding storage and clinical use of cocaine. Some surgeons simply use adrenaline-soaked patties, but the key to all methods is to allow at least 10–15 minutes for them to be effective.

Rhinoplasty and septorhinoplasty are most commonly performed under GA. The standard requirements are a stationary patient, dry surgical field, and smooth emergence from anaesthesia. A tracheal tube (usually a RAE tube) or a flexible reinforced laryngeal mask airway are most commonly used. Care must be taken when securing the airway device not to distort the upper lip. Blood contamination of the airway is minimized with meticulous surgical technique (dissection in the correct tissue plane), moderate controlled hypotension, and head-up positioning. If a throat pack is used, again, recommended safety strategies must be applied. Cranial nerves X and XII may be vulnerable to injury within the oropharynx, caused by compression from the airway device or throat pack, particularly during excessive head and neck manipulation. Care must therefore be taken to avoid excessive pressure that may result in the extremely

rare Tapia syndrome—paralysis of the hypoglossal and recurrent laryngeal branch of the vagus nerve.[48]

TIVA is well suited to the variations in magnitude of surgical stimulation, and may also facilitate a smooth emergence. A bolus of a longer-acting opioid towards the end of the procedure may also facilitate tracheal extubation without coughing or hypertension—particularly in combined osteotomy or turbinate surgery where there may be increased risk of bleeding. A cast is placed over the nose at the end of surgery, and care must be taken not to apply pressure to or alter the shape of this during emergence or postoperative recovery. Sometimes internal nasal splints or nasal packs are also placed, which may decrease or obstruct the nasal airway temporarily.

If a septal, temporalis fascia, or ear cartilage harvest have been required (or there is a concomitant septoplasty), postoperative pain is usually kept to a minimum by LA infiltration at the relevant anatomical sites. In ear cartilage harvest, postoperative pain may result from the pressure dressing (required for 2–5 days) applied to prevent conchal bowl haematoma. Rib grafts can be harvested from the medial part of the fifth to ninth ribs (generally the sixth or seventh is used). As the principal surgeon usually stands on the right-hand side of the patient, an assistant may harvest the bone from the left-hand side, or sometimes the opposing side to sleeping tendency is chosen. A Valsalva manoeuvre assists in detecting iatrogenic pneumothorax, in which case a chest drain may be required. Rib harvest may increase analgesic requirements postoperatively, and a continuous LA infusion (via a locally placed catheter) may be of benefit for the first 24 hours.

Otoplasty

Excessively protruding ears is one of the most common facial cosmetic complaints. It is most likely due to insufficient development of the ear cartilage, and/or incorrect position of the ear in relation to the skull. This can sometimes lead to emotional/psychological distress, especially in children, relating to teasing or bullying from peers, and surgical cosmetic correction may be offered. Although it can be performed at any age, it is preferable to complete the surgery before starting school if possible. Surgery is performed via an incision posterior to the pinna, which is subsequently barely detectable. The shape and position of the exterior ear and ear cartilage are altered, and once in the desired position, closed with absorbable sutures. In adults, this procedure may be performed under LA. In children, GA is required alongside LA infiltration, and a laryngeal mask airway usually provides sufficient airway protection (anaesthesia management of paediatric patients is discussed in detail in Chapter 11). Pain following the procedure is minimal, and aside from wearing a protective headband, no specific aftercare is required.

Facial augmentation

On-lay implants (implants that lie on top of the bone) may be inserted through small skin incisions to add volume to the face. Amenable areas are the malar region, chin, and mandible. The procedure can be undertaken under LA alone, LA plus sedation, or GA.

The least complicated method for chin augmentation (genioplasty) is to insert a suitably sized horseshoe-shaped silicone or porous high-density polyethylene implant. This shape of implant does not produce pressure on underlying bone and cause consequent atrophy. It is possible to insert the implant through a submental skin incision or an infralabial (labial sulcus) approach without visible scars. Genioplasty can also be performed by repositioning the bone itself. This operation is carried out intraorally, so that there are no visible skin scars. An incision through the gum on the inside of the lower lip allows access to the mandible, where an osteotomy can then be performed and secured with small metal plates and screws. A LA nerve block of the mental nerve with a long-acting LA and adrenaline reduces intraoperative bleeding and postoperative pain.

Liposuction

Liposuction is the aspiration of unwanted fat deposits from under the skin using a cannula. The procedure can reduce volume, induce skin retraction, and restore a youthful appearance. For facial aesthetics, it is usually performed to the neck or for facial contouring, and LA will normally suffice, unless it is undertaken as part of another surgical procedure. The tumescent anaesthesia technique of subcutaneous infiltration of high volumes of dilute LA (typically lidocaine 0.05% or 0.1%, 0.9% sodium chloride solution, and adrenaline) is used for anaesthesia, and hydrodissection to reduce blood loss (care must be taken to calculate the maximum doses to avoid toxicity). Only small volumes of fat are aspirated from the neck, such that complications associated with large volume liposuction from other areas of the body are less likely; however, awareness of the potential for venous thromboembolism, fat embolism, and fluid overload must be maintained.

Autologous fat transfer

Lipofilling is used in aesthetic surgery to provide volume or for smoothing of areas of the face subject to atrophy ('hollow' appearance), such as the cheek, periorbital region, and mandible. The fat is removed using targeted 'mini-liposuction' in one anatomical area, such as the abdomen or upper thigh. The Coleman technique is the gold standard method, divided into three stages: lipoaspiration under low pressure, centrifugation for 3 minutes at 2500–3000 rpm, and reinjection in three dimensions.[49] A tumescent anaesthesia technique is often used in conjunction with a GA, and the fat transfer may be performed alone or in combination with other procedures. The potential advantage of autologous fat grafting as opposed to synthetic fillers is that it is biocompatible, naturally integrating into tissues (and the local blood supply). The fat also contains adipose-derived stem cells, with potential regenerative properties. Surgeons may wish for patients to receive 1 week of oral antibiotics following surgery.

Considerations for non-surgical facial aesthetic procedures

Non-surgical aesthetic procedures, like Botox injection and dermal fillers, are very popular, with the number of patients undergoing such treatments rising every year. They are most often performed under topical anaesthesia, cold packs, or regional LA nerve blocks (e.g. infraorbital or mental nerves).

Botox

For Botox treatments of the face, no anaesthetic is necessary, as tiny needles (30–33 G) are used with only a small volume of injectate. However, treatments for hyperhidrosis in the hands or feet may require topical anaesthesia or a regional nerve block as they require larger volumes to be injected. Effects are seen within 72 hours and typically last 3 months. Complications are rarely seen; however, they may include haematoma formation, infection at the injection site, injection of the incorrect target muscle, and, extremely rarely, anaphylaxis.

Fillers

There are different types of filler, but currently hyaluronic acid is the most commonly used. Duration of desired effects depends upon the type of filler used. Pain during injection of dermal fillers varies with the injection site and the volume injected. One of the challenges is to find the best approach for each different patient and treatment, ranging from the application of ice packs or cooling sprays, to topical application of LA (e.g. lidocaine or prilocaine), to short-acting LA infiltration and regional nerve blocks. Localized oedema is relatively common, for 2–3 days post treatment. Complications are more common with permanent fillers, including tissue necrosis, granuloma formation, and foreign body inflammatory reactions.

Laser

The use of lasers in aesthetic practice is increasing. While surgery can improve the laxity of skin and shape of a facial feature, lasers may improve the tone, texture, pigmentation, and quality of the skin. In facial aesthetic practice, lasers are principally used for skin rejuvenation, but can be used for a wide variety of indications, including treatment of port-wine stains, facial telangiectasia, small-vessel disorders, vascular lesions, pigmented lesions, and tattoo and hair removal. The laser procedure may be performed alone, or in combination with other surgical/non-surgical procedures. The type of laser selected depends upon the particular lesion and the effect that is desired. While laser treatments are usually performed under topical or local/regional anaesthesia, anaesthetists may be required for paediatric cases, poorly tolerant adult patients, or for large lesions. As the treatments may also be carried out in the operating theatre as an adjunct to other operative procedures, anaesthetists must be familiar with the risks associated with laser use and the safety strategies employed.

Categories of laser

Lasers can be categorized as ablative or non-ablative, and fractionated or non-fractionated.[50] Ablative lasers are the most aggressive, vaporizing tissue and removing the whole epidermal layer. Consequently, they have the longest downtime period for healing with the greatest degree of discomfort, but the most effective results. Non-ablative lasers are gentler, inducing controlled tissue injury to the dermis, leaving the epidermis intact, and stimulating dermal remodelling and collagen production. The effects are more moderate, and the downtime for healing is significantly less compared with ablative therapies; however, repeated treatments are necessary to achieve the desired effect. Fractionated lasers target a small portion of the treatment area, whereas non-fractionated lasers act on the entire projected surface of the treated skin.[50] Non-ablative fractionated lasers may be considered to offer the best of both worlds—achieving effects close to ablative laser procedures with multiple treatments and shorter recovery times.

Radiofrequency therapy is another non-ablative therapeutic modality used for skin rejuvenation. It produces a controlled increase in tissue temperature in order to stimulate changes in collagen within skin cells. It has a high penetration depth, and with relatively low operating temperatures, it may spare the skin from damage.

Topical anaesthesia for laser surgery

There are several options for topical anaesthesia for facial laser therapies, dictated by the size of intended treatment area, the anatomical location, the skin depth required to be effective, the duration of LA required, and the safety profile of the LA. In common use is EMLA™ (Eutectic Mixture of Local Anaesthetic) topical cream, which contains 2.5% lidocaine, 2.5% prilocaine, and a fatty acid emulsifier. It reaches a depth of 3 mm at 60 minutes and 5 mm at 120 minutes. It produces vasoconstriction within the first 90 minutes and then rebound vasodilation and erythema.[51]

Cryoanaesthesia for laser surgery

This modality provides anaesthesia by cooling the epidermis, and may confer some thermal protection during laser therapy. Contact cooling involves direct application of a cooling system (e.g. cold water or ice) to the skin. Some lasers have an integrated cooling tip or 'finger'. Non-contact cooling is where the cooling effect is transferred via a gaseous medium, either by the evaporation of liquid (cold spray) or by the blowing of cold air onto the skin. Cryoanaesthesia can be used in conjunction with topical anaesthesia.[51]

Laser safety

All personnel should have appropriate training in the safe use of lasers in the medical environment.[52] Precautions mainly pertain to minimizing fire risk and the protection of patients and staff from the potentially damaging effects of lasers.

A fire risk exists when the three essential elements of the 'fire triad' are present—an oxidizer (oxygen or nitrous oxide), a fuel (tracheal tube, surgical drape, sponge or gauze, oxygen masks or nasal cannulae, alcohol-based skin preparations), and an ignitor (laser, electrocautery). Fire risk can be minimized by addressing each of the three 'fire triad' elements in turn. The lowest inspired oxygen concentration with the lowest flows should be used, and nitrous oxide should be avoided. Closed breathing circuits should be used where possible, and circuit leaks minimized. Surgical drapes should be well configured and vented to prevent oxygen pooling. Any surgical sponges or swabs should be kept moist, and alcohol-based skin preparations should be applied carefully to avoid pooling, allowed to air-dry, or avoided completely. Laser-safe equipment should be used, and only operated by a single trained practitioner. Tracheal tube cuffs should be inflated with water, with uncuffed tubes avoided, and laser-resistant tracheal tubes used if indicated (e.g. for surgery around the airway). The risks relating to laser surgery within the airway are not discussed in detail here as the lasers used for aesthetic purposes are typically employed externally. However, if the airway device being used during non-airway surgery is not laser resistant, it is advisable to protect it with aluminium foil or damp swabs when a laser is in use.

In the event of a laser fire, the laser should be deactivated immediately, any burning material removed, and the area should be flooded with 0.9% saline solution to extinguish the fire (a saline-soaked gauze or towel can be used to pat the area if it is small). A carbon dioxide fire extinguisher or fire blanket should be used if flames are not immediately controlled. In the event of an airway fire (involving the patient's airway or *in situ* airway device), gas flows should be discontinued and the airway device removed immediately, followed by flooding of the area with 0.9% saline. Airway control and manual ventilation should be re-established as soon as possible (usually with tracheal intubation), and the patient assessed for inhalational injury and airway burns.[53,54]

The eyes are particularly susceptible to damage from lasers, either directly or through reflection of the beam. The optical gain of the eye can result in a concentrated area of radiant energy falling on the cornea or retina, potentially resulting in permanent damage in a matter of seconds. Carbon dioxide lasers can cause serious corneal injury, whereas argon, KTP (potassium titanyl phosphate), and Nd:YAG (neodymium-doped yttrium aluminium garnet) lasers may burn the retina. The eyes of both the patient and operating theatre personnel should be protected by approved laser safety glasses appropriate to the type of laser in use (wavelength specific). Regular eyeglasses may provide sufficient protection, but contact lenses will not. Protective eyewear should be a good fit, undamaged with no surface reflections, incorporate side-shields, provide a damage threshold of >10 seconds, display permanent labels detailing the wavelength and optical density tolerance, and must be approved by the institution's laser safety officer. If patient protective eyewear interferes with the operative field, moistened sterile eye pads can be used to protect the eyes. Scleral/corneal protective shields are also available for surgery performed near or on the eyelids. All operating theatre windows must be covered with an opaque material that will absorb the appropriate wavelength of the particular laser, and specially designed warning signs should be displayed.[52,53]

During laser use, a bioaerosol of very small particles (smoke plume) may be released during the destruction of skin cells, which may contain hair, desiccated cells (viable and non-viable cellular material), prions, or other harmful matter. In addition to the smoke plume, noxious gaseous fumes or vapours can be emitted, which may have toxic or carcinogenic constituents.[52] Consequently, face masks should be worn by the laser operator and patient, and a smoke evacuator is recommended at the surgical site (operating theatre evacuation/ventilation systems are not effective in the removal of the smoke plume).

Revision surgery

Revision surgery of any type is not uncommon in facial cosmetic surgery. In revision surgery, the anaesthetist should prepare for the duration of the surgical procedure to be significantly prolonged, for any LA infiltration to be less effective due to scarring at the operative site, and for patient analgesic requirements to be considerably higher.

Acknowledgements

The author would like to thank the following for their valued contributions to the chapter: Mr W. N. A. Kirkpatrick, Consultant Craniofacial Plastic Surgeon, Chelsea and Westminster Hospital, London, UK; Mr N. Joshi, Consultant Oculoplastic Surgeon, Chelsea and Westminster Hospital, London, UK; Mr F. C. Bast, Consultant Rhinology and Facial-Plastic Surgeon, Guys' and St Thomas' Hospital, London, UK; Dr B. Norman, Consultant Anaesthetist, Chelsea and Westminster Hospital, London, UK.

REFERENCES

1. Royal College of Surgeons. Professional standards for cosmetic surgery. April 2016. https://rcseng.ac.uk/cosmeticsurgeryst andards

2. British Association of Aesthetic Surgeons. Cosmetic surgery statistics: dad bods and filter jobs. Updated 27 March 2019. https://baaps.org.uk/about/news/1535/cosmetic_surgery_stats_d ad_bods_and_filter_jobs

3. Klein AA, Meek T, Allcock E, Cook TM, Mincher N, Morris C, Nimmo AF, Pandit JJ, Pawa A, Rodney G, Sheraton T, Young P. Recommendations for standards of monitoring during anaesthesia and recovery 2021. *Anaesthesia*. 2021;**76**:1212–1223.

4. American Society of Anesthesiologists. ASA physical status classification system. Updated 23 October 2019. https://www. asahq.org/standards-and-guidelines/asa-physical-status-classif ication-system

5. Hartle A, McCormack T, Carlisle J, Pichel A, Woodcock T, Heagerty A. The measurement of adult blood pressure and management of hypertension before elective surgery. Joint Guidelines from the Association of Anaesthetists of Great Britain and Northern Ireland and the British Hypertension Society. *Anaesthesia*. 2016;**71**(3):326–337.

6. Grover R, Jones BM, Waterhouse N. The prevention of haematoma following rhytidectomy: a review of 1078 consecutive facelifts. *Br J Plast Surg*. 2001;**54**(6):481–486.

7. Nekhendzy V, Ramaiah VK. Prevention of perioperative and anesthesia-related complications in facial cosmetic surgery. *Facial Plast Surg Clin N Am*. 2013;**21**(4):559–577.

8. Ahlstrom KK, Frodel JL. Local anesthetics for facial plastic procedures. *Otolaryngol Clin North Am*. 2002;**35**(1):29–53.

9. Beck JI, Johnston KD. Anaesthesia for cosmetic and functional maxillofacial surgery. *Cont Educ Anaesth Crit Care Pain*. 2014;**14**(1):38–42.

10. Brunton G, Paraskeva N, Caird J, Schucan Bird K, Kavanagh J, Kwan I, et al. Psychosocial predictors, assessment, and outcomes of cosmetic procedures: a systematic rapid evidence assessment. *Aesth Plast Surg*. 2014;**38**(5):1030–1040.

11. American Society of Anesthesiologists. Continuum of depth of sedation: definition of general anesthesia and levels of sedation/analgesia. Amended 23 October 2019. https://www.asahq.org/ standards-and-guidelines/continuum-of-depth-of-sedation-def inition-of-general-anesthesia-and-levels-of-sedationanalgesia

12. Newton M, Blightman K. *Guidelines for the Provision of Anaesthesia Services (GPAS). Chapter 19: Guidance on the Provision of Sedation Services*. London: Royal College of Anaesthetists; 2016.

13. Forrester P. Anaesthesia and sedation. In: Jones BM, Grover R (eds) *Facial Rejuvenation Surgery*. Philadelphia, PA: Mosby Elsevier; 2008:11–16.

14. Academy of Medical Royal Colleges. Safe sedation practice for healthcare procedures: standards and guidance. 2013. https:// www.aomrc.org.uk/wp-content/uploads/2016/05/Safe_Sedation_ Practice_1213.pdf

15. Taghinia AH, Shapiro FE, Slavin SA. Dexmedetomidine in aesthetic facial surgery: improving aesthetic safety and efficacy. *Plast Reconstr Surg*. 2008;**121**(1):269–276.

16. McMorrow SP, Abramo TJ. Dexmedetomidine sedation: uses in pediatric sedation outside the operating room. *Pediatr Emerg Care*. 2012;**28**(3):292–296.

17. Tobias JD. Dexmedetomidine and ketamine: an effective alternative for procedural sedation? *Pediatr Crit Care Med*. 2012;**13**(4):423–427.

18. Pavlakovic L, Lee G. Anaesthesia for maxillofacial surgery. *Anaesth Intensive Care Med*. 2014;**15**(8):379–384.

19. Athanassoglou V, Patel A, McGuire B, Higgs A, Dover MS, Brennan PA, et al. Systematic review of benefits or harms of routine anaesthetist-inserted throat packs in adults: practice recommendations for inserting and counting throat packs. *Anaesthesia*. 2018;**73**(5):612–618.

20. Bailey CR, Nouraie R, Huitink H. Have we reached the end for throat packs inserted by anaesthetists? Editorial. *Anaesthesia*. 2018;**73**(5):535–548.

21. Nimmo AF, Absalom AR, Bagshaw O, Biswas A, Cook TM, Costello A, et al. Guidelines for the safe practice of total intravenous anaesthesia (TIVA). *Anaesthesia*. 2019;**74**(2):211–224.

22. Pal S, Kumar C. Anaesthesia for aesthetic surgery. In: Shaw I, Kumar CM, Dodds C (eds) *Oxford Textbook of Anaesthesia for Oral and Maxillofacial Surgery*, 1st ed, pp. 131–141. Oxford: Oxford University Press; 2010.

23. Heesen M, Klimek M, Imberger G, Hoeks SE, Rossaint R, Straube S. Co-administration of dexamethasone with peripheral nerve block: intravenous vs perineural application: systematic review, meta-analysis, meta-regression and trial-sequential analysis. *Br J Anaesth*. 2018;**120**(2):212–227.

24. Kurian A, Ward-Booth P. Blood transfusion and orthognathic surgery—a thing of the past? *Br J Oral Maxillofac Surg*. 2004;**42**(4):369–371.

25. Olsen JJ, Skov J, Ingerslev J, Thorn JJ, Pinholt EM. Prevention of bleeding in orthognathic surgery—a systematic review and meta-analysis of randomized controlled trials. *J Oral Maxillofac Surg*. 2016;**74**(1):139–150.

26. Christabel A, Muthusekhar MR, Narayanan V, Ashok Y, Loong Soh C, Ilganovan M, et al. Effectiveness of tranexamic acid on intraoperative loss in isolated Le Fort 1 osteotomies—a prospective, triple blinded randomized clinical trial. *J Craniomaxillofac Surg*. 2014;**42**(7):1221–1224.

27. Ker K, Edwards P, Perel P, Shakur H, Roberts I. Effect of tranexamic acid on surgical bleeding: systematic review and cumulative meta-analysis. *BMJ*. 2012;**344**:e3054.

28. Carlos E, Monnazzi MS, Castiglia YMM, Gabrielli MFR, Passeri LA, Guimaraes NC. Orthognathic surgery with or without induced hypotension. *Int J Oral Maxillofac Surg.* 2014;**43**(5):577–580.

29. Barak M, Yoav L, Abu el-Naaj I. Hypotensive anesthesia versus normotensive anesthesia during major maxillofacial surgery: a review of the literature. *ScientificWorldJournal.* 2015;**2015**:480728.

30. Prasant MC, Kar S, Rastogi S, Mukram Ali F, Mudhol A. Comparative study of blood loss, quality of surgical field and duration of surgery in maxillofacial cases with and without hypotensive anesthesia. *J Int Oral Health.* 2014;**6**(6):18–21.

31. Praveen K, Narayanan V, Muthusekhar MR, Baig MF. Hypotensive anaesthesia and blood loss in orthognathic surgery. *Evid Based Dent.* 2004;**5**(1):16.

32. Wesselink EM, Kappen TH, Torn HM, Slooter AJC, van Klei WA. Intraoperative hypotension and the risk of postoperative adverse outcomes: a systematic review. *Br J Anaesth.* 2018;**121**(4):706–721.

33. Vernooij LM, van Klei WA, Machina M, Pasma W, Beattie WS, Peelen LM. Different methods of modelling intraoperative hypotension and their association with postoperative complications in patients undergoing non-cardiac surgery. *Br J Anaesth.* 2018;**120**(5):1080–1089.

34. Popat M, Mitchell V, Dravid R, Patel A, Swampillai C, Higgs A. Difficult Airway Society Guidelines for the management of tracheal extubation. *Anaesthesia.* 2012;**67**(3):318–340.

35. Nair I, Bailey PM. Use of the laryngeal mask for airway maintenance following tracheal extubation. *Anaesthesia.* 1995;**50**(2):174–175.

36. Bates AS, Knepuk GJ. Systematic review and meta-analysis of the efficacy of hilotherapy following oral and maxillofacial surgery. *Int J Oral Maxillofac Surg.* 2015;**45**(1):110–117.

37. Glass GE, Waterhouse N, Shakib K. Hilotherapy for the management of perioperative pain and swelling in facial surgery: a systematic review and meta-analysis. *Br J Oral Maxillofac Surg.* 2016;**54**(8):851–856.

38. O'Doherty M, Joshi N. The 'bespoke' upper eyelid blepharoplasty and brow rejuvenation. *Facial Plast Surg.* 2013;**29**(4):264–272.

39. Scawn R, Gore S, Joshi N. Blepharoplasty basic for the dermatologist. *J Cutan Aesthet Surg.* 2016;**9**(2):80–84.

40. Mejia JD, Maria Ergo F, Nahai F. Visual loss after blepharoplasty: incidence, management and preventive measures. *Aesthet Surg J.* 2011;**31**(1):21–29.

41. Lee H, Quatela VC. Endoscopic browplasty. *Facial Plast Surg.* 2018;**34**(2):139–144.

42. Dobryansky M, Morrison CM, Zins JE. Patient draping and endotracheal tube positioning during facelift surgery. *Ann Plast Surg.* 2009;**63**(1):9–10.

43. Chaffoo RAK. Complications in facelift surgery: Avoidance and management. *Facial Plast Surg Clin N Am.* 2013;**21**(4):551–558.

44. Trussler AP, Hatef DA, Rohrich RJ. Management of hypertension in the facelift patient: results of a national consensus survey. *Aesthet Surg J.* 2011;**31**(5):493–500.

45. Ramanadham SR, Costa CR, Narasimhan K, Coleman JE, Rohrich RJ. Refining the anesthesia management of the face-lift patient: lessons learned from 1089 consecutive face lifts. *Plast Reconstr Surg.* 2015;**135**(3):723–730.

46. Samil E, Casselden E, Bast F, Whiteley W, Hopkins C, Surda P. Role of local anaesthetic nerve block in patients undergoing endonasal surgery—our experience of 48 patients. *Rhinol Online.* 2018;**1**:90–93.

47. Benjamin E, Wong DK, Choa D. 'Moffett's solution: a review of the evidence and scientific basis for the topical preparation of the nose. *Clin Otolaryngol Allied Sci.* 2004;**29**(6):582–587.

48. Lykoudis EG, Seretis K. Tapia's syndrome: an unexpected but real complication of rhinoplasty: case report and literature review. *Aesthet Plast Surg.* 2011;**36**(3):557–559.

49. Simonacci F, Bertozzi N, Pio Grieco M, Grignaffini E, Raposio E. Procedure, applications and outcome of autologous fat grafting. *Ann Med Surg (Lon).* 2017;**20**:49–60.

50. Preissig J, Hamilton K, Markus R. Current laser resurfacing technologies: a review that delves beneath the surface. *Semin Plast Surg.* 2012;**26**(3):109–116.

51. Gaitan S, Markus R. Anaesthesia methods in laser resurfacing. *Semin Plast Surg.* 2012;**26**(3):117–124.

52. Medicines and Healthcare products Regulatory Agency. *Lasers, Intense Light Source Systems and LEDs—Guidance for Safe Use in Medical, Surgical, Dental and Aesthetic Practices.* London: Medicines and Healthcare products Regulatory Authority; 2015.

53. Association of Anaesthetists of Great Britain & Ireland. 3-7 Patient fire. 2018. https://anaesthetists.org/Portals/0/PDFs/QRH/QRH_3-7_Patient_fire_v1.pdf?ver=2018-07-25-112714-097

54. Ward P. Airway fire. Anaesthesia tutorial of the week (tutorial 353). World Federation of Societies of Anaesthesiologists. 2017. https://resources.wfsahq.org/wp-content/uploads/353_english.pdf

10

Orthognathic surgery

Patrick A. Ward and Michael G. Irwin

Introduction

Orthognathic surgery involves the surgical repositioning of the mandible, maxilla, and/or the dentoalveolar segments, in order to correct malocclusion, craniofacial deformity, or skeletal disproportion (whether congenital, or acquired, e.g. post-traumatic injury, or following treatment of childhood malignancy). It is important to note that, while patients undergoing orthognathic procedures may have a significantly improved aesthetic facial appearance following the surgery, the fundamental purpose is to address underlying functional limitations that will lead to long-term health problems if not corrected. Significant malalignment of the maxilla, mandible, and/or associated dentition can lead to issues with occlusion, bite, chewing, speech, breathing, sleeping, oral and dental hygiene, and the health of the soft tissues, underlying bone, and temporomandibular joints. Untreated, these can lead to excessive erosion and damage, chronic pain syndromes, sleep apnoea and associated sequelae, impaired speech, and significant psychological harm. This type of surgery often represents the final step in a lengthy patient journey, since most of these techniques will not be undertaken until bone maturity, and because they are usually commenced only after more conservative management strategies have failed to correct the facial or dental disharmony. Treatments require extensive planning, are often performed as staged procedures, taking several years to achieve the final result, and involve a large multidisciplinary team.

Preoperative assessment, preparation, and planning

The majority of patients undergoing orthognathic surgery are young and healthy with dental malocclusion, who have reached bone maturity (i.e. late teens, early twenties) and have failed conservative orthodontic treatments. There are, however, a few patients with craniofacial anomalies and syndromes (e.g. Treacher Collins, Goldenhar, Crouzon, Apert, and Nager syndromes; cleft lip and palate) undergoing orthognathic procedures that pose additional challenges relating to airway management and their associated comorbidities. Additionally, there is now also a growing trend in orthognathic surgery to treat patients with severe obstructive sleep apnoea syndrome, such that the patient cohort is becoming increasingly complex, with a greater premorbid burden, placing an even greater importance upon thorough preoperative assessment, optimization, and planning.

A multidisciplinary team approach is essential throughout the patient journey and can involve dentists and dental hygienists; orthodontists; oromaxillofacial, otorhinolaryngology, neuro-, and plastic surgeons; anaesthetists; speech, language, and audiology specialists; psychologists and psychiatrists; dieticians and nutritionists; respiratory and sleep physicians (increasingly important given the evolution of sleep apnoea surgery); radiologists; intensivists; prosthetic specialists; and more.

The contribution from orthodontists, in particular, is fundamental. Having been involved with the patient from the outset with more conservative orthodontic treatment options, they are often the referring specialists to oromaxillofacial surgery, whom they will then work closely with to optimize the surgical outcome. The orthodontist will make dental impressions and occlusal records, create maxillary and mandibular surgical models to plan and guide the best surgical approach (Figs 10.1–10.3), utilize orthodontic braces and appliances to improve preoperative alignment and optimize postoperative dentoskeletal stability, and create bespoke occlusal wafers that are used intraoperatively to locate the dental arches in a pre-planned relationship, to help achieve the desired occlusion. There is an increasing role for computer-aided surgical simulation, or virtual surgical planning, combining three-dimensional tomographic data, digital photographic images, and virtual dental models to assist in accurately preparing these surgical splints and occlusal wafers (Fig. 10.4).

Specialist input from psychiatric and psychological teams is also extremely important. As already mentioned, the timing of surgery is aligned with the onset of bone maturity and, therefore, patients tend to be in their late teens, or early twenties, forming a unique patient cohort that should be recognized as having their own distinct psychosocial challenges. Patients may have undergone many treatments and hospital visits, developing a particular set of behaviours, perceptions, and expectations. Additionally, concerns over body image can be heightened in this age group, especially when there is significant craniofacial deformity, such that all anxieties should

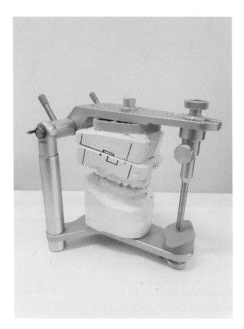
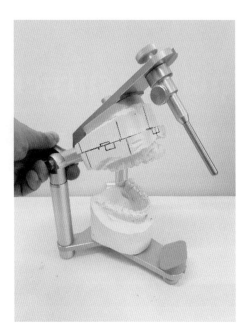
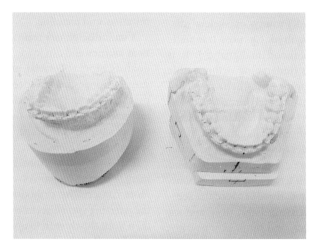

Figs 10.1–10.3 Occlusal records and models created preoperatively to assist in surgical planning.

be explored fully so that they can be optimally managed. Although rarely used, special mention should be made regarding patients treated with monoamine oxidase inhibitors, as there is potential for hypertensive crises in the context of the large volumes of local anaesthetic solutions containing adrenaline that is commonplace during orthognathic surgery. Caution is also warranted if large doses of local anaesthetics are planned to be used in patients taking tricyclic antidepressants because of their structural similarity to local anaesthetics, reduction of the seizure threshold, and propensity for bradycardia and hypotension. Perioperative management of psychoactive drugs should involve a multidisciplinary team approach, with careful consideration of if and when to discontinue medication, minimizing the risk of withdrawal, alternative short-term strategies to manage patients' psychiatric illness, clear planning for recommencement of patients' normal regimens, and involvement of patients' usual mental health support team.

Another subgroup of patients who merit special consideration are those who are taking anticoagulants and/or antiplatelet agents, including direct oral anticoagulants (such as apixaban and rivaroxaban), given the importance of minimizing bleeding intra- and postoperatively. Fortunately, the typical orthognathic patient rarely requires such agents; however, with the increasing trend of surgical intervention for sleep apnoea, this may become a more frequent occurrence (in those with cardiovascular comorbidity). Again, a multidisciplinary approach is indicated, with involvement of patient, surgeon, anaesthetist, haematologist, and cardiologist in order to fully explore the risk/benefit implications, to devise a clear plan for discontinuation of these drugs preoperatively, as well as bridging therapies if indicated.

As mentioned, there appears to be growing evidence to support the referral of patients with severe obstructive sleep apnoea for orthognathic intervention[1] and, with the rates of obesity now reaching epidemic levels in many countries, this trend is only likely to increase. Maxillomandibular advancement (bimaxillary osteotomy) may be effective in such patients, where the site of airway collapse is largely retrolingual, and more conservative strategies such as weight loss, non-invasive ventilation (continuous positive airway pressure (CPAP)), nasal surgery, tongue reduction surgery,

Descriptor	Meas.	Type	Mean	Sd	Patient	Graph	Comment
SNA		Deg	82.0	2.0	75.91	-(* |)+	Maxilla retruded
SNB		Deg	80.0	2.0	80.06	-(*)+	
ANB		Deg	2.0	2.0	-4.15	-(* |)+	Class III relationship
WITS		mm	0.0	1.0	-5.69	-(* |)+	Class III Skeletal problem
UI-PAL.PLANE		Deg	110.0	5.0	117.92	-(|*)+	Upper incisor proclined forward
LI to MAND		Deg	90.0	3.7	84.51	-(*|)+	Lower incisor too upright
Interincisal Angle	/1 to 1/	Deg	131.0	13.0	135.34	-(*)+	
PL-MAND PLANE		Deg	25.0	3.0	22.21	-(*)+	
UPPER FACE HEIGHT	N-ANS	%	45	3.0	43.0	-(*)+	
LOWER FACE HEIGHT	ANS-Gn	%	55.0	3.0	56.83	-(*)+	
RATIO		%	55.0	3.0	56.83	-(*)+	
LI-APOG		mm	1.0	2.0	2.45	-(*)+	
LOWER LIP TO E-LINE		mm	-2.0	2.0	-2.46	-(*)+	
Y AXIS	FH to S-Gn	Deg	59.4	3.8	49.08	-(*|)+	Horizontal growth tendency

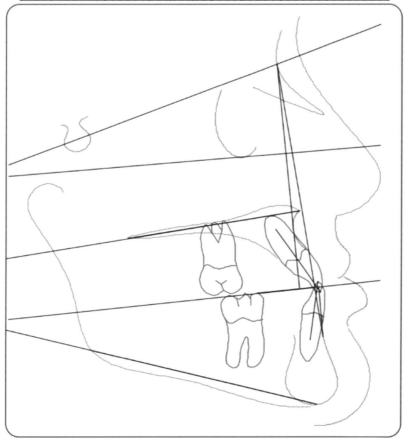

Fig. 10.4 Cephalometric tracing and Eastman analysis, utilized in surgical procedure planning.

and other soft tissue procedures such as uvulopalatopharyngoplasty have failed to improve symptoms. Careful preoperative assessment and planning is essential, with early involvement of respiratory/sleep physicians, combined with specific knowledge and understanding of sleep medicine, the associated metabolic syndrome, obstructive sleep apnoea and obesity hypoventilation syndrome.

Multidisciplinary craniofacial planning meetings can provide an ideal format for all of these diverse specialities to convene and discuss complex patients, to meet and establish a rapport with the patients in person (along with their next of kin), discuss relevant imaging, plan the best surgical approach, and, crucially, highlight and assess patients who may pose particular perioperative risk so that any necessary optimization can be undertaken, and so that

appropriate perioperative management strategies and postoperative care can be organized (e.g. planned postoperative critical care admissions for patients with severe obstructive sleep apnoea or those with predicted difficult airways). Patients identified as high risk can be directed towards the appropriate resources, and should, ideally, be assessed by an anaesthetist with a special interest and in-depth knowledge of these type of surgical procedures. It is unreasonable to expect all anaesthetists to be competent in all areas of anaesthesia and there is a move towards anaesthetic departments consisting of smaller teams of anaesthetists, each with subspeciality skills and knowledge (in this case, a small group of experts in oromaxillofacial anaesthesia and advanced airway management techniques).

Preoperative consent and premedication

High-risk cases should, ideally, have already been assessed, optimized, and a clear plan agreed between patient, surgeon, and anaesthetist. On the day of surgery, patients should be consented for general anaesthesia, with the discussion tailored to cover specific aspects relating to orthognathic surgery. Nasal intubation/nasotracheal tubes should be discussed, with the associated risks of postoperative sore throat, nasal discomfort, and nasal bleeding. If the use of more advanced airway techniques is indicated, such as awake/asleep fibreoptic intubation, submental intubation or tracheostomy, or airway exchange catheters/staged extubation strategies, these should be discussed in detail.

Patients should expect to have blurred vision on emergence due to the water-based lubricant used intraoperatively to protect the eyes (eye tapes/eye guards are frequently contraindicated as they compromise the surgical field and can affect the surgeon's perception of facial symmetry), and this can be particularly distressing if not mentioned preoperatively. Intraoperative use of hypotensive anaesthesia should be specifically discussed, if planned, and consent for blood transfusion obtained if blood loss is expected to be greater than usual (it is rare to require blood transfusion in orthognathic surgery). Salient postoperative points should be addressed, in particular the use of ice-packs/hilotherapy masks to reduce oedema and pain, the use of patient-controlled analgesia (rarely required), the sensation of numbness secondary to local anaesthetic infiltration (very common), and intermaxillary fixation, if being utilized (specifically, the limitations on communication, oral intake, etc. postoperatively).

Chlorhexidine mouthwash (e.g. Corsadyl*) should be administered to all patients preoperatively to reduce the risk of infection. Anxiolytic premedication is rarely indicated but may be required in young, particularly anxious patients. Caution should be taken with the increasing number of patients with obstructive sleep apnoea and their increased sensitivity to sedative medication. Pregabalin is generally safer than benzodiazepines and has additional analgesic properties.

Intraoperative management

Airway management

The patient's airway is 'shared' between anaesthetist and surgeon, therefore a good understanding of each other's requirements and good communication is essential. Oral tracheal tubes are generally contraindicated for orthognathic surgery as they preclude unobstructed surgical access to the oral cavity, maxilla, and mandible, and also prevent dental occlusion being utilized as a reference point for bony fixation. Consequently, nasotracheal intubation is the most common means of securing the airway to optimize surgical access.

For nasal intubation of the trachea, the nasal passages should be prepared with a local anaesthetic and vasoconstrictor spray (e.g. cophenylcaine) to reduce the risk of epistaxis, administered after induction (to prevent the unpleasant burning sensation) and prior to intubation. Various different local anaesthetic and vasoconstrictor combinations have been described, with limited evidence to support the efficacy of one over another.[2] Epistaxis usually results from minor mucosal tears in the anterior nasal septum, but can also occur from avulsion of nasal polyps, and from trauma to the turbinates, tonsils, adenoids, or posterior pharyngeal wall. Fortunately, epistaxis from nasotracheal intubation is usually mild and self-limiting. Pressure from the nasal tube itself can often tamponade the bleeding, but occasionally a nasal tampon or a Foley catheter (with cuff inflated after insertion) may be required. Submucosal placement and the formation of false passages with nasal tubes have been described, which has the potential for retropharyngeal abscess formation, and should be managed with prophylactic antibiotics.

Flexible reinforced/armoured nasal tubes are less likely to kink intraoperatively; however, the softer preformed north-facing polar nasal tubes are less traumatic to introduce and are more conveniently secured in position with tape and padding across the forehead. Nasotracheal tubes should certainly be well lubricated to aid passage, and sized appropriately for the patient to avoid trauma relating to an over-sized tube. The nasal airway should be assessed preoperatively, identifying any history of patency issues, septal deviation, nasal polyps, and so on in order to determine the preferred nostril for intubation. However, enquiry is poorly predictive and flexible nasendoscopy is rarely performed as an objective measure. Elective blind nasal intubation is generally not recommended due to the risk of causing airway trauma and bleeding and, for similar reasons, multiple attempts and the application of excessive force when navigating the nasotracheal tube through the nasal passages should be avoided. Serial dilatation of the nasal passages prior to intubation is not advocated as this also exposes the nasal mucosa to increased risk of trauma.

Asleep fibreoptic nasal intubation is probably best, least traumatic, and allows the anaesthetist to become very familiar with this technique, should it be required in more difficult circumstances. Nasal intubation can, however, usually be safely conducted with direct laryngoscopy or videolaryngoscopy (where mouth opening is not impaired), utilizing Magill forceps to assist in guiding the nasal tube if required. Awake nasal fibreoptic intubation may be required in patients presenting with very severe malocclusion or severe temporomandibular joint pathology who have significantly reduced mouth opening (as will some patients requiring revision surgery), which is unlikely to improve following induction of anaesthesia and neuromuscular blockade, such that an awake technique is the safest option (various approaches to awake fibreoptic intubation are discussed in detail in other chapters).

Thermo-softening of the nasal polar tube (in warm sterile water) is practised in some institutions to make the tube more malleable and less likely to cause trauma on insertion. However, this can make the tube more likely to twist and kink intraoperatively as the tube cools rapidly after removal from the water. Care should be taken to ensure that the nasal tube does not cause traction on the nasal tip/nostril, as this can lead to tissue necrosis in prolonged operations and can also distort the nasal septum during maxillary impaction. This passive positioning of the tube can be achieved by several strategies: securing the tube with tape at the nostril (although this may interfere with the surgical view); providing some 'slack' in the north-facing section of the tube; by securing the tube and breathing circuit on the forehead with a sponge (**Figs 10.5–10.7**) and additional tape around the head (**Figs 10.8 and 10.9**); and by supporting the weight of the breathing circuit using a tube support (orientated in an upside-down position) and breathing circuit ties. These ties also ensure that

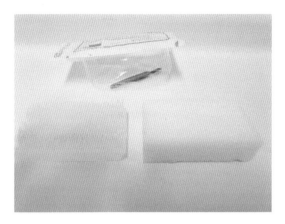

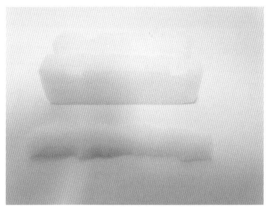

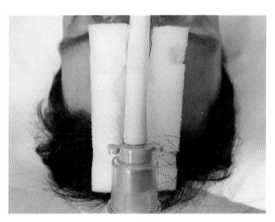

Figs 10.5–10.7 Positioning of polar nasal tube across the forehead using foam sponge from single-use surgical scrub brush (additional tape to secure nasotracheal tube not present in Fig. 10.7).

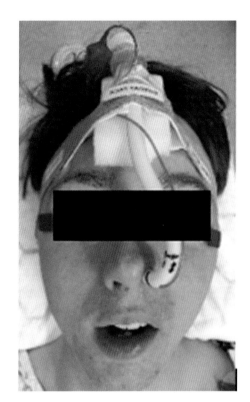

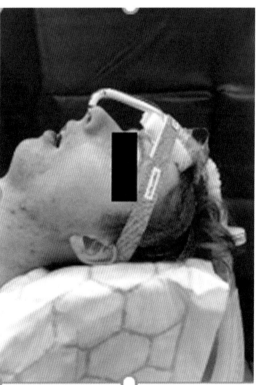

Figs 10.8 and 10.9 Passive positioning of nasotracheal tube, supported by foam block and tape around the head.

the breathing circuit is kept off the operating room floor away from the surgeon's feet, minimizing the risk of accidental occlusion or tracheal extubation. Considerable movement of the head and neck may be required, particularly during temporomandibular joint surgery, and the surgeon may also wish to undrape the face from time to time to assess facial symmetry. Therefore, the nasal tube, connections, and breathing circuit must be very secure. It is important to note that damage to the nasotracheal tube is also a recognized complication during maxillary osteotomy. Loss of tube integrity may be recognized immediately by the surgeon (audible air leak, gurgling, or smell of inhalational anaesthetic), or by failure to adequately ventilate the patient's lungs, or by appearance of blood in the nasal tube and breathing circuit. In this event, it may sometimes be possible

to compensate for small air leaks by packing with surgical swabs; however, an urgent tube exchange may be indicated. Performing a tube exchange in these circumstances may be very difficult, due to restricted access and impaired views, therefore exchange over an exchange catheter is advisable.

Occasionally, nasal intubation may not be possible and alternative strategies for securing the patient's airway and optimizing surgical conditions must be sought. Examples include when nasal passages are obstructed, particular craniofacial malformations, post-surgical intervention (e.g. sometimes after cleft palate repair, depending on the site of surgery), in naso-orbitoethmoidal or base of skull fractures, and in combined orthognathic and rhinoplasty cases.

One such strategy is retromolar intubation, where a reinforced tracheal tube is positioned in the retromolar space, which lies behind the most posterior molars, bounded anteriorly by the last molar and posteriorly by the anterior edge of the ascending mandibular ramus. It is less invasive than the other strategies and, usually, still enables occlusion of the teeth intraoperatively. It is normally performed using a flexible bronchoscope or Bonfils retromolar intubation fibrescope to optimize tube position.

Alternatively, submental intubation may be indicated (especially if the retromolar space is not adequate to allow dental occlusion). This provides unobstructed surgical access to both the nasal and oral cavities, while carrying fewer long-term complications than a surgical tracheostomy and better cosmetic outcome. In this case, the trachea is intubated with an oral tracheal tube (ideally an armoured reinforced tube), which is then passed, after removing the universal connector, through the anterior floor of the mouth via a small midline submental incision made by the surgeon. The universal connector may need to be removed in advance from some reinforced tubes (depending on the manufacturer) and replaced by the connector from a conventional, non-reinforced, tracheal tube (**Figs 10.10–10.12**). Alternatively, a Teleflex intubating laryngeal mask airway (iLMA; Teleflex Medical Europe Ltd, Ireland) tube is ideal for this procedure as it is flexible, reinforced, with a detachable universal connector (**Figs 10.13** and **10.14**). A dilator from a percutaneous tracheostomy set can then be used to assist in dilating the track along which the tracheal tube will pass, and then can be used to facilitate the safe transfer of the pilot balloon and tracheal tube through the submental aperture, in a two-stage process (**Figs 10.15–10.17**). If using the Teleflex iLMA tube, the iLMA introducer can, alternatively, be used to pull the tracheal tube through the submental incision (**Fig. 10.14**).

Finally, a surgical tracheostomy may still be indicated at the time of operation in some patients (very rare in orthognathic surgery). This may be the case when a prolonged period of ventilatory support is anticipated or when reintubation by other means would be impossible in the event of postoperative airway compromise (both submental intubation and surgical tracheostomy, are discussed in detail in Chapter 3).

Throat packs

The *routine* use of throat packs is a controversial area. Historically, throat packs have been used routinely in oral and maxillofacial surgery in an attempt to minimize the passage of blood, liquid nasal vasoconstrictors, secretions, and debris (e.g. bone chips, extracted teeth) down into the airway (theoretically reducing the potential risk of airway compromise, respiratory distress, laryngospasm at extubation of the trachea, and the so-called coroner's clot). Throat packs have also been utilized in an attempt to absorb any blood, with the intention of reducing its ingestion into the stomach, and minimizing the associated emetogenic effect. Throat packs can also be utilized to minimize cuff leak, stabilize the airway device *in situ*,

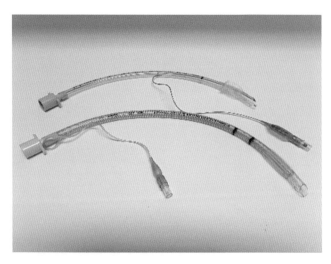
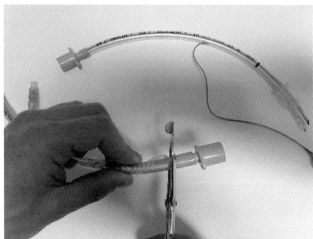
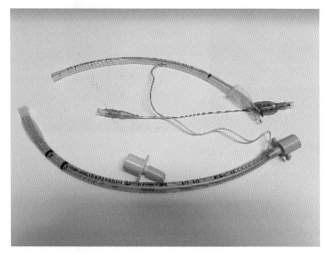

Figs 10.10–10.12 Removal of connector from reinforced tracheal tube and replacement with standard universal connector, to facilitate passage of reinforced tracheal tube through submental incision.

and may also confer some protection to the airway device from accidental damage by the surgeon. However, throat packs have been associated with significant complications, such as infection, bleeding, passage into the oesophagus or stomach, tears to the frenulum, trauma to the soft and hard palate, pharyngeal nerve injury, pharyngeal venous plexus compression ischaemia, death from accidental

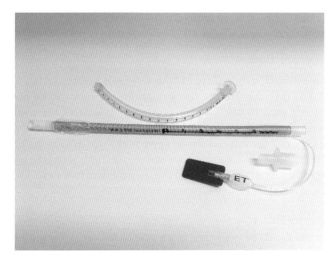

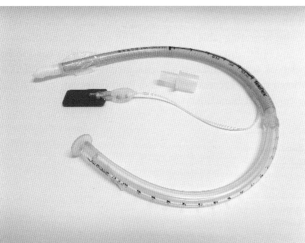

Figs 10.13 and 10.14 Teleflex iLMA tracheal tube with detachable connector and introducer that can be used to pull the tracheal tube through the submental incision.

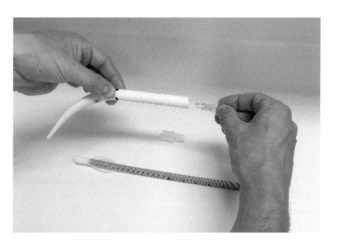

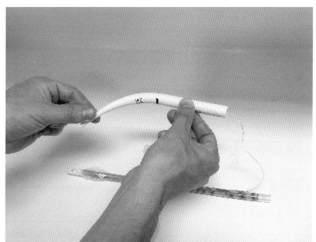

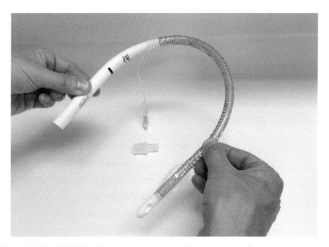

Figs 10.15–10.17 Pilot balloon inserted into lumen of percutaneous tracheostomy dilator, and dilator attached to Teleflex iLMA tracheal tube, to aid passage of pilot balloon and tube through submental incision.

retention at the end of surgery, critical airway obstruction, and hypoxia. Following National Patient Safety Agency alerts relating to accidentally retained throat packs (now considered a 'Never Event' by NHS England), guidance has been produced on minimizing this risk.[3] This guidance has evolved over time, with a range of recommendations made, including allocating responsibility for the throat pack to surgeon or anaesthetist (not both); highlighting the presence of the throat pack by utilizing high-visibility alert stickers in close proximity, on the airway device and/or on the patient; leaving a portion of the throat pack still visible from the mouth (usually precluded in oromaxillofacial surgery due to compromise of the surgical field and impaired surgical access); physically attaching the throat pack to the airway device, to ensure simultaneous removal; careful written documentation of its insertion and removal on the scrub count board and/or in patient notes and anaesthetic chart; formal inclusion of the throat pack in the swab count; the use of radio-opaque strips on the throat pack to facilitate radiological identification; removal by the same person who inserted it; and adaptation of the World Health Organization sign out to include removal of a throat pack as part of the checklist. Unfortunately, despite these recommendations, and others, there have still been significant safety concerns, and further critical incidents reported from their use. This led

to a systematic review of the routine insertion of throat packs by anaesthetists and a subsequent consensus statement from the Difficult Airway Society, the British Association of Oral and Maxillofacial Surgery, and the British Association of Otorhinolaryngology, Head and Neck Surgery.[4] The systematic review found that there is no evidence to support the routine use of throat packs and all available evidence relates to the harmful consequences of their use. Furthermore, with the advances in anaesthetic and surgical techniques (e.g. use of vasoconstrictor solutions), and availability of newer pharmacological agents (e.g. antifibrinolytic agents and remifentanil to reduce bleeding, antiemetics to reduce nausea and vomiting, etc.), the tendency for major bleeding and the associated negative sequelae has been significantly reduced. Interestingly, the systematic review also found that there was no available evidence on the best type of throat pack material, the optimum size (length or width), the ideal preparation (dry, damp, or wet), the recommended position for placement (anterior or posterior), or the best means of insertion of throat packs (blind finger placement or with Magill forceps under direct vision with a laryngoscope). Therefore, the consensus guidance is that throat packs should be avoided where possible, and should not be inserted routinely. If deemed absolutely necessary by the surgeon, the relevant national professional bodies have produced a protocol (**Fig. 10.18**) to be followed. In the case of oromaxillofacial surgery, where the throat pack lies within the operative field (as opposed to outside the operative field, e.g. in nasal surgery), the recommendation is that the surgeon should insert the throat pack, using a surgical swab (included in the surgical swab count), with placement assisted by the anaesthetist using laryngoscopy if required, and the surgeon should also remove the throat pack (and final swab count completed, before wakening the patient and extubating the trachea). Crucially, the anaesthetist is then responsible for examining the airway at the end of surgery, and meticulously suctioning under direct vision/videolaryngoscopic guidance, before extubation of the trachea.

Eye protection

As mentioned, standard eye pads/tapes/guards may be contraindicated as they may disrupt the surgical field or obscure the bony anatomy used by the surgeon as a guide to achieve symmetry. Therefore, a water-based eye lubricant should be used to protect the eyes, and the surgeon should apply steri-strips to keep the eyes closed without obscuring the bony contours. Patients should be consented specifically about blurred vision, secondary to the eye lubricant, at emergence.

Positioning

Patients should be orientated in a modest head-up supine position to aid venous drainage, minimize blood loss, and improve surgical access. The head should be kept in a stable position on a head ring, with the cervical spine supported appropriately. Alternatively, a specialist operating table (also utilized for ear, nose, and throat surgery and ophthalmic surgery) can be utilized, which has a shaped upper-back section and specially designed head rest that offers unrestricted surgical access to the head. Procedures can last 4–6 hours (e.g. combined bimaxillary osteotomy and genioplasty), therefore

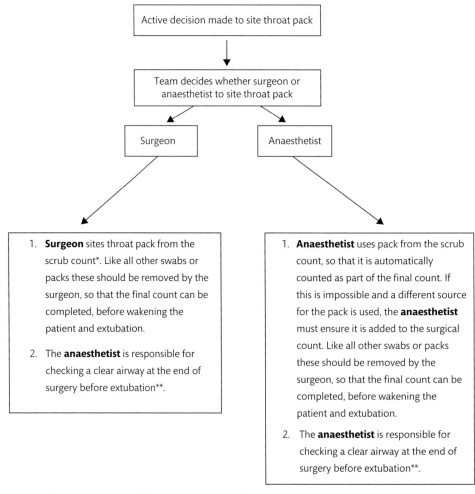

Fig. 10.18 Consensus protocol for throat pack use.[4] *The anaesthetist may be asked to assist, for example, with laryngoscopy; ** Notwithstanding cases where the jaw is wired, patient transferred ventilated to intensive care, etc, or where a pack is intentionally left *in situ*.

Athanassoglou, V, Patel, A, McGuire, B, et al. Systematic review of benefits or harms of routine anaesthetist-inserted throat packs in adults: practice recommendations for inserting and counting throat packs. Anaesthesia 2018; 73: 612– 8.

pressure areas must be meticulously protected with gel padding, and limbs placed in neutral positions. This is particularly important in the morbidly obese patient, where special consideration should also be made to safe manual handling (increasing the number of theatre staff assisting to ensure safe transfer and positioning, and utilizing hover mattresses when indicated).

Rather obviously, and as is the case for most oromaxillofacial procedures, the operating table is orientated with the 'head end' away from the anaesthetist, anaesthetic machine, and ventilator. Access to the shared airway by the anaesthetist intraoperatively is, therefore, extremely restricted (particularly in an emergency), adding additional importance to careful preoperative positioning and securing of the patient's head and neck, nasal tube, breathing circuit, and connections, in order to avoid injury, kinking, twisting, dislodging, or disconnection. Extensions to the breathing circuits and end-tidal carbon dioxide sampling line are recommended as they prevent excessive tension and aid with optimal positioning, minimizing inadvertent surgeon-related airway/breathing circuit issues.

Controlling blood loss

The midface is very vascular, therefore bleeding during orthognathic procedures from both bone and soft tissues can be extensive, particularly those involving the maxilla. During osteotomy, in particular, surgical haemostasis can be hard to achieve due to restricted access and difficulty in identification of the blood vessels as any bleeding rapidly obscures the surgical field. There are several strategies that can be employed to minimize surgical bleeding and optimize the surgical field. Simple strategies can be employed prophylactically, from the start of surgery. These include head-up positioning, avoidance of anything that may impair venous drainage or increase venous pressure (e.g. avoidance of coughing, tight drapes, high positive end-expiratory pressure), controlled ventilation (i.e. normocapnia), maintaining normothermia, relatively restrictive fluid administration regimens, the use of tranexamic acid (antifibrinolytic agent, usually 1 g administered following induction), and the liberal infiltration of local anaesthetic containing adrenaline prior to incision (maximum doses of local anaesthetic and adrenaline must be calculated preoperatively). These prophylactic measures are important; however, a brief period of deliberate moderate hypotension is often indicated when osteotomy cuts are made in the maxilla (which directly causes bleeding) and when the maxilla is down-fractured (particularly stimulating, indirectly causing bleeding) during a Le Fort I maxillary osteotomy. Bleeding occurs from branches of the maxillary artery, pterygoid, and greater palatine veins during the down-fracture, and can obscure the surgical field making further bony incision more difficult, and can be quite significant if not controlled (>500 mL blood loss). Often the down-fracture must be completed before surgical haemostasis can be achieved, making blood pressure control at this particular time crucial. A degree of deliberate hypotensive anaesthesia can be induced by various pharmacological agents, but most importantly must be employed in a safe, carefully monitored manner, in selected patients, only for the discrete period of maximal stimulus and blood loss and not for the whole duration of the operation. Good communication between surgeon and anaesthetist is essential, and advance warning that the maxilla is due to be 'taken down' enables the anaesthetist to ensure that the blood pressure is under meticulous control before this procedure is undertaken (further intricacies of hypotensive anaesthesia are discussed in detail in Chapter 7). With all these blood-conserving strategies employed, patients undergoing orthognathic surgery rarely require blood transfusion these days; however, those undergoing bimaxillary osteotomy should still have their haemoglobin level checked routinely preoperatively and an up-to-date group and save sample should be screened for atypical antibodies and availability made for rapid release of cross-matched blood units if required.

Trigeminocardiac reflex

Profound bradycardia, and even ventricular asystole, has, rarely, been described during down-fracture or mobilization of the maxilla, resulting from the parasympathetic response to traction on branches of the trigeminal nerve. As discussed above, good communication between surgeon and anaesthetist is, therefore, essential along with a high degree of vigilance. In the event of this reflex being provoked, surgical manipulation of the maxilla must be stopped immediately and anticholinergic medications administered as required.

Venous thromboembolism prophylaxis

Given the generally young and healthy patient cohort, postoperative venous thromboembolism is rare. However, with the increasing trend of treating patients with obstructive sleep apnoea, the average body mass index may start to rise and the incidence of venous thromboembolism may also increase. Hypotensive anaesthesia and a relatively restrictive fluid administration regimen (both designed to reduce blood loss), combined with the increasing use of antifibrinolytic agents and prolonged surgery, are all risk factors. Therefore, standard measures should be employed intraoperatively with graduated compression stockings and pneumatic compression devices, and postoperative low-molecular-weight heparin prophylaxis (usually the following morning after bimaxillary osteotomy to reduce bleeding risk, but to be considered on the same day of surgery for those with additional risk factors, e.g. morbid obesity).

Temperature control and measurement

Some orthognathic procedures can last several hours, therefore patients' core temperature should be monitored and patients should be actively warmed in order to maintain normothermia, using warmed intravenous fluids, fluid warmers, and forced air warmers. It is usually possible to utilize a nasopharyngeal temperature probe to monitor a patient's core temperature, placed via the free nostril that is not obscured by the nasotracheal tube; however, peripheral and rectal temperature probes obviate any potential issues with nasal placement. It is important to note that with only the head and neck exposed during these orthognathic procedures, and the rest of the body covered by the patient's surgical gown, a forced air warmer/blankets, and the surgical drapes, that it is very easy to overheat the patient during prolonged surgery, therefore it is always important to monitor the patient's temperature throughout.

Total intravenous anaesthesia and inhalational agents

Maintenance of anaesthesia can be conducted with total intravenous anaesthesia (TIVA) or inhalational agents, depending upon patient factors and anaesthetist preferences, with each technique, arguably, conferring potential pros and cons. Specifically for the orthognathic patient, TIVA reduces postoperative nausea and vomiting, produces a rapid and smooth emergence with swift recovery of protective airway reflexes (reducing laryngospasm and bronchospasm), and a speedy return to baseline cognition. Although processed electro-encephalogram monitoring is not essential, some anaesthetists prefer to use it and the type of surgery can pose some practical issues in obtaining reliable monitoring intraoperatively. Careful skin preparation with an alcohol-based wipe and securing of the adhesive monitoring strip across the forehead, together with a cooperative surgeon can usually circumvent these issues. Arguably, inhalational agents can be used to induce deliberate hypotension more easily (although the chapter authors don't recommend using excessive depth of anaesthesia to induce hypotension). The relative merits of TIVA versus volatile agents are beyond the scope of this chapter. Remifentanil can be used with both anaesthetic techniques and has become extremely popular and widely used due to its rapid onset and offset, and easily titratable properties, conferring a smooth anaesthetic during the intermittent peaks of surgical stimulus. Remifentanil can also be used to provide a smooth wake up for extubation of the trachea at the end of surgery (specific extubation strategies are discussed in detail later in the chapter).

Intraoperative analgesia

A multimodal approach to analgesia is indicated for orthognathic procedures. As discussed above, a remifentanil infusion is now the mainstay of intraoperative analgesia but must, of course, be combined with administration of longer-acting opioids, throughout the procedure or towards the end, to ensure adequate pain relief postoperatively. Given the high risk of postoperative nausea and vomiting following orthognathic surgery, opioid-sparing techniques are preferable.

The surgical team will infiltrate large volumes of dental local anaesthetic, typically lidocaine 2% with 1:80,000 epinephrine (Lignospan˚; Fig. 10.19), principally to minimize bleeding and optimize surgical conditions, but this also significantly reduces intraoperative analgesic requirements. Maxillary and mandibular local anaesthetic nerve blocks (e.g. inferior alveolar nerve block), performed at the start of surgery, can also be particularly beneficial, reducing the sympathetic response to surgery (attenuating spikes in blood pressure and reducing bleeding). Crucially, the maximum doses of local anaesthetic should be calculated and agreed preoperatively by the surgical and anaesthetic teams, in order to minimize the risk of local anaesthetic toxicity (7 mg/kg for lidocaine with adrenaline). Special consideration of the particularly high concentration of adrenaline

in dental local anaesthetic solutions should also be made, so as not to exceed the maximum recommended dosage of adrenaline, limiting usage to 300 micrograms per hour. In keeping with the general requirement for good communication between surgeon and anaesthetist in oromaxillofacial surgery, the surgeon should always inform the anaesthetist before infiltrating the local anaesthetic solution to prevent misinterpretation of a sudden increase in heart rate and blood pressure (resulting from the adrenaline), and especially in patients with cardiovascular comorbidities. In addition to lidocaine and adrenaline solutions, bupivacaine (Marcaine˚) 0.5% can be infiltrated at the end of surgery to reduce postoperative analgesic requirements (local anaesthetics and nerve blocks are also discussed in detail in Chapter 4).

Intravenous paracetamol and intravenous non-steroidal anti-inflammatory medications are widely used intraoperatively, and also provide the basis of most postoperative analgesic regimens. The transient hypotensive effect following administration of intravenous paracetamol can also be utilized to good effect by withholding administration until just before down-fracture of the maxilla, when controlled hypotension is desirable. Administration of non-steroidal anti-inflammatory drugs should generally be withheld until much of the orthognathic procedure is complete and maximal bleeding risk has passed or, alternatively, a cyclooxygenase (COX)-2 selective (coxib) drug selected.

Dexamethasone is a particularly useful adjunct to the advocated multimodal approach to analgesia, with positive effects in reducing the risk of trismus, reducing oedema (and the pain associated), its antiemetic properties, and in higher doses (equivalent to 8 mg), it has been shown to have beneficial effects on reducing postoperative analgesic requirements,[5] particularly for dental and orthognathic procedures. Magnesium, clonidine, and dexmedetomidine can also be used intraoperatively, being efficacious in both reducing opioid requirements and for inducing controlled hypotension, although the latter two agents may cause drowsiness on emergence, which may not be considered desirable in patients where there is concern regarding the ease of managing an airway or breathing complication at extubation (e.g. known difficult airway or intermaxillary fixation). Low-dose ketamine (0.25–0.5 mg/kg) can be a useful analgesic and opioid-sparing adjunct, particularly in longer, more extensive procedures.

Antiemetics

Orthognathic surgery is associated with a high incidence of postoperative nausea and vomiting, with specific risk factors including young patients, perioperative opioids, and inhalational anaesthetic agents. Of course, other factors such as female sex, non-smoking status, previous postoperative nausea and vomiting, motion sickness, excessive fasting and dehydration, inadequate pain relief, will also contribute. Intuitively, one might also include as a potentiating factor the presence of blood that has drained into the stomach perioperatively; however, the incidence of postoperative nausea and vomiting does not appear to be reduced by the presence of a throat pack. Multimodal prophylaxis is recommended with ondansetron and dexamethasone administered intraoperatively (particularly effective when administered together), with cyclizine available for treatment postoperatively and further ondansetron prescribed regularly for prevention. Clearly it is desirable to reduce postoperative nausea and vomiting in all patients, but it is particularly important

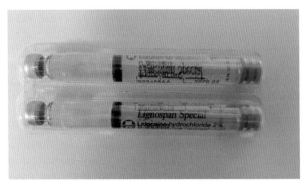

Fig. 10.19 Dental local anaesthetic, containing lidocaine 2% with 1:80,000 adrenaline.

in those undergoing orthognathic procedures, as retching and vomiting will increase venous pressure causing bleeding and may also potentially disrupt surgical sutures. Crucially, in those patients with intermaxillary fixation devices, vomiting can not only be extremely distressing, but can be potentially life-threatening, given the potential risk of acute airway obstruction and/or aspiration in such circumstances (specific management strategies are discussed later in the section on postoperative management).

Intraoperative fluid management

A generally liberal intravenous fluid administration regimen is advantageous, with early recommencement of oral fluid intake postoperatively, to reduce postoperative nausea and vomiting. However, for orthognathic cases where a relatively high degree of bleeding is expected, employing a relatively restrictive fluid policy up until maxillary down-fracture has occurred may be advantageous in minimizing blood loss, whereafter a more liberal approach can be resumed. Urinary catheterization is generally not indicated, even for longer cases such as combined bimaxillary osteotomy and genioplasty, but may be considered for cases that are expected to be more surgically challenging and prolonged. As discussed earlier, with current bleeding prevention strategies, blood transfusion is rarely required.

Antimicrobial prophylaxis

Postoperative infection is rare following orthognathic surgery. Nevertheless, in addition to preoperative rinsing of the oral cavity with chlorhexidine mouthwash, one dose of a broad-spectrum antibiotic is generally recommended at induction for most procedures (usually Augmentin* 1.2 g intravenously). Two postoperative antibiotic doses may also be requested by some surgeons for more complex procedures such as bimaxillary osteotomy, although practice will vary from centre to centre. Regular chlorhexidine mouthwash can also be continued for the first few days postoperatively.

Tracheal extubation and emergence

Extubation planning

An individualized tracheal extubation plan should be agreed for each patient, following discussion between the anaesthetist and surgeon, and considering the relative ease or difficulty with which the patient's airway was managed at induction, surgical concerns such as excessive swelling or bleeding, patient comorbidities, and specific risk factors, such as obstructive sleep apnoea.

Inspection and suctioning

The anaesthetist is responsible for assessing and preparing the airway prior to tracheal extubation and this should be undertaken before any intermaxillary fixation device (elastics or wiring) is undertaken. The anaesthetist should inspect the oropharynx to ensure that any throat pack has been removed (this should be a confirmatory check, as the throat pack should have already been removed by the operating surgeon by this stage of the operation, clearly announced to the theatre team at the time of removal, seen and confirmed by the anaesthetist, and carefully documented). The anaesthetist should then undertake meticulous suctioning of the oropharynx, under direct

vision, removing any clots that have accumulated during surgery (especially occult blood in the nasopharynx behind the soft palate, which has the potential for causing fatal airway obstruction, the so-called coroner's clot). Care must be taken not to apply excessive forward traction on the mandible during direct laryngoscopy as this may displace osteotomy segments. For similar reasons, it is rarely appropriate to exchange the nasotracheal tube for a supraglottic airway device, to facilitate smooth emergence, as this also requires manipulation of the mandible which is not desirable in patients after osteotomy. At this time, an appropriately sized nasopharyngeal airway can be inserted carefully via the un-intubated nostril, providing additional airway protection at extubation and emergence. A suction catheter can also be passed via this nasopharyngeal airway and the tip guided into the posterior nasopharynx under direct vision so that it is optimally placed for suctioning during emergence and postoperatively. The anaesthetist must be as confident as possible that surgical haemostasis has been achieved before any intermaxillary fixation devices are applied by the surgical team, and before extubation of the trachea is undertaken. This is particularly important if deliberate hypotension has been used intraoperatively and the blood pressure is now back to normal.

Nasopharyngeal adjuncts and smooth extubation

A smooth, no-cough, extubation is desirable to minimize straining and the associated surgical bleeding. However, even with good surgical haemostasis, further bleeding/ooze into the upper airway is not uncommon and, therefore, extubation of the trachea is most safely performed with the patient awake, with full return of protective airway reflexes. Clearly, extubation in these patients is a very carefully managed process, balancing the risk of coughing, disruption of suture lines, and bleeding in an awake patient with the potential for airway compromise in an obtunded patient. Slow and steady deflation of the nasotracheal cuff is advocated to reduce the stimulus to cough and a low-dose remifentanil infusion (preferably target controlled) can be used to facilitate smooth extubation in an awake patient. Remifentanil has little sedative effect and can be titrated to patient comfort while maintaining satisfactory spontaneous ventilation. The nasotracheal tube should be withdrawn slowly and gently to minimize the stimulus to cough and to prevent displacement of the sectioned nasal septum. It can also be only partially withdrawn and cut at the desired depth (**Figs 10.20** and **10.21**), such that it also acts as a nasopharyngeal airway, optimizing airway patency and oxygen delivery at extubation and emergence (i.e. at extubation, both nasal passages can be maintained by a nasopharyngeal airway device, with an optimally positioned suction catheter also *in situ*). These soft nasal airway devices are extremely well tolerated by patients, and can be removed safely in the post-anaesthesia care unit (PACU). During this process of extubation of the trachea, minimal head and neck movement is desirable, again to reduce the stimulus to cough. Therefore, placement of a Hudson mask (and hilotherapy mask) is recommended prior to lightening of anaesthesia and extubation of the trachea. Forceful airway manoeuvres (in particular, jaw thrust in mandibular surgery or chin lift in genioplasty surgery) and the application of a tight-fitting face mask are to be avoided in order to minimize pressure on the surgical plates, screws, and osteotomized segments. For patients in whom airway management was particularly complicated initially, or in whom there are concerns about adequacy of postoperative

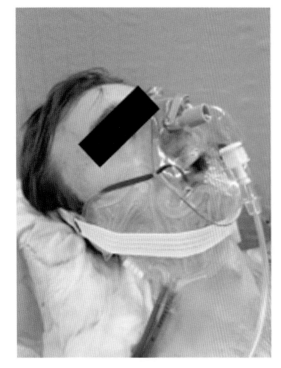

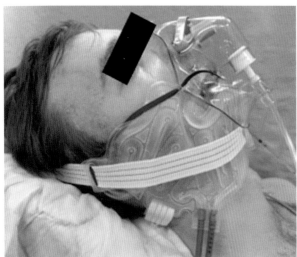

Figs 10.20 and 10.21 Nasotracheal tube withdrawn and cut at desired length, to act as a nasopharyngeal airway. Note: the Hudson mask and Hilotherapy mask were positioned carefully prior to lightening of anaesthesia and tracheal extubation.

oxygenation, airway patency, or the ease of reintubation, an airway exchange catheter can be employed and left *in situ* at extubation, to be removed safely later.

Postoperative management

Safe postoperative environment

After orthognathic surgery, patients should be cared for immediately postoperatively in a recovery area (PACU) near the operating theatre, with immediate access to the responsible anaesthetist and maxillofacial surgeon, by nursing staff who are experienced in managing this particular type of patient, especially those with obstructive sleep apnoea and/or intermaxillary fixation devices in place, where a particularly high degree of vigilance is required. Continuous capnography is important in enabling early recognition of complications.

Intermaxillary fixation devices

Rigid (wire) intermaxillary fixation devices are less common nowadays, but if the jaws have been wired together at the end of surgery, wire cutters must be immediately available at the bedside. Elastics, attached to arch bars or orthodontic brackets, are far more common and are used to facilitate the final jaw position. These can be cut easily with scissors for immediate access to the oropharynx (although if time allows, these can be plucked off swiftly with a finger, avoiding subsequent issues in locating and retrieving the elastic remnants). Anaesthetic, surgical, and nursing recovery staff should be familiar with the management of such airway emergencies, and should regularly practise simulated scenarios.

Nausea and vomiting

As mentioned earlier, postoperative nausea and vomiting is common, unless TIVA is used, despite perioperative multimodal antiemetic prophylaxis. Vomiting patients with intermaxillary fixation devices are at potential risk of aspiration and/or airway obstruction, and should be immediately sat upright and leant forwards as this promotes the passage of vomitus from the oropharynx via gaps in the fixation device on each side (if the patient is managed in the supine or semi-recumbent position, the gastric contents are more likely to overwhelm the oropharynx and be aspirated). Regular antiemetics should be prescribed and administered postoperatively.

Bleeding

As discussed earlier, minor epistaxis from traumatic nasotracheal intubation is not uncommon and usually self-limiting. Nasal bleeding can also occur following maxillary osteotomy, and this may require nasal packing with a tampon.

Positioning

Patients should be positioned in a moderate head-up position, to reduce swelling, aid venous drainage, and optimize respiratory mechanics. The nasopharynx should be suctioned as necessary via the *in situ* suction catheter (whose tip can be optimally positioned in the nasopharynx prior to extubation, as described earlier). The nasopharyngeal airways in each nostril can be removed after a short period, along with the suction catheter, when no longer required.

Respiratory support

If oxygen is required postoperatively, it should, ideally, be delivered with humidification to improve patient comfort and to prevent drying of blood and secretions in the nasopharynx. For patients with CPAP-dependent severe sleep apnoea, there is often symptomatic improvement postoperatively negating the need for additional respiratory support. However, if oxygen/CPAP is still necessitated, a high-flow humidified nasal oxygen delivery device (e.g. Optiflow™, Fisher and Paykel Healthcare Limited, Auckland, New Zealand), which also provides some positive airway pressure/small airways splinting is probably preferable to a tight-fitting traditional CPAP mask in patients after orthognathic surgery. Regular nebulized hypertonic saline every 4–6 hours can also be beneficial in reducing crusting of secretions and blood.

Analgesia

Generally speaking, orthognathic procedures, like most head and neck operations, are not too painful postoperatively. For minor procedures, regular paracetamol and ibuprofen or a coxib is normally sufficient. For moderate to major surgery (e.g. single jaw osteotomy), adding in regular codeine and oral morphine as required is usually adequate. Crucially, all oral analgesic medications should be in soluble/syrup formulation as capsules and tablets may be difficult to ingest. For two-jaw surgery such as bimaxillary osteotomy, a bolus-only fentanyl patient-controlled analgesia is recommended postoperatively, and for overnight the first night, being discontinued the following morning as the patient is converted onto the standard soluble oral regimen. Care must, of course, be taken with the severe sleep apnoeic patient and the risk of increased opioid sensitivity.

Reducing oedema

Along with nursing patients sitting upright, hilotherapy masks (Fig. 10.22) are very effective in reducing facial swelling, bruising, and relieving pain. The mask pumps cooled water through an anatomically fitted cuff at a controllable temperature. Simple ice packs are suitable for minor procedures such as dental extractions, but the hilotherapy mask confers significant advantages for moderate to major surgery, moulding to the patient's individual facial anatomy and having no limitation to the duration of use due to the temperature control (unlike ice packs). For bimaxillary osteotomy, hilotherapy masks may be worn for up to a week postoperatively (taken home by the patient on discharge), and have been associated with improved patient satisfaction and reduced length of hospital stay.

Dexamethasone is also effective in reducing postoperative oedema. Therefore, in addition to intraoperative administration, it can be given regularly for the first 24 hours postoperatively.

Fluid regimens

Early resumption of oral intake (free fluids) is important in reducing postoperative nausea and vomiting and improving comfort. Oral ice chips can be given in the PACU and provide some comfort to patients. For bimaxillary osteotomy, slow maintenance intravenous fluids are also recommended for the immediate postoperative period and overnight for the first night as oral intake is often inadequate. Hypotonic fluids (e.g. 5% glucose) and excessive crystalloids are not recommended intra- or postoperatively as they can exacerbate tissue and airway oedema.

Critical care

Routine postoperative admission to the intensive care unit or to a high dependency facility is no longer recommended, unless there

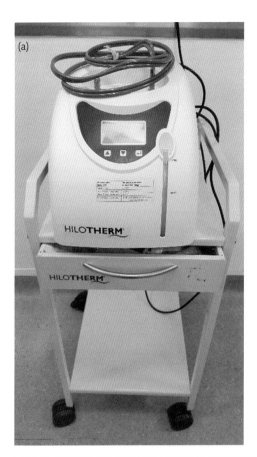

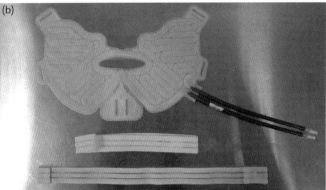

Fig. 10.22 Hilotherapy (a) machine and (b) mask, used for reducing oedema postoperatively.

are other pre-existing comorbidities that necessitate it, or there are particular concerns regarding excessive bleeding, oedema, or the potential for airway or breathing compromise, requiring additional monitoring and/or respiratory support. However, patients should be managed in a dedicated maxillofacial or head and neck surgical ward, where the nursing staff are experienced with such patients and can recognize potential complications early.

Enhanced recovery pathways

There is certainly the potential to develop pathways and protocols for patients undergoing orthognathic surgery, with the aim of ensuring best evidence-based practice, such that patient

Table 10.1 A typical postoperative drug prescription for bimaxillary osteotomy

Drug	Dose and frequency	Duration
Fentanyl	0–100 mcg IV (in 10–20 mcg boluses)	Recovery/PACU only
Fentanyl patient-controlled analgesia	20 mcg bolus IV, lockout 5 mins, no background infusion	Overnight first night only
Paracetamol	1 g QDS IV or PO liquid preparation	Continue, and take home on discharge, 1-week supply
Ibuprofen	400 mg TDS, PO liquid preparation	Continue, and take home on discharge, 1-week supply
Codeine	30 mg QDS, PO liquid preparation	Commence when patient-controlled analgesia discontinued, and take home on discharge for PRN use, 4–6-hourly, 1-week supply
Ondansetron	4 mg TDS IV	Regular for first 24 hours, changed to PRN after that
Cyclizine	50 mg TDS IV/IM	PRN only
Dexamethasone	8 mg BD IV	2 postoperative doses
Oxygen	2–10 L/min, inhalational, as required via Hudson mask or nasal cannulae as appropriate	Recovery/PACU only, rarely required on ward following discharge from recovery but should be humidified if needed
Hypertonic saline	5 mL 3% NaCl, sterile, nebulized, QDS	Regular for first 24–48 hours
Chlorhexidine mouthwash	QDS, PO (not swallowed)	Regular for first 24–48 hours
0.9% saline, compound sodium lactate, Plasma-Lyte®	60–100 mL/hr IV	Overnight first night
Augmentin	1.2 g TDS	2 doses only

BD, twice daily; IM, intramuscular; IV, intravenous; PO, oral; PRN, as required; QDS, four times daily; TDS, three times daily.

satisfaction, postoperative pain, incidence of nausea and vomiting, overall complication rates, and length of stay can be optimized. Constant audit and review of surgical and anaesthetic outcomes is essential to promote discussion, refinement of anaesthetic (and surgical) techniques, maintenance of high standards, and consistency in practice, leading to the generation of agreed protocols (e.g. bimaxillary osteotomy standardized postoperative prescription; Table 10.1). With appropriate preoperative planning and preparation (Fig. 10.23), good perioperative management, and adequate postoperative care and support, it should be possible/expected that patients undergoing single-jaw surgery are discharged home the same or the next day, and for those having

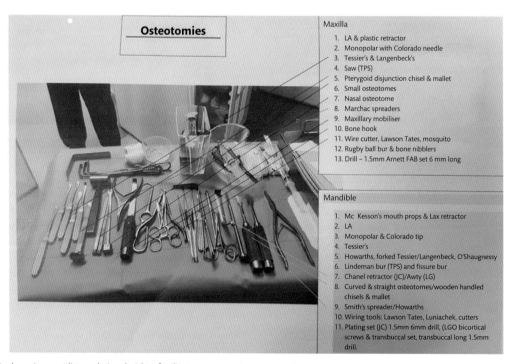

Fig. 10.23 A typical equipment list and visual aid to facilitate preoperative preparation.

Table 10.2 Orthognathic surgical procedures, with additional procedure-specific details

Operation	Procedure-specific details
Maxillary osteotomy	Le Fort I maxillary osteotomy Indications: maxillary–mandibular disproportion, obstructive sleep apnoea syndrome, post-cleft palate surgery, craniofacial abnormalities, skull base surgery Involves complete mobilization and repositioning of the maxilla Bleeding from down-fracture of the maxilla can be significant The inferior turbinates may also be trimmed, as necessary Postoperative intermaxillary fixation with elastics may be required
Mandibular osteotomy	Bilateral sagittal split mandibular ramus osteotomy Involves horizontal, vertical, and sagittal osteotomies to enable mobilization and repositioning of dentoalveolar segment of the mandible Indications: mandibular deficiency, prognathism, or asymmetry Postoperative intermaxillary fixation with elastics may be required
Bimaxillary osteotomy	Combination of Le Fort I maxillary osteotomy, followed by bilateral sagittal split mandibular ramus osteotomy ('bimax') Indications: used for optimal correction of significant maxillary–mandibular disproportion and other craniofacial deformities Postoperative intermaxillary fixation with elastics may be required
Genioplasty	Involves osteotomy of the mandibular symphysis Indications: augmentation or reduction of the chin, improving the chin profile and cosmetic appearance of the face Can be performed as the sole procedure, but is often combined with other osteotomies
Temporomandibular joint (TMJ) surgery	Procedures can include arthroscopy, arthrocentesis, meniscal surgery and arthrotomy for TMJ dysfunction, coronoidectomy for TMJ ankylosis, and even TMJ replacement for severe cases Mouth opening can range from mild restriction owing to muscle spasm in TMJ dysfunction (which usually relaxes after induction) to severely restricted, almost complete trismus, in patients with joint ankylosis, necessitating awake fibreoptic intubation Nasotracheal intubation and muscle relaxation are often necessary to optimize surgical access There is significant bleeding risk during TMJ replacement owing to the proximity of the carotid artery TMJ procedures are generally more painful than other orthognathic operations, requiring intravenous opioids, and patient-controlled analgesia postoperatively for TMJ replacement
Distraction osteogenesis	A relatively new technique used to generate new bone and soft tissue. Following a corticotomy or osteotomy, an adjustable distraction device is applied, which promotes bone formation between the surfaces of the bony segments as they are gradually separated by incremental traction, based upon the tension-stress principle Indications: severely deficient maxilla, midface hypoplasia (e.g. in Crouzon and Apert syndromes), deficient hypoplastic mandible, deficient maxillary alveolar bone prior to dental implant insertion Maxillary distraction osteogenesis is achieved through a Le Fort I osteotomy followed by placement of a distractor to achieve horizontal expansion (surgically assisted rapid palatal expansion (SARPE)) Midfacial advancement requires Le Fort II or Le Fort III osteotomy procedures, depending on the particular defect. Submental intubation is usually required. Once the distraction (halo) frame is attached, access to the airway can be significantly impaired, and even though the frames are designed to disarticulate, these patients can pose significant challenges to airway management at both intubation and extubation

two-jaw surgery (e.g. bimaxillary osteotomy), a 48-hour hospital stay should be the aim.

Specific orthognathic procedures

See Table 10.2 for procedure-specific details of commonly performed orthognathic procedures.

Conclusion

The principles that apply to anaesthesia for orthognathic procedures have been discussed. While Table 10.2 includes some procedure-specific additions, the general approach already described is universally applicable—careful multidisciplinary assessment, planning and optimization, attentive shared airway management necessitating cooperation and clear communication between surgeon and anaesthetist, strict control of blood loss, multimodal analgesia and antiemetic prophylaxis, safe and smooth extubation of the trachea, strategies to reduce postoperative oedema and bleeding, and specialist postoperative care facilities.

REFERENCES

1. Bettega G, Pépin JL, Veale D, Deschaux C, Raphaël B, Lévy P. Obstructive sleep apnea syndrome: fifty-one consecutive patients treated by maxillofacial surgery. *Am J Respir Crit Care Med.* 2000;**162**(2 Pt 1):641–649.
2. Katz RI, Hovagim AR, Finkelstein HS, Grinberg Y, Boccio RV, Poppers PJ. A comparison of cocaine, lidocaine with epinephrine, and oxymetazoline for prevention of epistaxis on nasotracheal intubation. *J Clin Anesth.* 1990;**2**(1):16–20.
3. Curran J, Ward M, Knepil G. Reducing the risk of retained throat swabs after surgery. National Patient Safety Agency. 2009. https://webarchive.nationalarchives.gov.uk/20171030130742/http://www.nrls.npsa.nhs.uk/resources/type/alerts/?entryid45=59853&p=2
4. Athanassoglou V, Patel A, McGuire B, Higgs A, Dover MS, Brennan PA, et al. Systematic review of benefits or harms of routine anaesthetist-inserted throat packs in adults: practice recommendations for inserting and counting throat packs. *Anaesthesia.* 2018;**73**(5):612–618.
5. N. H. Waldron NH, Jones CA, Gan TJ, Allen TK, Habib AS. Impact of perioperative dexamethasone on postoperative analgesia and side-effects: systematic review and meta-analysis, *Br J Anaesth.* 2013;**110**(2):191–200.

11

Paediatric surgery

Silky Wong and Theresa Wan-Chun Hui

Introduction

Anaesthesia for paediatric oromaxillofacial surgery involves the care of children with congenital craniofacial and developmental facial anomalies, cleft lip and palate, trauma, abnormal jaw growth, temporomandibular joint (TMJ) disorders, dentoalveolar conditions/anomalies, paediatric pathology, and obstructive sleep apnoea (OSA). Anaesthetists need to manage the specific needs of neonates, infants, and the growing child with special consideration of the anatomy, pharmacology, and physiology, along with behavioural factors which are different from adults.

Preoperative evaluation

The preoperative visit provides an opportunity to establish rapport and gain the confidence and acceptance of the patient and parents/carers. During the visit, a complete medical evaluation is required. History of respiratory compromise such as dependence on continuous positive airway pressure, bilevel positive airway pressure, or oxygen; airway obstruction like choanal stenosis or atresia; and snoring with OSA must be undertaken. Unlike in adults with OSA who are often obese, children with severe OSA may present as failure to thrive. In infants, there may be a history of difficulties with feeding. Tachypnoea, use of accessory muscles of respiration, subcostal retraction, and pectus excavatum indicate significant obstruction. Children with congenital syndromes requiring maxillofacial surgery may also have associated heart disease. Screening for cardiac defects and other coexisting congenital abnormalities should be undertaken as these can affect the perioperative anaesthetic management. History of recent upper respiratory tract infection, needle phobia, or problems with anaesthesia should be elicited. Anaesthesia in children with upper respiratory tract infection increases the risk of perioperative bronchospasm, laryngospasm, oxygen desaturation, and breath holding. Children with severe symptoms like purulent nasal secretions, fever, lethargy, moist cough, and wheezing will benefit from deferring elective surgery for at least 2 weeks.[1] For children with uncomplicated upper respiratory tract infection, the decision to postpone surgery is individualized and based on balancing both patient and surgical risks of developing complications with the benefit of proceeding to surgery. Investigations for a healthy child are not always required. However, if surgery is extensive, baseline investigations are indicated (including blood cross-matching).

Premedication

Sedation with premedication helps to smooth the induction process. While many older children do not need preoperative sedation, infants (around 6 months to 1 year old) and preschool age children who have developed stranger anxiety are often anxious upon entering the anaesthetic room/operating theatre. Moreover, many children with special educational needs and disabilities require sedation to allay their anxiety even after they reach adulthood.

Benzodiazepines are commonly used for this purpose. Midazolam given orally, 0.5–0.75 mg/kg with a maximum dose of 15 mg, half an hour before entering the anaesthetic room/operating theatre or intranasally, with doses of 0.2 mg/kg, has anxiolytic and amnesic effects.[2] Overdosing may cause respiratory depression. Some children exhibit paradoxical effects and become more agitated.

The highly selective α_2 agonist, dexmedetomidine, is equally effective[3-6] and does not cause respiratory depression. Intranasal administration has a rapid onset and high bioavailability. Dose ranges from 1 to 4 mcg/kg intranasally. This is often given in the preoperative receiving area with monitoring because it may cause bradycardia and hypotension.[5,7]

Ketamine is also an effective sedative premedication. When given intranasally at 5 mg/kg, though a little irritating, intramuscular injection or venous cannulation can be avoided. When the child is difficult to control, it can be given intramuscularly at doses of 3 mg/kg.[8]

Sedative premedication should not be substituted for psychological preparation during the preoperative visit. Preoperative preparation with skilled nurses and play therapists, visits to the operating theatre, and videos can help to allay anxiety. One must also consider the need for sedation and the presence of coexisting conditions and airway anomalies. Sedatives are contraindicated in children with potential airway obstruction and raised intracranial pressure because these children may not safely tolerate respiratory depressants. Local anaesthetic cream such as Eutectic Mixture of Local Anaesthetic (EMLA™) and amethocaine placed over a vein minimize the pain of inserting a venous catheter and is commonly prescribed with premedication.

Fasting

Preoperative fasting is to allow enough time for the stomach to empty and hence reduce the incidence of regurgitation of gastric contents into the trachea (and lungs). Fasting for prolonged periods increases thirst and irritability and results in detrimental physiological and metabolic effects. Traditionally, children have been permitted clear fluids until 2 hours, breast feeding until 4 hours, and formula feeds until 6 hours prior to surgery.[9] Accumulating evidence indicates that a more liberal clear fluid fasting regime does not affect the incidence of pulmonary aspiration[10] and 1 hour of clear fluid fasting did not alter gastric pH or residual volume as compared with 2 hours of fasting.[11] This has led to the recent recommendation of allowing and encouraging children to have clear fluids up to 1 hour before elective general anaesthesia in the UK, Europe, and Australia.[12] However, adherence to fasting guidelines must be emphasized as violations were identified as a potential cause of aspiration.[13]

Identification of the difficult airway and its management

A difficult airway in children can lead to potential serious complications. It is important to identify risk factors accurately and ascertain whether the difficulty is with tracheal intubation or ventilation, or both. The most serious of all is when there is an unanticipated difficult airway (in a retrospective study, 0.5% of paediatric intubations were classed as difficult, of which 20% were unanticipated).[14] In the American Society of Anesthesiologists closed claims analysis and perioperative cardiac arrest registry, claims in children were often due to cardiovascular events and airway incidents that were associated with inadequate ventilation, hypoxic brain damage, cardiac arrest, and death.[15–18]

At preoperative assessment, identification of a difficult airway is achieved through thorough history taking and physical examination.[19] The clinician must establish whether the child has noisy breathing, snoring, increased work of breathing, feeding intolerance, or apnoea. If the child has had previous anaesthesia, any previous difficulty with the airway management must be identified. The existence of any syndrome associations must be established, along with the position the child is most comfortable breathing in. During physical examination of the airway, it is prudent to look for features like midface hypoplasia, micrognathia or receding chin, large tongue, and poor dentition which indicate the possibility of difficult tracheal intubation (Figs 11.1 and 11.2).[20]

Unanticipated difficult tracheal intubation in children is unusual.[14] Most difficult airway cases are those with primary airway emergencies or specific syndromes like Pierre Robin Sequence, Goldenhar, Treacher Collins, achondroplasia, mucopolysaccharidoses, or craniofacial synostosis such as Apert, Crouzon, or Pfeiffer.[21] These syndromes are associated with various dysmorphic features like mandibular hypoplasia, retrognathia, facial asymmetry, limited mouth opening, and enlarged tongue.

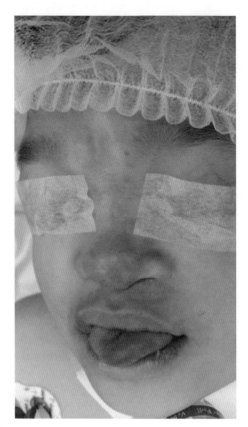

Fig. 11.1 Potential features of difficult airway management: a large tongue which is protruding out of the mouth.

Management of difficult intubation and ventilation varies greatly. Experience and familiarity with the equipment available will determine one's approach and it is important to have a backup plan.[21] A difficult intubation trolley which houses all airway management equipment should be in the operating theatre. To open the airway and optimize ventilation, the sniffing position should be maximized

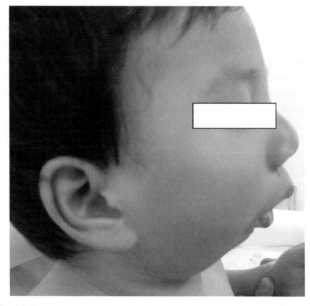

Fig. 11.2 Lateral view of a child showing mandibular hypoplasia.

using a shoulder roll or ramp. Most paediatric anaesthetists use the technique of spontaneous ventilation and intubation without muscle relaxation as their first-line management. This gives the greatest margin of safety because the child is breathing on his/her own. This technique, however, requires skill. Oversedation depresses breathing while inadequate sedation predisposes to laryngospasm during airway manipulation.

In recent years, with the introduction of sugammadex, use of the muscle relaxant rocuronium for better intubating conditions instead of a sedated but unrelaxed patient has been proposed by the Difficult Airway Society.[22] Neuromuscular blockade abolishes laryngeal reflexes, increases chest compliance, and facilitates face mask ventilation.[23,24] Rocuronium has a rapid onset and can be reversed rapidly with sugammadex. However, confirming the ability to perform effective face mask ventilation before paralysis may still be preferred by some anaesthetists in a child with an anticipated difficult airway.

In children with anticipated difficult mask ventilation, the goal is to maintain spontaneous breathing while adequately sedated for intubation. If the child's airway becomes obstructed, inserting an oral or nasopharyngeal airway into the posterior nasopharynx is often helpful. Where a paediatric nasopharyngeal airway is unavailable, a shortened uncuffed tracheal tube can be used as an alternative.[25]

For anticipated difficult tracheal intubation, laryngoscope blades of appropriate sizes and a supraglottic airway device must be available. In neonates and infants who have a relatively large and floppy epiglottis, a straight blade is often used to lift the epiglottis to obtain a good view of the larynx. Recently, videolaryngoscopy is being more widely used as backup or as first-line management. Local anaesthetic topicalization of the larynx with lidocaine may help to smooth the intubation procedure in a spontaneously breathing child.

Fibreoptic intubation is favoured as an alternative technique or as the primary technique when the airway is known to be difficult.[26] Awake tracheal intubation, which may be performed in cooperative adolescents, is impossible in infants or young children, and is not recommended. Asleep fibreoptic intubation requires skill due to the small airway size, partially collapsed soft tissue, and low threshold for oxygen desaturation. Such skill is acquired through training and practice. A nasopharyngeal airway or a small size tracheal tube inserted through one nostril into the posterior nasopharynx allows insufflation of oxygen while fibreoptic intubation is performed (Fig. 11.3). Alternatively, high flow nasal oxygen can be used to maintain oxygenation during fibreoptic intubation. Transnasal humidified rapid-insufflation ventilatory exchange (THRIVE) has been shown to safely prolong apnoeic oxygenation in children with healthy lungs and high flow nasal oxygen has been used successfully in spontaneously breathing children with abnormal airways who are at risk of apnoea during anaesthesia.[27] High-flow nasal oxygen can double the expected time to oxygen desaturation below 90% in healthy children. Total intravenous anaesthesia (TIVA) competency to maintain spontaneous breathing is an important adjunct for a successful high-flow nasal oxygen technique.[28]

Fibreoptic tracheal intubation assisted by direct/videolaryngoscopy has been described in the paediatric population. With this technique, the first anaesthetist controls the fibreoptic scope loaded with the tracheal tube. Meanwhile another anaesthetist uses the laryngoscope to push the tongue and other soft tissue away and facilitates the manipulation of the fibreoptic scope to gain access into the larynx. Another technique is to intubate via a supraglottic airway device. There are

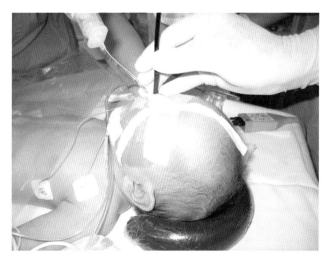

Fig. 11.3 Fibreoptic tracheal intubation of an infant, with insufflation of oxygen through a tracheal tube inserted into the nasopharynx via the left nostril.

devices specifically designed for this purpose such as the Air-Q® intubating laryngeal airway (Cookgas LLC, Mercury Medical, Clearwater, FL, USA). This method enables insufflation of oxygen, allows more time for manipulation of the tracheal tube without oxygen desaturation, and can be less stressful.[29,30]

For many anaesthetists, the ultimate backup plan is for the surgeon to perform tracheostomy. In infants and small children, crash tracheostomy is difficult to perform and is associated with significant morbidity. For management of unanticipated difficult intubation, difficult ventilation, and can't intubate, can't oxygenate situations, the Difficult Airway Society has useful guidelines.[31]

Induction of anaesthesia

Parental/carer presence at induction helps to allay the young child's anxiety. Either inhalation induction with sevoflurane or intravenous induction with propofol is appropriate. Gaseous induction is employed for children with needle phobia. However, establishment of intravenous access before induction is preferred in patients with an anticipated difficult airway. Some anaesthetists prefer spontaneous ventilation without muscle relaxation for tracheal intubation in young infants; others administer a neuromuscular blocking agent to facilitate intubation.

Tracheal tube selection

In the past, paediatric anaesthetists preferred to use uncuffed tracheal tubes in young children due to the fear the cuff may cause mucosal ischaemia and subsequent subglottic stenosis. Over the last decade, many have switched to using cuffed tracheal tubes with low-pressure cuffs that are designed specifically for use in children (e.g. microcuff tube).[32] This is beneficial as there is less leak at any time point throughout the procedure,[33,34] providing better ventilation. Compared to uncuffed tracheal tubes, there is less tube exchange; less perioperative respiratory events like laryngospasm and bronchospasm; and less stridor, sore throat, and hoarse voice postoperatively.[33,35] Although cuffed tracheal tubes are more expensive, the cost difference may be balanced by the fewer tube exchanges and lower fresh gas flows required due to reduced leak.[33]

Fluid management

During surgery, fluid management aims at providing basal metabolic requirements (maintenance fluids), compensating for preoperative fasting deficit and replacing losses from the surgical field. In children, volume and composition, tonicity, and glucose are important considerations. Maintenance fluids are given as isotonic crystalloid infusions. The common practice of '4–2–1' rule in calculating hourly infusion rate was evolved from Holliday and Segar's description of the relationship between physiological fluid losses and caloric expenditure:

- 4 mL/kg/hour for the first 10 kg body weight.
- 2 mL/kg/hour for the second 10 kg.
- 1 mL/kg/hour for each kg >20 kg thereafter.

Like in adults, infants and children mount a stress response secondary to surgery. This neurohormonal response promotes glycogenolysis and gluconeogenesis. The risk of perioperative hypoglycaemia is low except in neonates, young infants, those on total parenteral nutrition or certain metabolic diseases like glycogen storage disease, and prolonged surgery of >3 hours. Moreover, hyperglycaemia increases the risk of hypoxic–ischaemic brain damage and poor outcome.[36–38] Routine dextrose infusions are no longer recommended for healthy children undergoing surgery. In infants requiring glucose supplement, Plasma-Lyte® or Hartmann's solution with dextrose concentration of 12% are usually adequate, as infusions with higher concentrations of dextrose result in hyperglycaemia.[39–41]

Major maxillofacial surgery may be both prolonged and have extensive blood loss. The volume of blood loss is estimated and replaced with blood products and colloid. Regular point-of-care tests for measurements of haemoglobin, glucose, and electrolyte concentrations help guide the choice of fluids. Most children can drink early after maxillofacial surgery. Controversy exists regarding the choice and quantity of intravenous fluids for children who cannot tolerate oral fluids or in whom oral feeding is contraindicated in the postoperative period.[42] Intravenous fluids are usually infused at a rate of two-thirds of the hourly maintenance volume (because of the risk of increased antidiuretic hormone secretion) and 0.45% sodium chloride with glucose 5% may be safely administered. Whichever fluid is used, treatment should be individualized. There should be careful monitoring of patients with a minimum of daily blood tests for plasma electrolyte levels, weighing of the patient, and charting of fluid balance.

Analgesia

Multimodal analgesia is the regimen of choice. Dependent upon the type of surgical procedure, various combinations of local anaesthesia infiltration by the surgeon, nerve blocks, and non-opioid and opioid analgesics can be effective. Paracetamol is efficacious for mild pain in children and is opioid sparing in more major cases.[43] In those with low risk of bleeding, non-steroidal anti-inflammatory drugs (NSAIDs) can be given. These also reduce opioid consumption and the incidence of postoperative nausea and vomiting (PONV).[44] A NSAID in combination with paracetamol produces better analgesia than either alone.[45] Opioids, like morphine or oxycodone, can be used for severe pain.[46] However, careful titration of opioids according to the individual child's response is advised.

Postoperative nausea and vomiting

PONV, which causes dehydration and delayed discharge,[47] has a high incidence in children.[48] Oromaxillofacial surgery is associated with increased risk due to accidental ingestion of blood, and vomiting may disrupt the surgical site and/or cause airway obstruction, therefore preventive measures are mandatory. 5-Hydroxytryptamine type 3 antagonists, such as ondansetron, tropisetron, or granisetron, are used as first-line prevention. Dexamethasone is effective for preventing late PONV and has the added effect of decreasing oedema in the oropharyngeal region as well as reducing pain. The use of single antiemetics versus combination therapy depends upon the risk factors present (Table 11.1). Children at increased risk of PONV are given prophylactic intravenous ondansetron 0.15 mg/kg while in those at high risk of PONV, the addition of dexamethasone 0.15 mg/kg intravenously is recommended.[49] Metoclopramide is contraindicated for children aged <1 year of age and is only indicated as second-line therapy. Inhalational anaesthesia is more emetogenic than TIVA.[44] Hence, TIVA should be considered in high-risk patients. Stimulation of the P6 acupuncture point is also effective in preventing PONV and is best done before anaesthesia.[50,51]

The compromised airway in the postoperative period

All children with a potentially compromised airway should be fully awake before tracheal extubation. They must be closely monitored for respiratory obstruction, preferably in a high dependency unit. Where there is significant airway oedema from the surgery, tracheal

Table 11.1 Risk factors for postoperative nausea and vomiting in children

Patient factors	
Age	Age >3 years old–adolescent years
History	Previous history of PONV
Motion sickness	Positive motion sickness history
Sex	Postpubertal girls
Surgical factors	
Types of surgery	Adenotonsillectomy, strabismus surgery
Duration of surgery	>30 minutes
Anaesthetic factors	
Choice of drugs	Inhalational anaesthetic agents, anticholinesterase, and longer-acting opioids in the postoperative period

extubation should be deferred for 24–48 hours until it has subsided. In some patients, tracheostomy may be needed for postoperative respiratory care. Close monitoring and sedation of young infants (as well as paediatric arm splints, in some cases) may be required to prevent dislodgement of the tracheostomy tube.

Oromaxillofacial procedures

Cleft lip and palate

Cleft lip and palate are among the most common congenital anomalies and occur in about 1:600–700 live births.[52,53] Isolated cleft lip occurs in about 26% of cases, isolated cleft palate in 39% of cases, and both cleft lip and palate in 35% of cases.[53] These are further divided into syndromic and non-syndromic. More than 400 syndromes are associated with orofacial clefts. Common syndromes include Van der Woude syndrome,[54] DiGeorge syndrome,[55] Pierre Robin sequence,[56] and Down syndrome. Non-syndromic cleft lip with or without cleft palate (cleft lip, cleft palate, cleft lip and palate) is believed to be due to both environmental[57] and genetic factors.[58]

Children with orofacial clefts may have other congenital malformations even without a recognized syndrome. Congenital heart disease occurs in 5–10% of these patients.[59,60] Right ventricular hypertrophy and cor pulmonale may result from recurrent hypoxia secondary to airway obstruction. Chronic rhinorrhoea is common in infants with cleft palate due to nasal regurgitation during feeds.

Cleft lip is often repaired at 2–3 months of age whereas primary cleft palate repair occurs at 9–12 months old. Alveolar bone grafting is now widely considered an essential step for the repair of maxillary defects to stabilize the maxillary arch, to create support for permanent tooth eruption, to eliminate oral–nasal fistula, and to reconstruct the pyriform aperture. Optimal age for bone grafting is between 8 and 12 years old, before canine eruption.[61] Pharyngoplasty may be required for velopharyngeal incompetence. Sometimes rhinoplasty and maxillary osteotomy may be needed at 17–20 years of age (i.e. after the child has matured).

For anaesthesia in cleft surgery, preoperative assessment is important to identify two key issues: (1) any associated abnormalities and (2) the presence of predicted difficult airway management. The presence of syndromic facies like mandibular hypoplasia in Pierre Robin sequence should alert the anaesthetist to the possibility of difficult tracheal intubation. History of difficult breathing at birth and OSA are important clues. Rescheduling the surgery should be considered for infants with acute respiratory tract infection as adverse postoperative respiratory events after cleft palate repair have been reported to be 23%.[62]

Anaesthesia may be induced by intravenous or inhalation methods.[53,63] Where difficult intubation is suspected, maintenance of spontaneous ventilation until the airway is secured is generally advocated. Anticholinergic drugs such as atropine decrease secretions which, in turn, facilitates laryngoscopy and surgery. Dexamethasone 0.25–0.5 mg/kg may be given to decrease airway oedema. Tracheal intubation is usually performed using a south-facing oral Ring–Adair–Elwyn (RAE) tracheal tube. Alternatively, a wire-reinforced tube can be used. If the cleft defect is large, the laryngoscope blade may be lodged in the defect during laryngoscopy. Care should be taken to avoid the defect by placing the blade to one side or packing the defect with moist gauze. The tracheal tube fits under the tongue plate of the mouth gag during palate repair, and it should be securely taped to the lower lip during lip or palate repair. A throat pack is placed to prevent airway soiling with blood and secretions. The mouth gag that surgeons place may compress the tracheal tube, causing difficult ventilation intraoperatively. Good communication must be maintained with surgeons for repositioning the mouth gag in such an event.

Anaesthesia may be maintained with inhalational or intravenous agents. The goal is to allow the patient to awaken rapidly and smoothly at the end of surgery. Ultra-short-acting opioids like remifentanil (infusion) or short-acting fentanyl are commonly used.

At the end of surgery, the mouth should be carefully examined. Gentle suction should be undertaken, and all surgical packs removed under direct vision. Suctioning, if not done carefully, may cause rebleeding of the wound.[64] The trachea should be extubated awake and the patient closely observed postoperatively for 48 hours. The anaesthetist should be wary of excessive sedation from analgesics, airway obstruction due to tongue or laryngeal oedema,[65,66] and reduction of the pharyngeal space after closure of cleft palate. Where there is significant oedema, the patient should be transferred to the intensive care unit and extubation deferred until the swelling has subsided.

Cleft lip and palate correction surgeries are associated with intense postoperative pain. Incorporation of a multimodal analgesic approach reduces pain and aids recovery of these children. Infiltration of local anaesthetics by the surgeon has been used in both cleft lip and palate repair. Bilateral infraorbital nerve blocks reduce opioid requirements,[67] decrease emergence delirium,[68] and are superior to peri-incisional infiltration in cleft lip repair.[69] In cleft palate repair, palatal nerve block (nasopalatine, greater and lesser palatine)[70] or a bilateral suprazygomatic maxillary nerve block can reduce postoperative pain and favour early feeding[71] while intravenous paracetamol followed by regular oral paracetamol reduces postoperative morphine requirements.[72] NSAIDs reduce pain scores and the need for rescue opioids for up to 48 hours post-cleft palate repair, even more so when combined with paracetamol.[73] When opioids are used for postoperative analgesia, proper supervision in a high dependency unit is needed because of the concerns regarding sedation, respiratory depression, and consequent airway compromise.

Temporomandibular joint surgery

Temporomandibular joint ankylosis results in restricted or complete inability to open the mouth. Features of unilateral TMJ ankylosis include facial asymmetry, deviation of the mandible, and a hypoplastic mandible with receding chin on the affected side. In bilateral TMJ ankylosis, facial symmetry is maintained but there may be micrognathia from failure of the mandible to grow, a narrow maxilla, and protruding upper incisors, with limited (or non-existent) mouth opening. The child may suffer from OSA due to a small retruded mandible, malnutrition, and poor dental hygiene.

The aetiology of TMJ ankylosis may either be congenital or acquired. Acquired TMJ ankylosis may be caused by trauma, infection, systemic inflammatory disorders, irradiation, previous surgery, and neoplasm. The surgical techniques used to treat TMJ ankylosis are gap arthroplasty, interpositional arthroplasty, and joint reconstruction (Fig. 11.4).[74] Correction

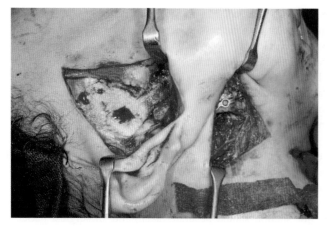

Fig. 11.4 An interpositional costochondral graft for a child with temporomandibular joint ankylosis.

of secondary deformities like facial asymmetry, occlusal canting, and micrognathic mandible may be performed concomitantly with the release of the ankylosis.[75–77]

The anaesthetic challenge in managing patients for surgical release of TMJ ankylosis lies in the management of the difficult airway. When mouth opening is limited, use of an oral airway or supraglottic airway and laryngoscopy becomes impossible. A nasal fibreoptic technique is often used.[78] Blind nasal intubation has also been used successfully.[79] Gaseous induction of the child is followed by instillation of a vasoconstrictor into the nares. A nasopharyngeal airway or a small size tracheal tube is placed into the pharynx to provide a means for insufflation of oxygen and anaesthetic agent. A cuffed reinforced tracheal tube or nasal RAE tube is preferred because it is not possible to pack the throat due to limited mouth opening. Elective tracheostomy is sometimes required in the child whose airway is precarious, to ensure safety perioperatively (**Fig. 11.5**).

Craniofacial procedures

One of the most common congenital craniofacial abnormalities requiring surgery is craniosynostosis where there is premature fusion of one or more cranial sutures. The restrictive nature of this

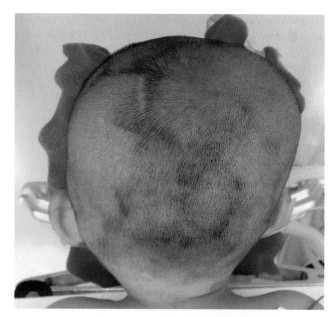

Fig. 11.6 Unilateral left lambdoidal craniosynostosis.

defect can lead to impaired brain growth, increased intracranial pressure, and psychologically devastating craniofacial deformities (**Figs 11.6** and **11.7**). Craniosynostosis occurs as an isolated condition in 80% of cases or as part of a syndrome in 20% of cases.[80] Mutation in genes coding for fibroblast growth factor receptors (FGFRs) or the *TWIST1* gene are responsible for the most common syndromes (**Table 11.2**).

In syndromic synostosis like Apert, Crouzon, and Pfeiffer syndromes, midface hypoplasia is an additional feature (**Figs 11.8** and **11.9**). Reconstruction of the cranium and midface involves several phased procedures (**Fig. 11.10**). Frontal orbital advancement and remodelling is undertaken in infancy to allow brain

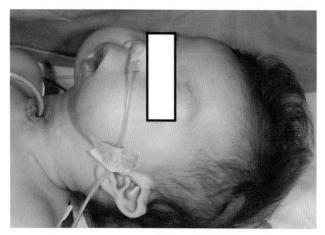

Fig. 11.5 Congenital temporomandibular joint ankylosis requiring surgical tracheostomy.

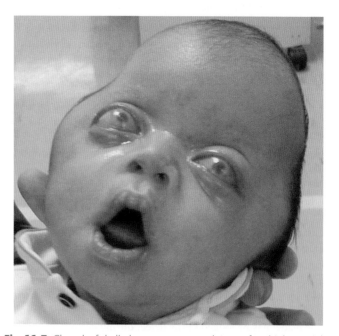

Fig. 11.7 Cloverleaf skull, due to premature closure of multiple cranial sutures.

Table 11.2 Syndromes most commonly associated with craniosynostosis

Disorder	Genetic mutation locus	Associated features
Apert syndrome	*FGFR2* (chromosome 10)	Midface hypoplasia, maxillary retrusion, proptosis, hypertelorism, syndactyly, cleft palate. May be associated with intellectual disability
Crouzon syndrome	*FGFR2* (chromosome 10)	Midface hypoplasia, maxillary retrusion, proptosis, hypertelorism, strabismus, beaked nose, often normal intelligence
Pfeiffer syndrome	*FGFR1* (chromosomal 8) *FGFR2* (chromosome 10)	Midface hypoplasia, maxillary retrusion, nasopharyngeal stenosis, proptosis, hypertelorism, strabismus, beaked nose, hearing loss, partial syndactyly, cartilaginous tracheal sleeve, broad thumbs and great toes, often normal intelligence
Saethre–Chotzen syndrome (acrocephalosyndactyly type III)	*TWIST1* (chromosome 7)	Short stature, hypertelorism, facial asymmetry, hearing loss, low frontal hairline, ptosis, mild partial syndactyly, usually normal intelligence

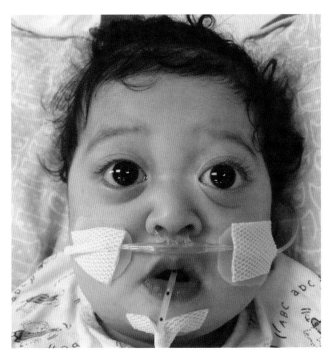

Fig. 11.8 Patient with Crouzon syndrome, showing midface hypoplasia and proptosis.

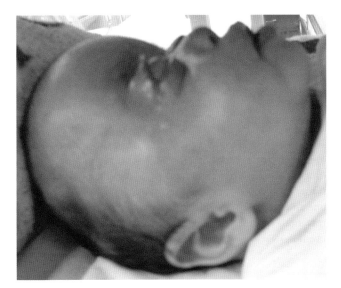

Fig. 11.9 Lateral view of a patient with Pfeiffer syndrome, demonstrating midface hypoplasia and exophthalmos.

growth and to protect the eyes in severe cases of exorbitism. Midface hypoplasia can be addressed at the time of cranial vault surgery with a monobloc advancement of the frontal bone, supraorbital bar, and midface, or staged—being undertaken later as a Le Fort III advancement. Orthognathic surgery is undertaken in young adulthood. A multidisciplinary approach involving plastic and reconstructive surgeons, neurosurgeons, maxillofacial surgeons, ear, nose, and throat surgeons, anaesthetists, orthodontists, orthoptists, speech therapists, and clinical psychologists is the key to success in craniofacial surgery.[81]

Orthognathic procedures

Le Fort III osteotomy

The Le Fort III osteotomy is a subcranial advancement of the lateral, inferior, and medial orbital elements including the zygoma and maxilla and is used to normalize orbital volume and restore projection of the zygoma. The monobloc procedure mobilizes the midface, brow, and forehead as a single unit that requires creating a

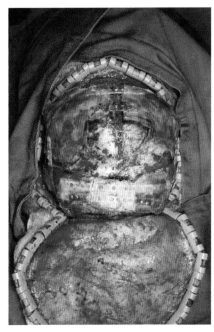

Fig. 11.10 Reconstruction of the cranium during craniosynostosis surgery.

communication between the intracranial and nasal cavities, whereas Le Fort III is completely extracranial.[82] Facial bipartition osteotomy, done in hypertelorism, allows three-dimensional correction of maxilla and orbits at the same time.

Distraction osteogenesis

Since the late 1990s, distraction osteogenesis using the Le Fort III or monobloc technique has been applied to midface advancement surgery. Distraction procedures utilize traditional patterns for osteotomies but generate new bone by allowing a period of healing followed by gradual advancement of the distraction segment by internal or external devices. The traditional use of bone graft is avoided.[83] However, a second operation is required to remove the external maxillary distraction device.

Anaesthesia for craniofacial and orthognathic procedures

Induction and airway management

Patients with congenital syndromes associated with craniofacial abnormalities may present a number of airway management challenges. Face mask ventilation can be difficult in patients with midface hypoplasia and proptosis. A suitable mask should be carefully selected to avoid injury to the eyes. An oropharyngeal airway is an effective adjunct for face mask ventilation in an obligate nose-breathing young infant who has choanal stenosis. About 50% of patients with Apert, Crouzon, or Pfeiffer syndrome develop OSA.[84] The role and indications for tracheostomy in these children with syndromes associated with OSA is unclear. In some centres, the presence of significant OSA is considered an indication for tracheostomy 1–2 weeks prior to definitive midfacial surgery,[85] while others prefer a more conservative approach with the use of continuous positive airway pressure. It is important to consider the effect of chronic airway obstruction on the child's cardiovascular system. Prior to surgery, all patients should have basal blood counts and cross-match done.

Gaseous induction with maintenance of spontaneous ventilation is often performed to minimize the risk of sudden loss of airway. An oropharyngeal or nasal airway is indicated if the child's airway obstructs during induction. Intravenous access can be difficult in young infants and particularly those with associated congenital limb abnormalities. It may be prudent to secure this before gaseous induction in those with severe OSA. Fentanyl and a non-depolarizing muscle relaxant should be administered after establishing intravenous access. Dexamethasone is administered at induction for its analgesic and antiemetic effects, and to minimize oedema.

Unlike mandibular hypoplasia, children with maxillary hypoplasia are less likely to be associated with a difficult tracheal intubation. However, in children who have undergone frontofacial advancement surgery, tracheal intubation may be more difficult as a result of the altered relationships between the maxilla and mandible and reduced TMJ movement.[86] For secondary surgery to remove the external maxillary distraction device (after distraction osteogenesis), the vertical bar can be removed to allow unobstructed access for direct laryngoscopy (**Fig. 11.11**).

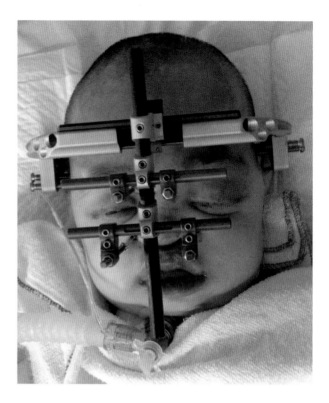

Fig. 11.11 Rigid external distraction (RED) device applied for distraction osteogenesis in midface advancement surgery. The vertical bar can be removed in the event of an airway emergency.

Intraoperative management

Major craniofacial surgery is associated with sudden cardiovascular changes and rapid blood loss. Two large peripheral intravenous catheters are essential. An arterial line is mandatory for close monitoring of blood pressure and blood sampling. A central venous line may be an appropriate measure in children requiring long-term venous access, particularly in cases where peripheral venous access proves limited.[82]

Maintenance of anaesthesia can be performed with an inhalational agent and oxygen/air mixture or TIVA with propofol and remifentanil infusion. Nitrous oxide is avoided when there is a cranial component to the surgery due to the risk of venous air embolism. There are now a number of commercial target-controlled infusion devices for propofol that incorporate pharmacokinetic algorithms which simplify TIVA in children, making it a viable option.[87]

Intraoperative fluids consist of routine maintenance fluids and replacement of blood loss. Estimation of blood loss is difficult and goal-directed fluid therapy using stroke volume variation or pulse pressure variation, together with regular point-of-care testing of haemoglobin and blood gases provide guidance in clinical management. A combination of opioids like fentanyl or morphine and intravenous paracetamol are administered for analgesia. Intravenous ondansetron and dexamethasone are recommended to prevent PONV.

Blood conservation

Various strategies for reducing homologous blood transfusion have been used. Preoperative autologous blood donation and acute normovolaemic haemodilution are difficult to achieve in young children because of their age and insufficient blood volume. Recombinant human erythropoietin and iron supplementation given weekly for 3–4 weeks prior to surgery increases the preoperative haemoglobin level and decreases transfusion requirements, particularly in those with pre-existing anaemia.[88–90] In children who cannot receive or do not respond to oral iron due to intolerance, poor adherence, or iron malabsorption, parenteral iron is a safe and effective means to treat iron deficiency.[91] Since the safe limits for hypotension in children are unknown, it has been suggested that hypotensive anaesthesia should not be used in paediatric midface advancement surgery.[82] Intraoperative blood salvage from the surgical site with reinfusion after processing can reduce homologous blood transfusion. In infants and young children, application of this technique is limited because of high priming volume and slow processing time. The safety of this cell salvage technique in operations where there may be microbiological contamination from the respiratory tract mucosa in the surgical field has also being questioned.[92] Antifibrinolytic agents have been shown to effectively decrease blood loss and exposure to allogeneic blood transfusion in children undergoing craniosynostosis surgery,[88,93] major orthopaedic surgery,[94] and cardiac surgery[95] and is therefore recommended in craniofacial surgery where there is a significant risk for perioperative transfusion.

Prophylactic or therapeutic administration of tranexamic acid, an antifibrinolytic agent, is a well-tolerated and effective strategy to reduce bleeding, decrease the requirement for allogeneic blood product transfusion, and improve patient outcomes.[96,97] It has a good safety profile.[98] Patients may develop hypotension with fast intravenous administration, but convulsions occur only with very high doses. Although the optimal dose regimen is not established, a loading dose of between 10 and 30 mg/kg followed by 5–10 mg/kg/hr maintenance infusion have been used in paediatric trauma and surgery.[99] Absolute contraindications include hypersensitivity, active thromboembolic disease, and fibrinolytic conditions with consumption coagulopathy.

Postoperative management

Children should be nursed in a high dependency area after major craniofacial surgery. In a multicentre observational study comprising 72 patients, 52% of the Le Fort III and 73% of the monobloc patients were kept intubated in the intensive care unit after surgery.[82] Head-up position is recommended to decrease local swelling. Analgesia should be multimodal, with an intravenous opioid (morphine or fentanyl) infusion or patient/nurse-controlled analgesia, regular paracetamol, and NSAID. Nausea or vomiting should be treated with antiemetics.

Surgery for trauma

Paediatric facial injuries are usually minor, and fracture is rare compared to adults. However, when it occurs, it is associated with severe injury and disability. Concomitant head, cervical spine, and ocular injuries need to be considered. Motor vehicle accidents, falls from height, and sport-related injuries are the leading causes. It is estimated that <1% of maxillofacial trauma occurs in children <5 years of age.[100] Greater flexibility of bones, underdeveloped sinuses, unerupted teeth, the presence of protective fat pads, and less involvement in high-velocity road traffic accidents make children less prone to injury.[101] Cranial and central facial injuries are more common among toddlers and infants, and mandibular injuries are more common among adolescents. Treatment is usually conservative for facial injury with minimal manipulation to prevent growth disturbance. Surgical intervention is indicated only for the repair of severely displaced and comminuted fractures that are likely to cause functional impairment, aesthetic deformity, or both.[102]

Anaesthetic management requires immediate assessment of the airway. Even an unobstructed airway should be carefully monitored, as increasing oedema, swelling, and haematoma may later cause compromise. Depending on the degree of obstruction, simple measures like clearing the airway, optimizing positioning, and insertion of an oropharyngeal airway will suffice. Obstruction from bi-mandibular fractures can be relieved by anterior traction on the jaw or tongue. Successful tracheal intubation can be achieved using several different techniques (as described in the earlier section on difficult airway management), depending on the type of injury and patient condition. When anatomical disruption makes intubation difficult or impossible, a surgical airway is lifesaving.

Minor oromaxillofacial procedures

Tongue tie

Tongue tie (ankyloglossia) is an anomaly comprising an abnormally short lingual frenulum. Tongue tie occurs in about 4% of newborns and may be associated with feeding and speech problems.[103] There is no consensus on the optimum timing and the indications for tongue tie surgery. This operation is a short procedure where the surgeon performs frenulotomy under local or general anaesthesia. A simple approach to anaesthesia, without airway instrumentation, is to allow the child to spontaneously breathe sevoflurane/oxygen via a face mask. Once the child is anaesthetized, local anaesthetic is applied topically, and the surgeon performs the frenulotomy. The anaesthetist should be wary of laryngospasm if the patient is not in a sufficiently deep plane of anaesthesia, and close cooperation between the surgeon and anaesthetist is required. Alternatively, a supraglottic airway may be used by some anaesthetists, though tracheal intubation is seldom required. Simple oral analgesics are sufficient for postoperative pain management.

Dental surgery

Children may present for dental procedures such as teeth scaling and polishing, extraction, or drainage of dental abscess (and its complication Ludwig's angina). Most young children will need general anaesthesia for extensive and lengthy dental procedures.

For dental abscess, it is important to assess the airway before surgery to ensure it is not compromised. Trismus is unusual and may relax upon induction of anaesthesia if the infection is superficial. If the infection has spread to the submasseteric area, relaxation of the trismus is unlikely and fibreoptic intubation will be required.

Many anaesthetists insert a nasotracheal tube if both left and right sides are to be manipulated. Nasotracheal tubes have less chance of dislodgement, but increased risk of epistaxis and sinusitis. Some anaesthetists intubate the trachea orally with a south-facing RAE tube, taped to the opposite side if only one side is to be manipulated.

A throat pack (if required) should be placed after the patient is asleep. A study comparing propofol versus sevoflurane-based anaesthesia for dental procedures showed less PONV and less nursing interventions with propofol, although a similar rate of postoperative delirium.[104] Careful suctioning and removal of the throat pack should be done before awake tracheal extubation. Simple analgesics suffice for postoperative pain.

Conclusion

Anaesthesia for oromaxillofacial surgery in children can be challenging. The type of anaesthesia required for children of different age groups, comorbidities, and severity of operation may vary greatly and needs to be tailored to each child. Anaesthetists should always be prepared for the possibility of difficult intubation and ventilation, massive fluid shifts, and prolonged procedures. A multidisciplinary approach is essential for satisfactory outcome.

REFERENCES

1. Regli A, Becke K, von Ungern-Sternberg BS. An update on the perioperative management of children with upper respiratory tract infections. *Curr Opin Anaesthesiol.* 2017;**30**(3):362–367.
2. Mostafa MG, Morsy KM. Premedication with intranasal dexmedetomidine, midazolam and ketamine for children undergoing bone marrow biopsy and aspirate. *Egypt J Anaesth.* 2013;**29**(2):131–135.
3. Ghai B, Jain K, Saxena AK, Bhatia N, Sodhi KS. Comparison of oral midazolam with intranasal dexmedetomidine premedication for children undergoing CT imaging: a randomized, double-blind, and controlled study. *Paediatr Anaesth.* 2017;**27**(1):37–44.
4. Jun JH, Kim KN, Kim JY, Song SM. The effects of intranasal dexmedetomidine premedication in children: a systematic review and meta-analysis. *Can J Anaesth.* 2017;**64**(9):947–961.
5. Yuen VM, Hui TW, Irwin MG, Yuen MK. A comparison of intranasal dexmedetomidine and oral midazolam for premedication in pediatric anesthesia: a double-blinded randomized controlled trial. *Anesth Analg.* 2008;**106**(6):1715–1721.
6. Zub D, Berkenbosch JW, Tobias JD. Preliminary experience with oral dexmedetomidine for procedural and anesthetic premedication. *Paediatr Anaesth.* 2005;**15**(11):932–938.
7. Yuen VM, Irwin MG, Hui TW, Yuen MK, Lee LH. A double-blind, crossover assessment of the sedative and analgesic effects of intranasal dexmedetomidine. *Anesth Anal.* 2007;**105**(2):374–380.
8. Gyanesh P, Haldar R, Srivastava D, Agrawal PM, Tiwari AK, Singh PK. Comparison between intranasal dexmedetomidine and intranasal ketamine as premedication for procedural sedation in children undergoing MRI: a double-blind, randomized, placebo-controlled trial. *J Anesth.* 2014;**28**(1):12–18.
9. Practice guidelines for preoperative fasting and the use of pharmacologic agents to reduce the risk of pulmonary aspiration: application to healthy patients undergoing elective procedures: an updated report by the American Society of Anesthesiologists Task Force on Preoperative Fasting and the Use of Pharmacologic Agents to Reduce the Risk of Pulmonary Aspiration. *Anesthesiology.* 2017;**126**(3):376–393.
10. Andersson H, Zaren B, Frykholm P. Low incidence of pulmonary aspiration in children allowed intake of clear fluids until called to the operating suite. *Paediatr Anaesth.* 2015;**25**(8):770–777.
11. Schmidt AR, Buehler P, Seglias L, Stark T, Brotschi B, Renner T, et al. Gastric pH and residual volume after 1 and 2 h fasting time for clear fluids in children. *Br J Anaesth.* 2015;**114**(3):477–482.
12. Thomas M, Morrison C, Newton R, Schindler E. Consensus statement on clear fluids fasting for elective pediatric general anesthesia. *Paediatr Anaesth.* 2018;**28**(5):411–414.
13. Pfaff KE, Tumin D, Miller R, Beltran RJ, Tobias JD, Uffman JC. Perioperative aspiration events in children: a report from the Wake-Up Safe Collaborative. *Paediatr Anaesth.* 2020;**30**(6):660–666.
14. Karsli C, Pehora C, Al-Izzi A, Mathew P. A retrospective review of pediatric difficult airways: once easy, not always easy. *Can J Anaesth.* 2016;**63**(6):776–777.
15. Morray JP, Geiduschek JM, Caplan RA, Posner KL, Gild WM, Cheney FW. A comparison of pediatric and adult anesthesia closed malpractice claims. *Anesthesiology.* 1993;**78**(3):461–467.
16. Mamie C, Habre W, Delhumeau C, Argiroffo CB, Morabia A. Incidence and risk factors of perioperative respiratory adverse events in children undergoing elective surgery. *Paediatr Anaesth.* 2004;**14**(3):218–224.
17. Jimenez N, Posner KL, Cheney FW, Caplan RA, Lee LA, Domino KB. An update on pediatric anesthesia liability: a closed claims analysis. *Anesth Anal.* 2007;**104**(1):147–153.
18. Bhananker SM, Ramamoorthy C, Geiduschek JM, Posner KL, Domino KB, Haberkern CM, et al. Anesthesia-related cardiac arrest in children: update from the Pediatric Perioperative Cardiac Arrest Registry. *Anesth Anal.* 2007;**105**(2):344–350.
19. Adewale L. Anatomy and assessment of the pediatric airway. *Paediatr Anaesth.* 2009;**19** Suppl 1:1–8.
20. Santillanes G, Gausche-Hill M. Pediatric airway management. *Emerg Med Clin North Am.* 2008;**26**(4):961–975, ix.
21. Bew S. Managing the difficult airway in children. *Anaesth Intensive Care Med.* 2006;**7**(5):172–174.
22. Frerk C, Mitchell VS, McNarry AF, Mendonca C, Bhagrath R, Patel A, et al. Difficult Airway Society 2015 guidelines for management of unanticipated difficult intubation in adults. *Br J Anaesth.* 2015;**115**(6):827–848.
23. Warters RD, Szabo TA, Spinale FG, DeSantis SM, Reves JG. The effect of neuromuscular blockade on mask ventilation. *Anaesthesia.* 2011;**66**(3):163–167.
24. Sachdeva R, Kannan TR, Mendonca C, Patteril M. Evaluation of changes in tidal volume during mask ventilation following administration of neuromuscular blocking drugs. *Anaesthesia.* 2014;**69**(8):826–831.
25. Masters IB, Chang AB, Harris M, O'Neil MC. Modified nasopharyngeal tube for upper airway obstruction. *Arch Dis Child.* 1999;**80**(2):186–187.
26. Brooks P, Ree R, Rosen D, Ansermino M. Canadian pediatric anesthesiologists prefer inhalational anesthesia to manage difficult airways. *Can J Anaesth.* 2005;**52**(3):285–290.
27. Humphreys S, Lee-Archer P, Reyne G, Long D, Williams T, Schibler A. Transnasal humidified rapid-insufflation ventilatory exchange (THRIVE) in children: a randomized controlled trial. *Br J Anaesth.* 2017;**118**(2):232–238.
28. Humphreys S, Schibler A. Nasal high-flow oxygen in pediatric anesthesia and airway management. *Paediatr Anaesth.* 2020;**30**(3):339–346.
29. Walker RW. The laryngeal mask airway in the difficult paediatric airway: an assessment of positioning and use in fibreoptic intubation. *Paediatr Anaesth.* 2000;**10**(1):53–58.
30. Walker RW, Allen DL, Rothera MR. A fibreoptic intubation technique for children with mucopolysaccharidoses using the laryngeal mask airway. *Paediatr Anaesth.* 1997;**7**(5):421–426.

31. Difficult Airway Society. Difficult Airway Society 2015 guidelines for cannot intubate and cannot ventilate (CICV) in a paralysed anaesthetised child aged 1 to 8 years 2015. https://das.uk.com/guidelines/paediatric-difficult-airway-guidelines

32. Weiss M, Dullenkopf A, Gerber AC. [Microcuff pediatric tracheal tube. A new tracheal tube with a high volume-low pressure cuff for children]. *Anaesthesist*. 2004;**53**(1):73–79.

33. Chambers NA, Ramgolam A, Sommerfield D, Zhang G, Ledowski T, Thurm M, et al. Cuffed vs. uncuffed tracheal tubes in children: a randomised controlled trial comparing leak, tidal volume and complications. *Anaesthesia*. 2018;**73**(2):160–168.

34. Shah A, Carlisle JB. Cuffed tracheal tubes: guilty now proven innocent. *Anaesthesia*. 2019;**74**(9):1186–1190.

35. Weiss M, Dullenkopf A, Fischer JE, Keller C, Gerber AC; European Paediatric Endotracheal Intubation Study GROUP. Prospective randomized controlled multi-centre trial of cuffed or uncuffed endotracheal tubes in small children. *Br J Anaesth*. 2009;**103**(6):867–873.

36. Elkon B, Cambrin JR, Hirshberg E, Bratton SL. Hyperglycemia: an independent risk factor for poor outcome in children with traumatic brain injury. *Pediatr Crit Care Med*. 2014;**15**(7):623–631.

37. Drummond JC, Moore SS. The influence of dextrose administration on neurologic outcome after temporary spinal cord ischemia in the rabbit. *Anesthesiology*. 1989;**70**(1):64–70.

38. Duckrow RB, Beard DC, Brennan RW. Regional cerebral blood flow decreases during chronic and acute hyperglycemia. *Stroke*. 1987;**18**(1):52–58.

39. Nishina K, Mikawa K, Maekawa N, Asano M, Obara H. Effects of exogenous intravenous glucose on plasma glucose and lipid homeostasis in anesthetized infants. *Anesthesiology*. 1995;**83**(2):258–263.

40. Dubois MC, Gouyet L, Murat I, Saint-Maurice C. Lactated Ringer with 1% dextrose: an appropriate solution for peri-operative fluid therapy in children. *Pediatr Anesth*. 1992;**2**(2):99–104.

41. Tosh P, Rajan S, Barua K, Kumar L. Comparison of intraoperative glycemic levels in infants with the use of ringer lactate with supplemental 1% versus 2% dextrose as maintenance fluid. *Anesth Essays Res*. 2019;**13**(4):631–635.

42. Paut O, Lacroix F. Recent developments in the perioperative fluid management for the paediatric patient. *Curr Opin Anaesthesiol*. 2006;**19**(3):268–277.

43. Anderson BJ. Paracetamol (acetaminophen): mechanisms of action. *Paediatr Anaesth*. 2008;**18**(10):915–921.

44. Michelet D, Andreu-Gallien J, Bensalah T, Hilly J, Wood C, Nivoche Y, et al. A meta-analysis of the use of nonsteroidal antiinflammatory drugs for pediatric postoperative pain. *Anesth Anal*. 2012;**114**(2):393–406.

45. Anderson BJ. Comparing the efficacy of NSAIDs and paracetamol in children. *Paediatr Anaesth*. 2004;**14**(3):201–217.

46. Wilson-Smith EM. Systemic analgesics in children. *Anaesth Intensive Care Med*. 2010;**11**(6):217–223.

47. Ali U, Tsang M, Igbeyi B, Balakrishnan S, Shackell K, Kotzer G, et al. A 4 year quality improvement initiative reducing post-operative nausea and vomiting in children undergoing strabismus surgery at a quaternary paediatric hospital. *Paediatr Anaesth*. 2019;**29**(7):690–697.

48. Rose JB, Watcha MF. Postoperative nausea and vomiting in paediatric patients. *Br J Anaesth*. 1999;**83**(1):104–117.

49. Martin S, Baines D, Holtby H, Carr AS. APAGBI guidelines on the prevention of post-operative vomiting in children. 2016. https://www.apagbi.org.uk/sites/default/files/inline-files/2016%20APA%20POV%20Guideline-2.pdf

50. Dune LS, Shiao SY. Metaanalysis of acustimulation effects on postoperative nausea and vomiting in children. *Explore (NY)*. 2006;**2**(4):314–320.

51. Zhang Y, Zhang C, Yan M, Wang N, Liu J, Wu A. The effectiveness of PC6 acupuncture in the prevention of postoperative nausea and vomiting in children: A systematic review and meta-analysis. *Paediatr Anaesth*. 2020;**30**(5):552–563.

52. Kobayashi GS, Brito LA, Meira JGC, Alvizi L, Passos-Bueno MR. Genetics of cleft lip and cleft palate: perspectives in surgery management and outcome. In: Alonso N, Raposo-Amaral CE (eds) *Cleft Lip and Palate Treatment*, pp. 25–35. Cham: Springer; 2018.

53. Tremlett M. Anaesthesia for cleft lip and palate surgery. *Curr Anaesth Crit Care*. 2004;**15**(4):309–316.

54. Schutte BC, Sander A, Malik M, Murray JC. Refinement of the Van der Woude gene location and construction of a 3.5-Mb YAC contig and STS map spanning the critical region in 1q32–q41. *Genomics*. 1996;**36**(3):507–514.

55. Devriendt K, Fryns JP, Mortier G, van Thienen MN, Keymolen K. The annual incidence of DiGeorge/velocardiofacial syndrome. *J Med Genet*. 1998;**35**(9):789–790.

56. Wan T, Chen Y, Wang G. Do patients with isolated Pierre Robin Sequence have worse outcomes after cleft palate repair: a systematic review. *J Plast Reconstr Aesthet Surg*. 2015;**68**(8):1095–1099.

57. Mirilas P, Mentessidou A, Kontis E, Asimakidou M, Moxham BJ, Petropoulos AS, et al. Parental exposures and risk of nonsyndromic orofacial clefts in offspring: a case-control study in Greece. *Int J Pediatr Otorhinolaryngol*. 2011;**75**(5):695–699.

58. Kohli SS, Kohli VS. A comprehensive review of the genetic basis of cleft lip and palate. *J Oral Maxillofac Pathol*. 2012;**16**(1):64–72.

59. Barbosa MM, Rocha CM, Katina T, Caldas M, Codorniz A, Medeiros C. Prevalence of congenital heart diseases in oral cleft patients. *Pediatr Cardiol*. 2003;**24**(4):369–374.

60. Reena, Bandyopadhyay KH, Paul A. Postoperative analgesia for cleft lip and palate repair in children. *J Anaesthesiol Clin Pharmacol*. 2016;**32**(1):5–11.

61. Alonso N, da Silva Freitas R, Amundson J, Raposo-Amaral CE. Bone graft in alveolar cleft lip and palate. In: Alonso N, Raposo-Amaral CE (ed) *Cleft Lip and Palate Treatment*, pp. 247–261. Cham: Springer; 2018.

62. Jackson O, Basta M, Sonnad S, Stricker P, Larossa D, Fiadjoe J. Perioperative risk factors for adverse airway events in patients undergoing cleft palate repair. *Cleft Palate Craniofac J*. 2013;**50**(3):330–336.

63. Steward DJ. Anesthesia for patients with cleft lip and palate. *Semin Anesth Periop Med Pain*. 2007;**26**(3):126–132.

64. Oosthuizen A. Anaesthesia for cleft lip and palate surgery. *S Afr J Anaesth Anal*. 2017;**23**(2):128–133.

65. Patane PS, White SE. Macroglossia causing airway obstruction following cleft palate repair. *Anesthesiology*. 1989;**71**(6):995–996.

66. Chan MT, Chan MS, Mui KS, Ho BP. Massive lingual swelling following palatoplasty. An unusual cause of upper airway obstruction. *Anaesthesia*. 1995;**50**(1):30–34.

67. Rajamani A, Kamat V, Rajavel VP, Murthy J, Hussain SA. A comparison of bilateral infraorbital nerve block with intravenous fentanyl for analgesia following cleft lip repair in children. *Paediatr Anaesth*. 2007;**17**(2):133–139.

68. Wang H, Liu G, Fu W, Li ST. The effect of infraorbital nerve block on emergence agitation in children undergoing cleft lip surgery

under general anesthesia with sevoflurane. *Paediatr Anaesth.* 2015;**25**(9):906–910.

69. Prabhu KP, Wig J, Grewal S. Bilateral infraorbital nerve block is superior to peri-incisional infiltration for analgesia after repair of cleft lip. *Scand J Plast Reconstr Surg Hand Surg.* 1999;**33**(1):83–87.

70. Jonnavithula N, Durga P, Madduri V, Ramachandran G, Nuvvula R, Srikanth R, et al. Efficacy of palatal block for analgesia following palatoplasty in children with cleft palate. *Paediatr Anaesth.* 2010;**20**(8):727–733.

71. Mesnil M, Dadure C, Captier G, Raux O, Rochette A, Canaud N, et al. A new approach for peri-operative analgesia of cleft palate repair in infants: the bilateral suprazygomatic maxillary nerve block. *Paediatr Anaesth.* 2010;**20**(4):343–349.

72. Nour C, Ratsiu J, Singh N, Mason L, Ray A, Martin M, et al. Analgesic effectiveness of acetaminophen for primary cleft palate repair in young children: a randomized placebo controlled trial. *Paediatr Anaesth.* 2014;**24**(6):574–581.

73. Mireskandari SM, Makarem J. Effect of rectal diclofenac and acetaminophen alone and in combination on postoperative pain after cleft palate repair in children. *J Craniofac Surg.* 2011;**22**(5):1955–1959.

74. Kennett S. Temporomandibular joint ankylosis: the rationale for grafting in the young patient. *J Oral Surg.* 1973;**31**(10):744–748.

75. Andrade NN, Raikwar KR. Management of patients with obstructive sleep apnoea induced by temporomandibular joint ankylosis: a novel 2-stage surgical protocol and report of 5 cases. *Asian J Oral Maxillofac Surg.* 2009;**21**(1):27–32.

76. Feiyun P, Wei L, Jun C, Xin X, Zhuojin S, Fengguo Y. Simultaneous correction of bilateral temporomandibular joint ankylosis with mandibular micrognathia using internal distraction osteogenesis and 3-dimensional craniomaxillofacial models. *J Oral Maxillofac Surg.* 2010;**68**(3):571–577.

77. Munro IR, Chen YR, Park BY. Simultaneous total correction of temporomandibular ankylosis and facial asymmetry. *Plast Reconstr Surg.* 1986;**77**(4):517–529.

78. Kilmartin E, Grunwald Z, Kaplan FS, Nussbaum BL. General anesthesia for dental procedures in patients with fibrodysplasia ossificans progressiva: a review of 42 cases in 30 patients. *Anesthes Anal.* 2014;**118**(2):298–301.

79. Marhatta MN, Acharya SP. Blind nasal intubation in a child with ankylosis of temporomandibular joint. *Nepal Med Coll J.* 2008;**10**(4):271–274.

80. Buchanan EP, Xue AS, Hollier LH, Jr. Craniofacial syndromes. *Plast Reconstr Surg.* 2014;**134**(1):128e–153e.

81. Sawh-Martinez R, Steinbacher DM. Syndromic Craniosynostosis. *Clin Plast Surg.* 2019;**46**(2):141–155.

82. Glover CD, Fernandez AM, Huang H, Derderian C, Binstock W, Reid R, et al. Perioperative outcomes and management in midface advancement surgery: a multicenter observational descriptive study from the Pediatric Craniofacial Collaborative Group. *Paediatr Anaesth.* 2018;**28**(8):710–718.

83. Yu JC, Fearon J, Havlik RJ, Buchman SR, Polley JW. Distraction osteogenesis of the craniofacial skeleton. *Plast Reconstr Surg.* 2004;**114**(1):1E–20E.

84. Moore MH. Upper airway obstruction in the syndromal craniosynostoses. *Br J Plast Surg.* 1993;**46**(5):355–362.

85. Thomas K, Hughes C, Johnson D, Das S. Anesthesia for surgery related to craniosynostosis: a review. Part 1. Paediatric anaesthesia. 2012;**22**(11):1033–1041.

86. de Beer D, Bingham R. The child with facial abnormalities. *Curr Opin Anaesthesiol.* 2011;**24**(3):282–288.

87. Anderson B, Houghton J. Ankle biters: how to use TIVA in children. In: Wong GTC, Irwin MG, Lam SW (eds) *Taking on TIVA: Debunking Myths and Dispelling Misunderstandings,* pp. 111–123. Cambridge: Cambridge University Press; 2019.

88. Escher PJ, Tu A, Kearney S, Wheelwright M, Petronio J, Kebriaei M, et al. Minimizing transfusion in sagittal craniosynostosis surgery: the Children's Hospital of Minnesota Protocol. *Childs Nerv Syst.* 2019;**35**(8):1357–1362.

89. Vega RA, Lyon C, Kierce JF, Tye GW, Ritter AM, Rhodes JL. Minimizing transfusion requirements for children undergoing craniosynostosis repair: the CHoR protocol. *J Neurosurg Pediatr.* 2014;**14**(2):190–195.

90. Meara JG, Smith EM, Harshbarger RJ, Farlo JN, Matar MM, Levy ML. Blood-conservation techniques in craniofacial surgery. *Ann Plast Surg.* 2005;**54**(5):525–529.

91. Crary SE, Hall K, Buchanan GR. Intravenous iron sucrose for children with iron deficiency failing to respond to oral iron therapy. *Pediatr Blood Cancer.* 2011;**56**(5):615–619.

92. Anderson S, Panizza B. Are cell salvage and autologous blood transfusion safe in endonasal surgery? *Otolaryngol Head Neck Surg.* 2010;**142**(3 Suppl 1):S3–S6.

93. Lu VM, Goyal A, Daniels DJ. Tranexamic acid decreases blood transfusion burden in open craniosynostosis surgery without operative compromise. *J Craniofac Surg.* 2019;**30**(1):120–126.

94. McNicol ED, Tzortzopoulou A, Schumann R, Carr DB, Kalra A. Antifibrinolytic agents for reducing blood loss in scoliosis surgery in children. *Cochrane Database Syst Rev.* 2016;**9**:CD006883.

95. Hassan M, Hasan K, Salam A, Razzak A, Ferdous S, Maruf F, et al. Effect of tranexamic acid after cardiac surgery in children. *Cardiovasc J.* 2009;**1**(2):189–192.

96. Goobie SM, Meier PM, Pereira LM, McGowan FX, Prescilla RP, Scharp LA, et al. Efficacy of tranexamic acid in pediatric craniosynostosis surgery: a double-blind, placebo-controlled trial. *Anesthesiology.* 2011;**114**(4):862–871.

97. Dadure C, Sauter M, Bringuier S, Bigorre M, Raux O, Rochette A, et al. Intraoperative tranexamic acid reduces blood transfusion in children undergoing craniosynostosis surgery: a randomized double-blind study. *Anesthesiology.* 2011;**114**(4):856–861.

98. Goobie SM, Cladis FP, Glover CD, Huang H, Reddy SK, Fernandez AM, et al. Safety of antifibrinolytics in cranial vault reconstructive surgery: a report from the pediatric craniofacial collaborative group. *Paediatr Anaesth.* 2017;**27**(3):271–281.

99. Goobie SM, Faraoni D. Tranexamic acid and perioperative bleeding in children: what do we still need to know? *Curr Opin Anaesthesiol.* 2019;**32**(3):343–352.

100. Haug RH, Foss J. Maxillofacial injuries in the pediatric patient. *Oral Surg Oral Med Oral Pathol Oral Radiol Endod.* 2000;**90**(2):126–134.

101. Ferreira PC, Amarante JM, Silva PN, Rodrigues JM, Choupina MP, Silva AC, et al. Retrospective study of 1251 maxillofacial fractures in children and adolescents. *Plast Reconstr Surg.* 2005;**115**(6):1500–1508.

102. Mukherjee CG, Mukherjee U. Maxillofacial trauma in children. *Int J Clin Pediatr Dent.* 2012;**5**(3):231–236.

103. Klockars T, Pitkaranta A. Pediatric tongue-tie division: indications, techniques and patient satisfaction. *Int J Pediatr Otorhinolaryngol.* 2009;**73**(10):1399–1401.

104. Konig MW, Varughese AM, Brennen KA, Barclay S, Shackleford TM, Samuels PJ, et al. Quality of recovery from two types of general anesthesia for ambulatory dental surgery in children: a double-blind, randomized trial. *Paediatr Anaesth.* 2009;**19**(8):748–755.

12

Infection

Adam R. Duffen and David J. A. Vaughan

Introduction

This chapter describes the anaesthetic management of patients presenting for surgery with oral and dental infections, including the pathophysiology, associated complications, clinical assessment, and management options (including antimicrobials), and an overview of the key aspects of managing patients with sepsis.

Infection of the oral cavity, including dental caries, dental abscesses, and gingivitis, is the commonest disease in the world. Management of the majority of these conditions does not usually require an anaesthetist. In the minority, however, where simple management with oral hygiene and antibiotics fail, more serious localized infection may develop, or infection may become systemic (leading to sepsis), necessitating operative intervention and/or supportive management in the critical care unit. Indeed, infections of the head and neck make up a significant proportion of the emergency workload in oromaxillofacial surgical units.

Epidemiology

Globally, despite great improvements in oral health, oral disease is still a major public health problem.[1] Dental caries affects nearly all adults and between 60% and 90% of children worldwide, with particularly high rates in developed countries. Improved public health, through health promotion[2] and the widespread addition of fluoride to drinking water and toothpaste, has led to a reduction in tooth decay (from 46% to 28% in adults, between 1998 and 2009). There are social variations in tooth decay prevalence, with those in professional occupations being 11% less likely to be affected.[3]

Most serious dental infections are preventable with regular dental care. However, there is some evidence that the incidence of hospital admissions from severe odontogenic infection may have increased in the UK. Analysis of hospital statistics between 1998 and 2006 showed a doubling of admissions for drainage of dental abscesses. It has been suggested that this may be a consequence of reduced access to routine dental care,[4] although it may also reflect the increasing reticence of community dental physicians to treat these issues, for medicolegal and possibly remunerative reasons.

Oral disease can be associated with other chronic conditions or health-related risk factors. Patients presenting with odontogenic infections will therefore have a higher incidence of diabetes, obesity, smoking, and drug and alcohol misuse. Poor nutritional status may be a causative factor or a direct consequence of the condition.

Pathophysiology

Dental caries is caused by the action of acid-producing bacteria on the dental enamel, causing it to dissolve. Bacteria can enter the tooth through a carious cavity and then pass through the dentine and into the pulp (**Fig. 12.1**). Infection may track through the pulp to the root apex and into the alveolar bone forming a periapical abscess.

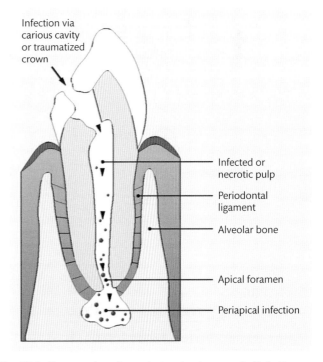

Infection via carious cavity or traumatized crown

Infected or necrotic pulp

Periodontal ligament

Alveolar bone

Apical foramen

Periapical infection

Fig. 12.1 Cross-section of a tooth showing the spread of infection.

Table 12.1 Classification of dental abscesses

Type of abscess	Tissue affected
Periapical	Infection at the apex of the root
Periodontal	Infection begins at the periodontal pocket and affects the ligament
Gingival	Infection involves only the gum tissue, and not the tooth
Pericoronal	Infection involves the soft tissues surrounding the crown
Combined periodontic-endodontic	Infection originates from both the dental pulp and the periodontal tissues

Alternatively, infection may enter via a broken tooth, resulting from extensive periodontal disease, or failed root canal treatment. Periapical abscesses are the most common type of dental abscess. Other types of abscess can be classified according to the anatomical location of the tissue affected (**Table 12.1**).[5]

Infection that enters via the pulp may resolve, cause a pulpitis, become localized and form a periapical abscess, or can spread through the cortical plate and into surrounding tissue. The position of the tooth influences the likely spread of an abscess formed at that site. **Fig. 12.2** shows the position of the paediatric and adult teeth, and the location of the incisors, canines, premolars, and molars.[6]

Infection follows the path of least resistance, spreading along the fascial planes, and into adjoining structures (**Fig. 12.3**). Pus arising from the lower teeth (mandibular) may drain outwards, intraorally

(from incisors, canines, and premolars) or extraorally through the skin or submandibular tissue (from second and third molars). Infection arising from the upper teeth (maxillary) may spread into the maxillary sinuses or infraorbital soft tissue.[7] In addition, infection may spread deeper into the facial or deep neck spaces, or via the venous circulation into the cranium. Both phenomena can have serious consequences. The fascial spaces are potential areas which open as a consequence of pressure from spreading infection. The spread through these spaces is determined by muscle, bone, and fascial attachments. The spread into the different planes can be either from mandibular or maxillary dental infections,[8] and the clinical consequences of the spread is directly related to the fascial plane that is involved.[9] The clinical effects of these infections are summarized in **Table 12.2**.

Microbiology

Dental caries is thought to be caused by serotypes of *Streptococcus mutans* (*S. cricetus*, *S. rattus*, *S. ferus*, and *S. sobrinus*) most commonly, although lactobacilli also contribute to enamel decay, by production of acid.

Odontogenic infections are usually polymicrobial and caused by the organisms that are present in the normal oral flora (**Table 12.3**).[10] Over 460 unique bacterial taxa have been identified in dental infections. They are commonly caused by a combination of facultative anaerobes and strict anaerobes.

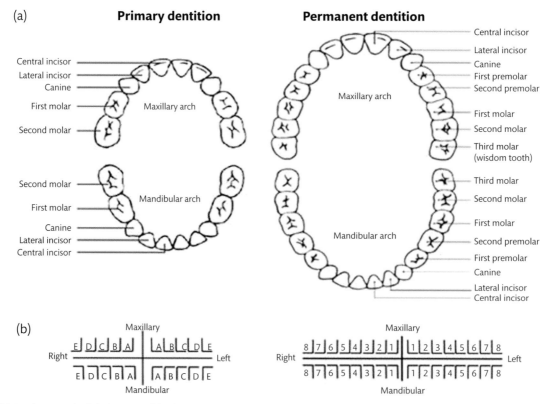

Fig. 12.2 (a) Paediatric and adult dentition. (b) Palmer notation, indicating the position of paediatric and adult teeth.

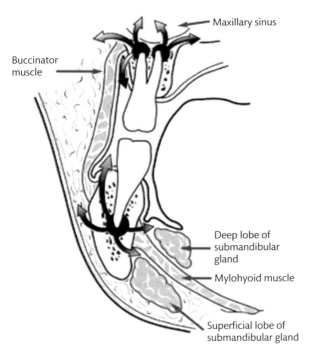

Fig. 12.3 Spread of odontogenic infection through the fascial planes.

Antimicrobials

Patients with uncomplicated dental abscesses who are systemically well do not usually require antibiotic treatment. In more severe cases, with systemic signs or severe localized infections,

Table 12.2 Clinical consequences of spread of infection according to the fascial plane involved

Maxillary spaces	
Infraorbital space (canine)	Cavernous sinus spread
	Cavernous sinus thrombosis
Buccal space	Facial swelling
Infratemporal space	Trismus
Mandibular spaces	
Parapharyngeal space:	
Anterior	Trismus, dysphagia, displacement of the tonsil and pharyngeal wall
Posterior	Displacement of posterior pharyngeal wall, thrombosis of internal jugular vein
Retropharyngeal space	Airway obstruction at the pharynx
	Torticollis
	Lymphadenopathy
Buccal space	Facial swelling
Sublingual space	Drooling, dysphagia, Ludwig's angina
Submandibular space	Trismus, Ludwig's angina
Masticator space	Trismus
Submasseteric space	Marked trismus
Carotid space	Vocal cord paralysis, Horner's syndrome
Pretracheal space	Dysphagia, airway obstruction, mediastinitis

Table 12.3 Common causative organisms in odontogenic infections

Facultative anaerobes	Strict anaerobes
Streptococcus viridans—mitis, oralis, salivarius, mutans	*Prevotella* (most common)
Streptococcus milleri	*Fusobacterium* species
Staphylococcus aureus	*Porphyomonas* species
Staphylococcus epidermidis (coagulase-negative strains)	*Bacteroides* species
	Clostridium species

early antibiotics are justified.[11] Signs of severe infection include pyrexia, lymphadenopathy, cellulitis, and diffuse swelling. Early antibiotics should also be considered for patients at a high risk of complications, including those that are immunocompromised or diabetic.

Antibiotic therapy alone, without surgical intervention, may not be effective because of poor antibiotic penetration into the abscess cavity, ineffectiveness at low pH levels, and the inoculum effect (where an increased inhibitory concentration of an antibiotic is seen with an increase in the number of organisms inoculated, as with beta-lactam antibiotics).[12]

Antibiotic selection is ideally guided by sensitivity results from bacterial culture tests. However, a major limitation of culture tests is that the majority of oral microflora do not grow on conventional culture media.[10] Strict sampling techniques are necessary to ensure contamination from normal oral flora does not give spurious results. Sampling of purulent material gives poor yields of strict anaerobes. Consequently, the antibiotic is often selected to cover a range of causative organisms.

First-line antibiotic choice is guided by local microbiology protocols, but traditionally has been co-amoxiclav, due to its high sensitivity against the majority of causative organisms (up to 90% in one microbiology study).[13] The clavulanic acid binds and inhibits beta-lactamase enzymes expanding the spectrum of activity of the penicillin. In penicillin-allergic patients, options include azithromycin or macrolides (e.g. erythromycin), although the latter has high resistance among anaerobic organisms (in the same microbiology study, only 60% of organisms were sensitive).[13] Metronidazole is highly active against most anaerobes and can be used in combination with other first-line agents. Clindamycin confers additional benefits including good oral absorption and high penetration into bone. Table 12.4 summarizes the antibiotic options for dental infections, and the relative drug sensitivity of the bacteria.

Table 12.4 Antibiotic options for the management of dental infections

Antibiotic choice	Relative sensitivity of the cultures
First-line agent	Co-amoxiclav (90% sensitivity)
Penicillin allergic	Azithromycin (90%) +/– metronidazole (85%)
Other agents	Erythromycin (60%)
	Clindamycin (60%)
	Ciprofloxacin (70%)

Antibiotic prophylaxis

Historically, dental procedures have been viewed as conferring a risk of bacteraemia, where oral organisms enter the bloodstream, causing a risk of colonization of vulnerable sites and resulting, particularly, in infective endocarditis. More recently, the UK National Institute for Health and Care Excellence (NICE) has assessed the evidence for prophylactic antibiotics in this group of patients.[14] They identified high-risk patients as those with the following conditions:

- Acquired valvular heart disease with stenosis or regurgitation.
- Hypertrophic cardiomyopathy.
- Previous infective endocarditis.
- Structural congenital heart disease.
- Valve replacement.

However, NICE also stated that antibiotic prophylaxis against infective endocarditis is not recommended routinely for patients undergoing dental procedures. This conclusion is based upon the lack of evidence of a causal link between dental treatment and endocarditis, and even less evidence suggesting that prophylaxis may be of any benefit. NICE recommends that healthcare professionals offer those at risk clear and consistent information about prevention, including an explanation of why antibiotic prophylaxis is no longer routinely advised, the importance of maintaining good oral health, and highlighting symptoms that may indicate infective endocarditis and when to seek expert help.

When considering the value of antibiotics for prophylaxis, it is also crucial to take into account the potential harm that can be caused by anaphylaxis to these agents (antibiotics are commonly implicated), and the importance of antibiotic stewardship in reducing microbial resistance.[15] Conversely, patients presenting with severe infections, requiring anaesthetic care, are likely to be on antibiotics prior to surgery, making the need for prophylactic antibiotics for prevention of postoperative infections less likely (discussed in more detail later in the section on secondary infections).

Clinical assessment

Many patients with dental abscesses can be managed in the community, with surgical drainage under local anaesthetic and administration of appropriate antibiotics. More serious infections, including those where systemic symptoms have developed, are likely to require hospital management. This may include urgent or emergency surgery under general anaesthesia and, in some cases, require ongoing care in the critical care unit. Even for patients not requiring immediate surgery, the anaesthetic team is often involved from the point of admission due to concerns of airway compromise with worsening infection ('watchful waiting').

Preassessment

Patients presenting with odontogenic infections pose a number of challenges to the anaesthetist. The most common presenting symptoms are pain and facial swelling; however, if the infection progresses it can lead to trismus, dysphagia, stridor, and cardiovascular collapse (if sepsis ensues). This range of presentations precludes a

Table 12.5 Considerations when assessing patients with a potentially difficult airway

Questions to consider when evaluating the anticipated difficult airway	
1	Will I be able to mask ventilate?
2	Will I be able to perform laryngoscopy, directly or indirectly?
3	Will I be able to intubate the trachea?
4	Is there a significant aspiration risk?
5	Can I access the front of neck if required?

single simple approach to the management of these patients. The occurrence of potentially life-threatening complications, albeit uncommon, means thorough preoperative assessment is essential in avoiding delayed diagnosis of any of these sometimes rapidly progressive conditions.

The patient population typically comprises younger adults. Comorbidities relating to drug and alcohol misuse are more common and should be specifically sought, along with other risk factors such as smoking, diabetes, and obesity. Patients can present late, dehydrated, and malnourished due to several preceding days of inadequate fluid intake and poor nutrition due to dysphagia.

An 'ABCD' approach to initial assessment is best practice. A detailed airway assessment is critical as this will guide airway management planning and the urgency of any interventions. Table 12.5 outlines the specific questions that must be considered when evaluating the potentially difficult airway.[16]

An assessment of mouth opening, measured as interincisor gap, may indicate the feasibility of performing laryngoscopy, with a distance of <3 cm being a non-reassuring sign. Some videolaryngoscope blades require as little as 1.8 cm for insertion, and supraglottic airway devices have been successfully inserted in patients with <2 cm of mouth opening. Other airway assessment tools, including the Mallampati grade, thyromental distance, jaw protrusion, and neck movement, all assess different aspects of the airway and its dynamic response to movement. Although there is a lack of predictive power of any individual test, they should heighten awareness of the potential for difficulty and allow appropriate planning. Previously documented airway management technique and grade of laryngoscopy can be helpful, although in the acute circumstances, previous grading may be falsely reassuring.

Cardiorespiratory physiological parameters are important in assessment of the patient's current fluid status. Respiratory rate, blood pressure, and heart rate, along with an assessment of conscious level, can be used to identify those with systemic involvement requiring urgent intervention (risk scoring systems are discussed in detail later in the chapter). Awareness of the symptoms and signs of rarer complicating conditions ensures that these are not missed, including eye signs (orbital cellulitis, cavernous sinus thrombosis), chest pain (mediastinitis), and haemoptysis (Lemierre's syndrome), leading to more rapid diagnosis and treatment of these conditions.

In the acute setting, swelling and distortion of tissues can be very painful, and analgesia should be optimized. A multimodal approach to analgesia is advocated, although strong opioids are often required. Dental nerve blocks can offer a means of providing local anaesthesia, although poor tissue penetration, an acidic environment inhibiting transfer of active drug into the nerve, and restricted intraoral access often mean they are ineffective.

Management of the uncomplicated patient

Patients with an uncomplicated dental abscess, no significant medical history, and an unobstructed airway may be managed in a conventional manner, which may include:

- Intravenous induction of anaesthesia using a rapid sequence technique (if indicated).
- Nasotracheal intubation, to facilitate surgical access.
- Use of a throat pack, to prevent spread of pus and debris.
- Antibiotic administration (as discussed earlier).
- Intraoperative optimization of patient temperature and blood pressure.
- Standard tracheal extubation.
- Admission to a surgical ward for postoperative observation.

Management of the patient with serious complications

Dental abscesses and other oral infections can cause a number of rare, but serious, complications that are associated with significant morbidity and mortality, and pose particular challenges to the anaesthetist (Table 12.6). An 'ABCD' approach to assessment is essential in minimizing issues during the management of these conditions.

Airway complications and their management

The effects of infection on the airway can be subdivided into those causing immediate airway compromise and those that make tracheal intubation under general anaesthesia more challenging.[17]

Airway compromise

Infection causing airway compromise is an anaesthetic emergency and requires rapid assessment and management to avoid complete airway obstruction and respiratory arrest. Patients can present with a combination of respiratory and systemic signs, including dyspnoea, cyanosis, stridor, wheeze, agitation, confusion, or unconsciousness. The spectrum of presenting symptoms is wide and the decision regarding the need to secure the airway is made on the overall patient condition and response to initial treatment (Table 12.7). Emergency management of the obstructing airway requires experienced senior support to minimize the high risk of morbidity associated. Ludwig's angina is one such aetiology associated with airway compromise, and is discussed in **Box 12.1**.

Table 12.6 Serious complications associated with oral infections

Airway complications	Airway compromise Difficult tracheal intubation and extubation
Systemic effects	Sepsis Acute respiratory distress syndrome
Spreading infection	Maxillary sinusitis Orbital cellulitis and abscess Brain abscess Descending necrotizing mediastinitis Cervical necrotizing fasciitis Cavernous sinus thrombosis Lemierre's syndrome

Table 12.7 Airway complications associated with oral infections

Infective causes of airway compromise	Infective causes of difficult tracheal intubation

- Airway oedema, causing mechanical obstruction and increased tissue friability
- Spreading infections:
  - Epiglottitis
  - Peritonsillar abscess
  - Retropharyngeal abscess
  - Ludwig's angina
	- Trismus
	- Osteomyelitis
	- Abscess of the floor of the mouth

When the patient's airway is at risk of obstruction, and requires immediate intervention, several approaches to airway management are available (Table 12.8). When selecting the most appropriate technique, it is important to consider separately the feasibility of face mask ventilation, the feasibility of laryngoscopy, and the feasibility of tracheal tube placement. The oedema and distorted anatomy associated with odontogenic infections often confer potential difficulties with both face mask ventilation and laryngoscopy, and therefore an awake technique is often chosen.

In a retrospective study of 36 patients with Ludwig's angina, standard tracheal intubation attempts failed in 55% and resulted in acute airway loss requiring emergency tracheostomy.[19] This high level of morbidity associated with standard tracheal intubation attempts has led to awake fibreoptic tracheal intubation or surgical airway being considered 'plan A' of the airway management strategy. In a further study of 93 patients with late presentation of Ludwig's angina, 65% of patients underwent surgical tracheostomy under local anaesthesia.[18] Awake fibreoptic tracheal intubation has been shown to have a high success rate[20]; nevertheless, oedema and immobility of tissues can cause significant distortion of airway anatomy such that navigation of the fibrescope can be challenging, and experience with the device is essential to ensure safe practice. Copious secretions, pus, blood, and a compressed airway can cause supraglottic or glottic obstruction on passing the scope, therefore the difficulties in securing the airway via this method should not be underestimated.

The particular technique chosen to secure the airway is also dependent upon the clinical skills of the anaesthetic team managing the patient. Whichever method is chosen, the case should

---

Box 12.1 Ludwig's angina

Ludwig's angina is a potentially fatal, rapidly progressive infection of the tissues of the floor of the mouth. The term angina is derived from the Greek word meaning 'strangling' and the eponym relates to the German physician who first described the condition in 1836.

Infection occurs bilaterally, involving more than one deep neck space around the mandible. As with other odontogenic infections the aetiology is polymicrobial and starts with a gangrenous, putrid infiltration often with very little pus initially.[18] The infection is most commonly odontogenic (90%), but other causes include trauma to the floor of the mouth, recent tooth extraction, peritonsillar abscess, and postprocedural infection following frenulum piercing. The infection can lead to a board-like swelling of the submandibular tissues and elevation of the tongue, leading to drooling, dysphonia, and ultimately to airway obstruction.

Management of the condition requires a combination of antimicrobial treatment, urgent airway management, and surgery. Patients may be severely septic at presentation.

Table 12.8 Options for airway management in the compromised airway

Awake	Flexible fibreoptic
	Videolaryngoscopy
	Surgical airway (cricothyroidotomy/tracheostomy)
Asleep	Flexible fibreoptic
	Videolaryngoscopy
	Direct laryngoscopy

be managed collaboratively, with the surgical team present and immediately ready to perform an emergency tracheostomy or cricothyroidotomy if irretrievable airway compromise occurs. A stepwise airway strategy should be communicated clearly to the entire team, to ensure a shared approach in the event that the initial airway management plan is unsuccessful ('preparing to fail').[21] Ensuring all rescue devices are immediately available and operational ensures valuable time is not lost if the clinical situation deteriorates. Transnasal humidified rapid-insufflation ventilatory exchange (THRIVE) has been shown to prolong safe apnoea time in patients with difficult or partially obstructed airways.[22] As long as a patent airway can be maintained, THRIVE may provide greater time for direct or videolaryngoscopy views to be optimized and for tracheal intubation to be safely achieved, although currently there are no large-scale studies relating to this technique in this particular patient population.

Difficult tracheal intubation

Rather more commonly than the life-threatening airway compromise described above, standard approaches to tracheal intubation may be impaired by infection causing trismus. Trismus is reduced opening of the jaw and is usually caused by spasm of the muscles of mastication. Both odontogenic and non-odontogenic infections can cause trismus and it is one of the presenting features of tetanus following infection by *Clostridium tetani*.

Trismus and an interincisor gap of <2.5 cm correlates with increased difficulty in tracheal intubation, such that nasotracheal intubation using a fibrescope is often the technique of choice. In this particular clinical situation, where airway compromise is not imminent, more time is available to plan the approach to airway management, and to undertake additional investigations. These might include computed tomography (CT) imaging of the head and neck, and flexible nasendoscopy.

CT images can assist in identifying the level of any airway swelling, help quantify the severity of any obstruction, and can demonstrate any extension into the deep neck spaces. Early CT imaging is therefore recommended, where the clinical situation permits, as this will guide surgical management,[23] as well as assisting in the diagnosis of abscess formation and those at risk of complications such as vascular compromise or osteomyelitis.[24] The airway dimensions (patency) can also be quantified, which may guide the type and size of tracheal tube selected, or indeed alter the approach to airway management (e.g. opting for an awake technique if the potential risk of airway compromise is deemed high). Flexible nasendoscopy facilitates evaluation of the airway above the glottis, allowing visualization of any airway oedema or compression. It is a dynamic investigation

which enables assessment during normal and deep breathing. It can swiftly provide valuable information in the acute setting, which again, may be used to inform the choice of airway management technique. Virtual endoscopy combines these two investigations, generating reconstructed three-dimensional images of the airway, as assessed by a 'virtual' endoscope.[25]

Sepsis

Sepsis is associated with significant morbidity and mortality. In the UK, there are approximately 123,000 cases of sepsis per year and around 36,800 deaths, making sepsis the second highest cause of death after cardiovascular disease.[26] The incidence is increasing as life expectancy increases, although patients without serious pre-existing comorbidities are more likely to survive.

Sepsis associated with odontogenic infections is common. In one study, 61% of patients with a primary odontogenic infection had sepsis on admission to hospital, as defined by systemic inflammatory response syndrome criteria.[7] In this study, 95% of patients required surgical incision and drainage as part of their management plan and 9% were admitted postoperatively to the critical care unit.

Recognition of sepsis is the first critical step in enabling timely intervention. Sepsis is a multisystem condition and remains difficult to define. The third international consensus definitions task force defined sepsis as a 'life-threatening organ dysfunction due to a dysregulated host response to infection.'[27] A gold standard diagnostic test for sepsis does not exist. Screening tools such as the systemic inflammatory response syndrome criteria have been used previously to define sepsis, and allowed for early detection by identifying simple clinical measurements. The quick Sequential (Sepsis-related) Organ Failure Assessment (qSOFA) has been shown to detect sepsis with greater sensitivity (Table 12.9). Patients scoring ≥2 points in the presence of infection accounted for 70% of deaths and 70% of prolonged critical care stays from sepsis, thereby correlating with severity of illness. The presence of serum lactate levels of 2.0 mmol/L or higher does not form part of this scoring system but may be useful in identifying those with qSOFA scores of 1 who are at a higher overall risk of morbidity from sepsis.

To improve sepsis outcomes following identification, treatment should be rapid and targeted to improve organ perfusion. The 'Surviving Sepsis' campaign was developed to reduce mortality from the condition by a process of building awareness, education, and the implementation of management guidelines.[28] Care bundles (Table 12.10), which comprise time-dependent management aims, have also been shown to improve survival. These aims were simplified into the 'Sepsis Six' resuscitation bundle, which includes:

- Delivering high-flow oxygen to maintain oxygen saturations >94%.
- Taking blood cultures.
- Administering empirical intravenous antibiotics.

Table 12.9 qSOFA criteria in the presence of infection

Criteria for defining qSOFA score: total score of 3, 1 point gained for each criterion present	
Respiratory rate	≥22 breaths per minute
Systolic blood pressure	≤100 mmHg
Altered mental status (Glasgow Coma Score)	<15

Table 12.10 'Surviving Sepsis' time-dependent care bundle

'Surviving Sepsis' campaign care bundles	
To be completed within 3 hours	
1	Measure lactate level
2	Obtain blood cultures, prior to administration of antibiotics
3	Administer broad-spectrum antibiotics
4	Administer 30 mL/kg crystalloid for hypotension or if lactate ≥4 mmol/L
To be completed within 6 hours	
5	Institute vasopressor medication (for hypotension that does not respond to initial fluid resuscitation) to maintain a mean arterial pressure ≥65 mmHg
6	In the event of persistent arterial hypotension despite volume resuscitation (septic shock) or initial lactate ≥4 mmol/L (36 mg/dL): • Measure central venous pressure (CVP)[a] • Measure central venous oxygen saturation (ScvO$_2$)[a]
7	Remeasure lactate if initial lactate was elevated[a]

[a] Targets for quantitative resuscitation include a CVP of ≥8 mmHg, ScvO$_2$ of ≥70%, and normalization of lactate levels.

- Measuring serum lactate and full blood count.
- Starting intravenous fluid resuscitation.
- Commencing accurate urine output measurement.

These steps should be commenced within 1 hour, and together have been shown to reduce mortality by 50%. Patients who are refractory to initial treatment may require invasive monitoring, targeted fluid resuscitation, and critical care management.

In certain circumstances, patients presenting with sepsis require immediate surgical management, such as those with necrotizing fasciitis. Other cases may benefit from a period of stabilization and optimization prior to undergoing surgical exploration. If an abscess is present, surgical drainage is necessary to treat the source of the sepsis, and surgery should therefore be expedited, but patients should be resuscitated following the aforementioned guidance prior to any surgical procedure.

The response to initial treatment and continued assessment of oxygenation and serum lactate guide prognosis. A failure of lactate levels to decrease following initial therapy is indicative of a poor outcome.[29] The detailed management of sepsis is beyond the scope of this chapter but patients are best managed in a critical care environment. Acute respiratory distress syndrome and multiorgan failure can occur as a consequence of sepsis or odontogenic infections alone and may require invasive ventilation and additional organ support.

Spreading infection

Maxillary sinusitis and orbital cellulitis

Infection arising in the root apices of the maxillary teeth may spread into the maxillary sinuses or infraorbital soft tissues. Maxillary sinusitis can cause fever, pain, and tenderness, and requires treatment with antibiotics, as well as potentially requiring surgical drainage (endoscopically or intraorally).

Odontogenic infections can spread to cause orbital cellulitis or an orbital abscess. Spread can be through the local fascial planes, haematogenous or via involvement of the paranasal sinuses,[30] and manifests as eyelid swelling, reddening, proptosis, and altered vision. Early visual assessment is needed to avoid a delay in diagnosis

and treatment which can lead to severe and permanent visual loss. CT images showing gas within the orbit is strongly suggestive of an orbital abscess which may require drainage.

Dental cysts and osteomyelitis

Undrained dental abscesses may eventually resolve, leaving a fluid-filled cyst within the bone. These can lead to recurrent infection, and patients may present for surgical excision of the cyst. Alternatively, dental abscesses may progress to cause an osteomyelitis in either the mandible or maxilla. This is characterized by pain, swelling, fever, dental loss, and formation of fistulae[31] and sequestrum (necrotic bone). This may be diagnosed using standard radiography (showing radiolucent regions of bony destruction) or via CT imaging (showing erosions of the medullary and cortical bone).[13] Management often involves protracted courses of antibiotics. Oral osteomyelitis can become chronic if it is refractory to treatment for >1 month, leading to bony destruction and deformity. The best treatment option for chronic osteomyelitis is a combination of antimicrobial therapy and surgical excision and reconstruction. Involvement of the mandible will compromise mouth opening and could lead to difficult tracheal intubation.

Intracranial abscess

Although rare, dental infections can spread to cause an intracranial abscess. Direct spread tends to cause a solitary abscess, whereas haematogenous spread usually results in multiple foci.[13] There is often a latent period of days to weeks before the cerebral symptoms of headaches, malaise, and apathy appear. Signs and symptoms will vary depending on the site of the lesions and the presence of any mass effect.[32] Treatment involves the use of antimicrobials which, if odontogenic infections are suspected, should cover anaerobic organisms, and may also include surgical intervention.

Descending necrotizing mediastinitis

The fascial planes of the neck are contiguous with those of the mediastinum. Consequently, downward spread of infection from dental infections can occur very rapidly. Acute inflammation of the connective tissues in the middle thoracic cavity defines mediastinitis. In 20% of cases, a diffuse polymicrobial infection can occur, known as descending necrotizing mediastinitis (DNM).[33] Retrosternal or pleuritic pain may suggest spread, and early CT scanning of the neck and chest can aid diagnosis. The diagnostic criteria for DNM are described in **Table 12.11**. Management of this condition necessitates a multidisciplinary approach, broad-spectrum antibiotics covering Gram-positive and anaerobic organisms, critical care admission, and often repeated transthoracic surgical drainage. Early surgery is thought to be advantageous, but evidence for the optimal timing

Table 12.11 Diagnostic criteria for descending necrotizing mediastinitis

1	Clinical manifestation of severe infection
2	Characteristic radiographic findings—gas in the tissues, an air-fluid level, mediastinal widening
3	Documentation of DNM at operation
4	Establishment of relationship between oropharyngeal infection and DNM

of surgery is still lacking. Although rare, the condition is associated with significant morbidity and a prolonged course in critical care. The mortality rate remains high at 18% despite improvements in diagnosis and management.

Cervical necrotizing fasciitis

Cervical necrotizing fasciitis, a condition of progressive necrotizing infection along the deep neck space planes, is an associated cause of mediastinitis. It carries a high mortality particularly when associated with septic shock (36–64%)[33] and requires extensive debridement of necrotic tissue.

Cavernous sinus thrombosis

Periapical abscesses affecting the maxillary incisors and canine teeth can spread via the facial vein into the cranium. Because of the absence of valves within the cavernous sinus, bidirectional spread of infection and thrombi can occur,[13] leading to septic thrombosis of the cavernous sinus. Seven per cent of all cavernous sinus thromboses are of dental origin. Patients present with headache, fever, periorbital oedema, exophthalmos, and chemosis. Treatment involves high-dose broad-spectrum antibiotics, systemic anticoagulation, and surgical management of the causative infection. Fewer than 40% of patients have a full recovery, 20% may die secondary to meningitis or sepsis, and those who survive may suffer impaired vision, hemiparesis, and seizures.

Lemierre's syndrome

Lemierre's syndrome is described as thrombophlebitis of the internal jugular vein and subsequent haematogenic spread of infection via septic emboli.[34] These emboli can cause lesions in the lung (which can present with haemoptysis and pleuritic chest pain) and other remote sites. Endocarditis or pericarditis are rare manifestations. Prompt, aggressive surgical exploration and debridement is mandatory. Mortality rates range from 4% to 12%.

Tracheal extubation and postoperative management

Patients who have followed a complicated course due to their infection may require a higher degree of planning, observation, and care postoperatively. Those that have developed organ dysfunction as a result of sepsis from an odontogenic infection may require organ support in a critical care environment. Such patients may require respiratory support (particularly if acute respiratory distress syndrome ensues), circulatory support in the form of meticulous fluid management, inotrope and vasopressor medications, renal replacement therapy in the context of acute kidney injury or severe acidosis, and other supportive measures (including, in particular, antimicrobials based upon positive cultures and continuous input from microbiology colleagues). Detailed postoperative management of these patients is beyond the scope of this chapter.

A decision regarding the appropriateness and optimum timing of tracheal extubation must be made in every patient. Ongoing tracheal intubation and mechanical ventilation may sometimes be required solely for airway support, but is often necessary as part of ongoing supportive measures. Tracheal extubation is unlikely to be undertaken while significant sepsis-related haemodynamic compromise

persists, while severe complications continue to be treated, or when recurrent surgery is anticipated. The decision regarding tracheal extubation must therefore be judged on a case-by-case basis, and be agreed by the surgical, anaesthetic, and critical care teams together.

When considering tracheal extubation, the ability to oxygenate and reintubate the trachea must be considered. The Difficult Airway Society provides guidance on preparing for a potentially difficult tracheal extubation (**Fig. 12.4**).[35] The cuff leak test (deflation of the cuff to assess air leak around the tracheal tube), is widely used in an attempt to predict successful tracheal extubation, but this has not been shown to reliably identify those patients who will require tracheal reintubation.[36] If after assessing and optimizing the patient it is felt safe to remove the tracheal tube, options include an awake extubation, or an advanced extubation technique, such as exchange for a laryngeal mask airway, use of an airway exchange catheter, or tracheal extubation on remifentanil. If the airway is still considered 'at risk', a surgical tracheostomy should be considered, otherwise tracheal extubation should be postponed to allow further time for oedema/bleeding to reside and/or concurrent therapies to improve the likely chance of a successful tracheal extubation in due course.

Secondary infections

Infections of the oral cavity can be a complicating factor following elective oromaxillofacial procedures. Procedures that involve incising the oral mucosa are considered 'clean-contaminated' due to the abundance of bacteria and potential pathogens in the oral cavity.[37] Surgical site infections can complicate both elective and emergency procedures, having a deleterious effect on outcomes, and potentially requiring further treatments. Reported infection rates range from 10% to 15% following intraoral surgery.

Antibiotic prophylaxis is recommended before invasive surgery to minimize the rates of postoperative infection. Common antibiotics include co-amoxiclav, cephalosporins, or clindamycin. Studies have assessed the potential benefit of extended courses of postoperative antibiotics; however, there is little consensus on the value of this. One study comparing 3-day versus 1-day postoperative regimens for orthognathic surgery showed a reduction of surgical site infections from 17.6% to 7.0%. However, with a number needed to treat of 10 in this study, the benefit of reduced infection may not outweigh the risks of anaphylaxis or antibiotic-related infections such as *C. difficile*. The World Health Organization guidelines on the prevention of surgical site infection state that antibiotics should be given within 120 minutes prior to surgical incision and that there is insufficient evidence to recommend prolonged antibiotic use after surgery.[38] Often local guidelines exist regarding antibiotic prophylaxis for specific surgical procedures.

Surgery requiring reconstruction with either a tissue flap or revascularized osteocutaneous flap are of particular concern with regard to postoperative infection, with infection being cited as the leading cause of flap failure in some studies.[39] Infection of a free flap can cause breakdown of the vascular anastomosis, leading to catastrophic haemorrhage, requiring emergency surgery.

When prostheses are used in reconstructive procedures, postoperative infection can lead to failure of the implant. One study into temporomandibular joint prostheses found a prosthesis infection rate of 1.6%. When a prosthesis becomes infected, it usually necessitates a

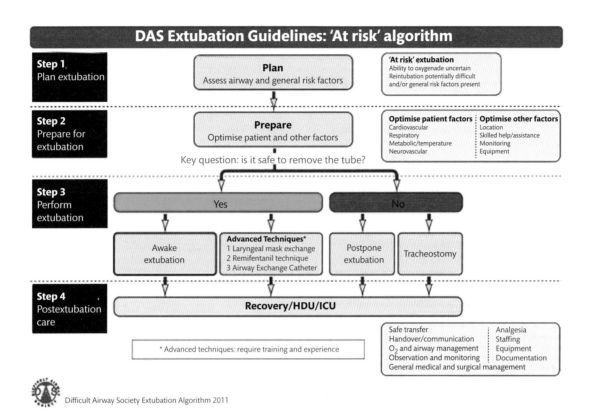

Fig. 12.4 Difficult Airway Society tracheal extubation guidelines.
Popat M, Mitchell V, Dravid R, Patel A, Swampillai C, Higgs A. Difficult Airway Society Guidelines for the management of tracheal extubation. Anaesthesia. 2012; 67(3): 318–40. doi: 10.1111/j.1365-2044.2012.07075.x.

prolonged in-patient stay on intravenous antibiotics, punctuated by multiple surgical procedures, in order to address the infection. Early aggressive treatment may reduce the risk of acute infection evolving into a chronic process.

Conclusion

Patients with oral or dental infections pose a number of particular challenges—potentially difficult airway management, combined with emergency surgery, and a high incidence of pre- and postoperative morbidity. These are stressful and demanding high-risk cases that require a collaborative approach to management, with early involvement of an experienced anaesthetic and surgical team, so that the best patient outcomes can be achieved.

REFERENCES

1. Petersen PE, Bourgeois D, Ogawa H, Estupinan-Day S, Ndiaye C. The global burden of oral disease and risks to oral health. *Bull World Health Organ.* 2005;**83**(9):661–669.
2. National Institute for Health and Care Excellence. Oral health promotion: general dental practice. NICE guideline [NG30]. 2015. https://www.nice.org.uk/guidance/ng30
3. White D, Pitts N, Steele J, Sadler K, Chadwick B. Disease and related disorders—a report from the Adult Dental Health Survey 2009. The Health and Social Care Information Centre. 2011. https://digital.nhs.uk/data-and-information/publications/statisti
cal/adult-dental-health-survey/adult-dental-health-survey-2009-summary-report-and-thematic-series
4. Thomas SJ, Hughes C, Atkinson C, Ness AR, Revington P. Is there an epidemic of admissions for surgical treatment of dental abscesses in the UK? *BMJ.* 2008;**336**(7655):1219–1220.
5. American Academy of Periodontology. Parameter on acute periodontal disease. *J Periodontol.* 2000;**7**(5):863–866.
6. Abeyundara L, Creedon A, Soltanifar D. Dental knowledge for the anaesthetist. *BJAnaesth Educ.* 2016;**16**(11):362–368.
7. Handley T, Devlin M, Koppel D, McCaul J. The sepsis syndrome in odontogenic infection. *J Intensive Care Soc.* 2009;**10**(1):21–25.
8. Norton NS. Cervical fascia. In: *Netter's Head and Neck Anatomy for Dentistry*, pp. 460–472. Philadelphia, PA: Saunders Elsevier: 2007.
9. Murray AD. Deep neck infections. Medscape. 30 April 2020. http://emedicine.medscape.com/article/837048-overview
10. Shweta, Krishna Prakash S. Dental abscess: a microbiological review. *Dent Res J (Isfahan).* 2013;**10**(5):585–591.
11. National Institute for Health and Care Excellence. Dental abscess. NICE Clinical Knowledge Summary. 2018. https://cks.nice.org.uk/topics/dental-abscess/
12. Gould J. Dental abscess medication. Medscape. 22 January 2019. http://emedicine.medscape.com/article/909373-medication#2
13. Bahl R, Sandhu S, Singh K, Sahai N, Gupta M. Odontogenic infections: microbiology and management. *Contemp Clin Dent.* 2014;**5**(3):307–311.
14. National Institute for Health and Care Excellence. Prophylaxis against infective endocarditis: antimicrobial prophylaxis against infective endocarditis in adults and children undergoing interventional procedures. NICE clinical guideline [CG64]. 2016. https://www.nice.org.uk/guidance/cg64

15. Hossaini-zadeh M. Current concepts of prophylactic antibiotics for dental patients. *Dent Clin North Am.* 2016;**60**(2):473–482.

16. Crawley SM, Dalton AJ. Predicting the difficult airway. *Br J Anaesth Educ.* 2015;**15**:253–257.

17. Bali RK, Sharma P, Gaba S, Kaur A, Ghanghas P. A review of complications of odontogenic infections. *Natl J Maxillofac Surg.* 2015;**6**(2):136–143.

18. Botha A, Jacobs F, Postma C. Retrospective analysis of etiology and comorbid diseases associated with Ludwig's angina. *Ann Maxillofac Surg.* 2015;**5**(2):168–173.

19. Parhiscar A, Har-El G. Deep neck abscess: a retrospective review of 210 cases. *Ann Otol Rhinol Laryngol.* 2001;**110**(11):1051–1054.

20. Ovassapian A, Tuncbilek M, Weitzel EK, Joshi CW. Airway management in adult patients with deep neck infections: a case series and review of the literature. *Anesth Analg.* 2005;**100**(2):585–589.

21. Frerk C, Mitchell VS, McNarry AF, Mendonca C, Bhagrath R, Patel A, et al. Difficult Airway Society 2015 guidelines for management of unanticipated difficult intubation in adults. *Br J Anaesth.* 2015;**115**(6):827–848.

22. Patel A, Nouraei SAR. Transnasal humidified rapid-insufflation ventilatory exchange (THRIVE): a physiological method of increasing apnoea time in patients with difficult airways. *Anaesthesia.* 2015;**70**(3):323–329.

23. Kim YJ, Kim JD, Ryu HI, Cho YH, Kong JH, Ohe JY, et al. Application of radiographic images in diagnosis and treatment of deep neck infections with necrotizing fasciitis: a case report. *Imaging Sci Dent.* 2011;**41**(4):189–193.

24. Gonzalez-Beicos A, Nunez D. Imaging of acute head and neck infections. *Radiol Clin North Am.* 2012;**50**(1):73–83.

25. Ahmad I, Millhoff B, John M, Andi K, Oakley RJ. Virtual endoscopy—a new assessment tool in difficult airway management. *Clin Anesth.* 2015;**27**(6):508–513.

26. NHS England. Improving outcomes for patients with sepsis. 2015. https://www.england.nhs.uk/wp-content/uploads/2015/08/Sepsis-Action-Plan-23.12.15-v1.pdf

27. Seymour CW, Liu VX, Iwashyna TJ, Brunkhorst FM, Rea TD, Scherag A, et al. Assessment of clinical criteria for sepsis for the Third International Consensus Definitions for Sepsis and Septic Shock (Sepsis-3). *JAMA.* 2016;**315**(8):762–774.

28. Dellinger RP, Levy MM, Rhodes A, Annane D, Gerlach H, Opal SM, et al. Surviving Sepsis campaign: international guidelines for management of severe sepsis and septic shock: 2012. *Crit Care Med.* 2013;**41**(2):580–637.

29. McCrate Protus B. Evidence of effectiveness of BMJ Best Practice. *J Med Libr Assoc.* 2014;**102**(3):224–225.

30. Youssef OH, Stefanyszyn MA, Bilyk JR. Odontogenic orbital cellulitis. *Ophthal Plast Reconstr Surg.* 2008;**24**(1):29–35.

31. Slough CM, Woo BM, Ueeck BA, Wax MK. Fibular free flaps in the management of osteomyelitis of the mandible. *Head Neck.* 2008;**30**(11):1531–1534.

32. Azenha MR, Homsi G, Garcia IR Jr. Multiple brain abscess from dental origin: case report and literature review. *Oral Maxillofac Surg.* 2012;**16**(4):393–397.

33. Prado-Calleros HM, Jiménez-Fuentes E, Jiménez-Escobar I. Descending necrotizing mediastinitis: systematic review on its treatment in the last 6 years, 75 years after its description. *Head Neck.* 2016;**38**(1):E2275–E2283.

34. Noy D, Rachmiel A, Levy-Faber D, Emodi O. Lemierre's syndrome from odontogenic infection: review of the literature and case description. *Ann Maxillofac Surg.* 2015;**5**(2):219–225.

35. Popat M, Mitchell V, Dravid R, Patel A, Swampillai C, Higgs A. Difficult Airway Society Guidelines for the management of tracheal extubation. *Anaesthesia.* 2012;**67**(3):318–340.

36. Shin SH, Heath K, Reed S, Collins J, Weireter LJ, Britt LD. The cuff leak test is not predictive of successful extubation. *Am Surg.* 2008;**74**(12):1182–1185.

37. Davis CM, Gregoire CE, Davis I, Steeves TW. Prevalence of surgical site infections following orthognathic surgery: a double-blind, randomized controlled trial on a 3-day versus 1-day postoperative antibiotic regimen. *J Oral Maxillofac Surg.* 2016;**75**(4):796–804.

38. World Health Organization. Global guidelines on the prevention of surgical site infection. 2016. https://www.who.int/gpsc/ssi-prevention-guidelines/en/

39. Smolka W, Lizuka T. Surgical reconstruction of maxilla and midface: clinical outcome and factors relating to postoperative complications. *J Craniomaxillofac Surg.* 2005;**33**(1):1–7.

13

Trauma

Rebecca Thurairatnam and Fauzia Mir

Introduction

Maxillofacial trauma forms a significant proportion of major trauma injuries. It affects patients across all age groups. Any severe trauma involving maxillofacial structures can have profound, life-changing consequences, with four of the five sensory modalities (sight, smell, taste, and hearing) potentially affected. Significant injuries can also cause aesthetic changes which drastically affect a patient's identity, their social interactions, and their quality of life.

Epidemiology and aetiology

Maxillofacial trauma accounts for a significant proportion of major trauma patients, reported to be as high as 16% in one retrospective regional study of major trauma cases in Australia.[1] The most common causes of maxillofacial trauma include road traffic accidents, interpersonal violence, sports-related injuries, falls (particularly in extremes of age), and industrial accidents.[2–4] Trauma is more common in men, with a mean age of 25 years.[5] Alcohol-related injuries are common, and must be considered as part of patient assessment and treatment.[5]

Classification of fractures

Maxillofacial fractures can be classified anatomically, comprising lower, middle, and upper thirds of the facial structures. Trauma can also be classified according to blunt versus penetrating injuries. Fractures involving the maxillary region of the face are most frequent,[4] while other common fractures involve the mandible, followed by zygomatic and nasal structures.[2,7] Of interest to the anaesthetist, certain maxillofacial injuries can directly or indirectly affect airway patency and therefore their subsequent management.

Lower third

Lower-third fractures involve the mandible, teeth, temporomandibular joint, and skull base. Trauma in this region is likely to cause more than one fracture.[8] Airway compromise can be profound, such as with bilateral anterior mandibular fractures, where in an obtunded patient the tongue can obstruct the airway in the supine position.[9] Other potential risks to the airway include the presence of haematomas or foreign bodies, such as avulsed or fractured teeth.[9]

Middle third

The middle third involves the maxilla, zygoma, and lower half of the naso-orbitoethmoidal complex. This area acts as a 'crumple zone' to protect the brain from injury and is most frequently involved in facial trauma.[10] Haemorrhage in this area can be severe, resulting in both airway and haemodynamic compromise. Fractures in this region can be further subdivided according to the Le Fort classification, I–III (Fig. 13.1), although this is largely academic since it is possible to have a combination of some or all subtypes, along with frequent involvement of the mandible[8] (Fig. 13.2). In Le Fort I, fracturing of the maxilla causes separation from the face. Le Fort II involves the maxilla and nasal complex fracturing from the facial bones, causing increased mobility, relative to Le Fort I. Le Fort III injuries involve the whole midface dissociating from the base of the skull and facial bones. Le Fort fractures may cause airway compromise via maxillary prolapse, oedema, or haemorrhage.[8]

Upper third

The upper third comprises the frontal bone, sphenoid, and upper half of the naso-orbitoethmoidal complex. Trauma here can cause injuries to the eyes and the paranasal sinuses. Injuries to the frontal sinus can cause pneumatization of surrounding tissues and craniofacial surgical emphysema, which, if severe, can cause airway obstruction. One case report describes this particular injury with subsequent pneumomediastinum.[11] Severe fractures can involve the anterior skull base, with associated neurological injury and subsequent infection through dural tears and leakage of cerebrospinal fluid (CSF). Though not an absolute contraindication, caution must be taken with the use of nasopharyngeal airways, nasotracheal tubes, nasogastric tubes, and nasopharyngeal temperature probes.[12]

Blunt trauma

Blunt craniofacial trauma can be associated with severe haemorrhage, though in isolation is unlikely to result in circulatory shock. Options for management include anterior and posterior nasal

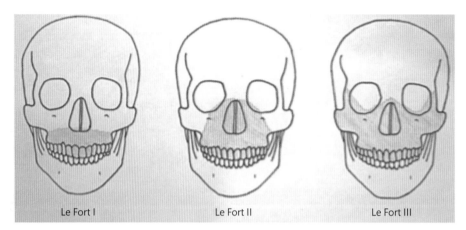

Fig. 13.1 Le Fort classification of facial fractures.
Morosan M, Parbhoo A, Curry N. Anaesthesia and common oral and maxilla-facial emergencies. *Continuing Education in Anaesthesia, Critical Care and Pain.* 2012;12(5):257–262.

packing (Fig. 13.3), the use of angiography and arterial emboliza-tion, and operative strategies such as fracture reduction (including intermaxillary fixation) and arterial ligation.[13,14] General principles of Advanced Trauma Life Support (ATLS) management regarding the control of haemorrhage and correction of coagulopathy are also applicable, including the use of pharmacological agents such as tran-examic acid, the prevention of hypothermia (including judicious administration of warmed fluids), and the guided use of blood prod-ucts, according to coagulation studies (laboratory clotting studies and/or point-of-care testing).

Penetrating trauma

Penetrating trauma can be caused by gunshot wounds and stabbing injuries. The extent of the injury is dependent upon factors such as

force and velocity, that is, the energy transfer to surrounding tis-sues. Tissue disruption and subsequent oedema can be extensive, particularly with high-speed injuries. Injuries sustained from gun-shots are more likely to require expedited surgical intervention.[13] Signs that would warrant urgent anaesthetic support, imaging, and possible surgical exploration include the presence of haemodynamic instability, or a pulsatile or expanding haematoma. Also, the pres-ence of airway compromise, subcutaneous emphysema, air bubbling through the wound, or neurological deficits are concerning signs.[15] In the haemodynamically stable patient, computed tomography (CT) angiography is widely used to assess the extent and severity of

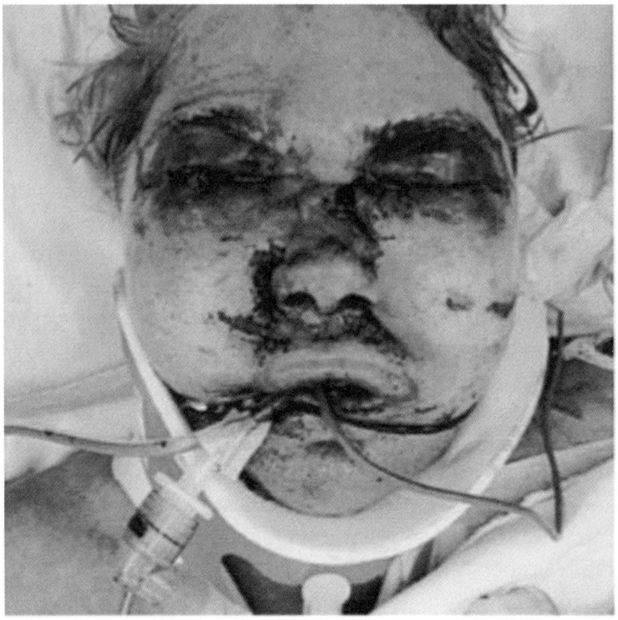

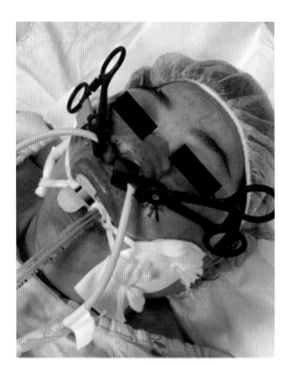

Fig. 13.3 Major haemorrhage caused by closed maxillofacial trauma, treated by anterior and posterior nasal packing.
Hsu F-Y, Mao S-H, Chuang AD-C, Wong Y-C, Chen C-H. Shock Index as a Predictor for Angiographic Hemostasis in Life-Threatening Traumatic Oronasal Bleeding. *International Journal of Environmental Research and Public Health.* 2021; 18(21):11051. https://doi.org/10.3390/ijerph182111051.

Fig. 13.2 Severe midfacial trauma showing gross oedema and necessity for early definitive airway management.
Lynham AJ, Hirst JP, Cosson JA et al. Emergency department management of maxillofacial trauma. *Emergency Medicine Australasia.* 2004;16:7–12.

injuries. Structured clinical examination, regardless of the zone of injury, is crucial to determine which patients warrant CT angiography or indeed surgical exploration.[15] Caution should be applied with the use of a cervical spine collar in the trauma patient as this may mask an expanding haematoma.

Associated injuries

Associated injuries are extremely common in patients presenting with severe maxillofacial trauma, given the proximity to vital structures and the magnitude of forces involved, so they must be actively sought and excluded, according to ATLS principles. The incidence of associated injuries varies in the literature, ranging from 35% up to 80% in severe traumatic injuries.[6,7] Concomitant injuries can be missed—up to 22% in one retrospective study.[6] Associated injuries can involve structures in the neck as well as ophthalmic, pharyngeal, and oesophageal trauma. Associated neurological injuries include traumatic brain injury, skull fractures, and dural tears, with resulting CSF leaks.

Traumatic brain injury

Maxillofacial injuries are associated with traumatic brain injury.[7] If injuries involve the orbit and midface structures, traumatic brain and skull injuries are more likely.[7] Traumatic brain injuries are more common in patients >50 years of age,[16] those with injuries sustained from road traffic accidents, and those in association with combined maxillary and mandibular fractures.[17]

Dural tears and cerebrospinal fluid leaks

This can occur with fractures involving the midface and superior structures. Signs of a CSF leak include otorrhoea and rhinorrhoea. Presentation may be delayed initially owing to initial tissue swelling, which then subsides to reveal a fluid leak. Leaks often resolve around the time of fracture reduction and stabilization; however, persistent cases require neurosurgical repair. Clinical diagnosis of a CSF leak can be challenging due to the similarity in appearance to a mixture of blood and saliva (known as the 'target sign').[18] Clinical features of a persistent CSF leak include postural headache (with improvement in symptoms in the supine position), neck pain, visual disturbance, tinnitus, and cranial nerve palsies. For radiological identification and localization, high-resolution CT or magnetic resonance imaging is used.[19] Antibiotic prophylaxis is often administered to reduce the risk of meningitis, although its effectiveness is still considered controversial and may be associated with antibiotic resistance.[18] Although possible CSF contamination can occur with nasal intubation, a nasotracheal tube is preferable during surgical correction of some facial injuries (specialist advice should be sought from neurosurgical colleagues if there is any doubt).

Cervical spine injury

Cervical spine trauma must also be considered in the context of maxillofacial trauma. The reported incidence varies in the literature between 2% and 4%, with up to 25% delayed diagnosis in patients presenting with severe maxillofacial trauma.[20,27] In any obtunded patient presenting with severe maxillofacial trauma, radiological evaluation of the cervical spine is required. Given the high risk of

associated injuries, airway management should routinely include manual cervical spine immobilization, as part of ATLS principles.

Oesophageal injury

Oesophageal injury, including perforation, is associated with very high morbidity and a mortality of up to 20%. Trauma-related injuries to the oesophagus are most commonly located in the proximal oesophagus and can result from both penetrating (most commonly, including iatrogenic injury) and blunt injuries.[21,22] Signs include odynophagia and dysphagia, as well as persistent vomiting and dyspnoea when eating. There may also be the presence of craniofacial emphysema and pneumomediastinum, causing retrosternal chest pain and dyspnoea.[11] If suspected, radiological evaluation (utilizing CT imaging, with water-soluble contrast for swallow studies in order to minimize the risk of mediastinitis), as well as oesophagoscopy, is warranted.[22] Surgical correction, along with antibiotics and insertion of a neck drain, is usually required, together with parenteral nutrition. Voice quality, including hoarseness, may indicate concomitant laryngeal injury.

Ocular injury

The incidence of ocular injury associated with maxillofacial trauma is variably reported in the literature, with an incidence of up to 70%.[23] It is commonly associated with frontal bone fractures. Any suspicion of globe rupture, retinal detachment, penetrating injuries, reduced visual acuity, corneal injury, or pupillary deformity requires urgent assessment by an ophthalmologist.[20]

Iatrogenic trauma

Iatrogenic trauma includes dental damage or avulsion from anaesthetic or surgical airway management,[24] ocular injuries (typically from mask ventilation), airway soft tissue injuries from throat pack insertion, and epistaxis (usually from nasotracheal intubation). Temporomandibular joint dysfunction from direct laryngoscopy and/or jaw thrust manoeuvre has also been reported,[24,25] as well as jaw dislocation from the use of supraglottic airway devices (SADs). Diagnostic and therapeutic interventions can also result in oesophageal rupture.[21]

Emergency airway management

ATLS principles should apply when managing maxillofacial trauma, including undertaking a structured primary survey. Early airway assessment and establishing a secure airway (with appropriate cervical spine stabilization) are essential. A relatively low number of patients require emergency airway management in the context of maxillofacial trauma (reported in one study as <2% of cases[10]). The assessment and optimization of respiratory function, followed by control of haemorrhage and optimization of coagulation should also take place. Utilizing the standardized ATLS approach assists in systematically identifying and treating potentially life-threatening injuries, since severe maxillofacial injuries are rarely in isolation. These assessments should be undertaken simultaneously as part of a well-drilled multidisciplinary trauma team. Management of maxillofacial trauma may warrant specialist input in the emergency setting, including otolaryngology, maxillofacial surgery, ophthalmology, and neurosurgery.

Recognition of acute airway obstruction in maxillofacial trauma

There are specific injuries in the context of maxillofacial trauma that should be identified as posing an immediate risk to airway patency, as described by Hutchinson et al.[9] Tongue base prolapse, caused by bilateral mandibular body fractures, can be fatal if unrecognized, particularly in the context of reduced consciousness in the supine patient. Maxillary prolapse posteriorly and inferiorly can also cause nasopharyngeal obstruction. Direct tracheal or laryngeal trauma can result in cervical airway obstruction, through displacement and swelling of structures. Structures may be difficult to identify, and tracheal intubation may be extremely difficult, regardless of whether direct laryngoscopy is possible.[9] The presence of foreign bodies, blood, vomitus, bony fragments, and fractured teeth can also cause direct airway obstruction.[9] Haemorrhage can directly cause airway obstruction, but also contributes to the difficulty in airway management through difficult mask ventilation and difficult direct and indirect laryngoscopy (fibreoptic and videolaryngoscopic views can be significantly impaired in the presence of bleeding). Haemorrhage also provides additional challenges of potential circulatory collapse at induction of anaesthesia and coagulopathy.[9] Soft tissue oedema can cause delayed airway obstruction and should be considered when deciding whether emergency tracheal intubation is indicated, and in the assessment of suitability for extubation of the trachea after surgical correction.[9]

Additional considerations in emergency airway management

Full stomach

All trauma patients should be considered to have a full stomach. Gastric emptying is impaired in the context of acute trauma, pain, and opioid administration. Blood and secretions are also likely to have been swallowed by the patient. Rapid sequence induction with cricoid pressure is therefore recommended by ATLS.[26]

Cervical spine injury

Studies have shown a 2–4% incidence of cervical spine fractures in patients sustaining blunt maxillofacial trauma.[27] Cervical spine immobilization, through manual in-line stabilization, should be performed until the cervical spine can be cleared radiologically and clinically.

Conscious level

There is an association between traumatic brain injury and maxillofacial trauma. Patients may have a reduced Glasgow Coma Score (GCS) from traumatic brain injury, or from hypoxia due to airway or respiratory compromise. Traumatic brain injury itself may warrant tracheal intubation to minimize secondary brain injury. A GCS of ≤8 warrants the establishment of a secure airway.

Level of experience and difficult airway equipment availability

Communication issues, lack of preparation, and human factors continue to play a significant role in airway-related critical incidents, such as those identified in the UK Fourth National Audit Project.[28] Senior clinicians should provide support in the management of a potentially difficult airway. Clinicians should also use equipment they are familiar with to minimize possible adverse effects or complications. A clear escalation plan for the management of failed tracheal intubation should be defined and preparations for airway rescue should be undertaken prior to induction of anaesthesia, following established algorithms such as those proposed by the Difficult Airway Society (DAS).[29] If techniques required for airway management are beyond the scope of the attending anaesthetist, expert help should be sought prior to induction of anaesthesia.[26]

Options for emergency airway management

Direct conventional laryngoscopy

Direct conventional laryngoscopy is still the most common method employed to secure the airway, as part of a rapid sequence induction, with the use of cricoid pressure to reduce the risk of aspiration of gastric contents. Manual in-line stabilization, as part of ATLS principles, must be performed as part of securing the airway to reduce cervical spinal injury.

Fibreoptic tracheal intubation

Fibreoptic scopes offer an indirect view of the vocal cords to facilitate tracheal intubation. However, with the presence of severe airway haemorrhage or foreign bodies, this technique is not always appropriate in maxillofacial trauma. Adequate local anaesthetic topicalization can also be difficult to achieve in the presence of secretions and blood in the airway. An awake technique may also not be tolerated in the obtunded patient with traumatic brain injury or in the intoxicated patient.

Nasotracheal intubation

Nasotracheal intubation may be required, particularly in the context of persistent trismus post-induction (discussed in detail later in the preoperative assessment and planning section). However, caution should be applied with nasotracheal intubation in patients with midface fractures or fractures of the base of the skull.[30] Case reports have described the inadvertent placement of nasotracheal tubes intracranially, though this is extremely rare.[31] A fibreoptic-assisted technique for nasotracheal intubation confers the advantages of a port for suctioning and for local anaesthetic administration; however, the scope must be the appropriate length to facilitate guiding the tracheal tube into the trachea.

Videolaryngoscopy

Videolaryngoscopy is increasingly being used in emergency airway management, particularly as cervical spinal movements should be minimized in the trauma patient, and this can be achieved with videolaryngoscopy.[32] There are several different models available and it is important for anaesthetists to familiarize themselves with the specific equipment in their local emergency department and operating theatres. Studies have demonstrated success rates >90% during first intubation attempts. Rigid stylets specific to the blade can be used to increase manoeuvrability and to aid tracheal intubation (although the gum elastic bougie can still be used).

Supraglottic airway devices

In the emergency setting, SADs are often used as bridging techniques to provide oxygenation and ventilation in the event of failed tracheal intubation. The DAS has emphasized the benefits of second-generation SADs, which have been found to provide a more effective supraglottic seal with lower ventilatory pressures.[29] Some SADs also provide an additional port for the placement of an orogastric tube, to enable suctioning of gastric contents to minimize pulmonary aspiration risk. The SAD can also serve as a conduit for tracheal intubation. The use of SADs in maxillofacial trauma may not always be appropriate, however. They do not provide protection from pulmonary aspiration and the presence of foreign bodies may preclude their use. The nature of some maxillofacial injuries may also affect the ease of insertion of the device, while fixed restriction of mouth opening may preclude their insertion entirely. Therefore, not all stages of the DAS failed intubation algorithm may be applicable in maxillofacial trauma, such that airway strategy and planning may include support from surgical colleagues at the outset, with an emphasis on prioritizing oxygenation of the patient at all times.

Combitubes

These are double-lumen tubes designed to be inserted blindly into the oesophagus and trachea. They have been associated with severe injuries to local structures, causing considerable morbidity, including mediastinitis,[26] and are not recommended in this context.

Front of neck airway

A front of neck airway is often performed as an emergency, in the event of failed tracheal intubation and failed oxygenation. The most recent DAS guidelines support the use of a scalpel cricothyroidotomy (scalpel–bougie–tube) as a standardized approach that requires minimal expertise and utilizes readily available equipment.[29] Certain clinical presentations may warrant the formation of a surgical tracheostomy under local anaesthesia, performed by surgical teams prior to induction of anaesthesia, although this may not always be possible in the trauma setting due to reduced consciousness and inability to cooperate under local anaesthesia, cardiovascular instability, or lack of availability of the necessary surgical expertise.

Airway guidelines and maxillofacial trauma

The updated DAS guidelines were published in 2015 to reflect changing and emerging strategies in the management of difficult airways and failed tracheal intubation. Some of the key changes are relevant to maxillofacial trauma, where difficulties in airway management must be anticipated. The 'ABCD' algorithm reflects the need to have a structured approach to management of the unanticipated difficult airway. Two key aspects are emphasized in greater detail in the updated guideline—adequate planning and preparation as part of plan A is essential, and that oxygenation must be prioritized at all stages of management. Videolaryngoscopy should be utilized if appropriate in plan A. The use of second-generation SADs (that provide a better seal at higher ventilatory pressures, provide a conduit for subsequent intubation, and sometimes a port for insertion of a gastric drainage tube) should be utilized in plan B. Cricoid pressure is still recommended in emergency airway management, although in the event of difficult SAD insertion or difficult mask ventilation, cricoid pressure should be released or removed completely. Gentle mask ventilation with ongoing cricoid pressure is now considered appropriate if the risk of aspiration of gastric contents is deemed to be low.[29]

There are important caveats in the context of maxillofacial trauma—the use of SADs, mask ventilation, and videolaryngoscopy may not be possible in the presence of marked deformity, haemorrhage, or oedema. A front of neck airway may be the most appropriate first-line option to secure the airway in this context. These options are explored in more detail below.

Videolaryngoscopy

Videolaryngoscopy is increasingly utilized across anaesthesia, emergency medicine, and intensive care, both as a first-line airway management technique and as a rescue technique, following failed direct laryngoscopy. A retrospective analysis of >340,000 patients demonstrated increasing use of videolaryngoscopy after failed direct laryngoscopy, being used in 80% of cases in 2012 compared with 30% in 2004.[33] The C-MAC® (Karl Storz, Tuttlingen, Germany) has also been shown to be more successful as a rescue device relative to direct laryngoscopy following failed tracheal intubation in the emergency department.[32] A Cochrane systematic review found an improved glottic view and decreased incidence of failed tracheal intubation, particularly in patients with predicted difficult airways (although the number of tracheal intubation attempts, and time for successful intubation were not known).[34] An improved glottic view with videolaryngoscopy may be of particular benefit in maxillofacial trauma patients with cervical spine immobilization. However, an adequate view does not necessarily correlate with ease of tracheal intubation or time to intubation, as described in a quantitative review and meta-analysis by Mihai et al.[35] Success rates also rely upon operators having reasonable experience of videolaryngoscopy.[36] Although improved intubation success rates with videolaryngoscopy are apparent, there is not yet enough evidence for them to be considered a first-line technique in emergency airway management. A comprehensive airway assessment must still be performed when utilizing videolaryngoscopy, as successful tracheal intubation still relies upon the patient having adequate mouth opening (and other favourable anatomical features). The presence of blood or foreign bodies may also preclude their use in significant maxillofacial trauma, due to the glottic view being obscured (as with fibreoptic scopes). A recent systematic review and meta-analysis identified that anaesthetists experienced in the use of videolaryngoscopy were more successful at securing difficult airways,[10] therefore it is important that anaesthetists gain experience through frequent use of the specific type of videolaryngoscope available at their institution to gain mastery and to minimize complications.

Front of neck airway

The DAS guidelines from 2015 identified scalpel cricothyroidotomy (scalpel–bougie–tube) as the preferable technique to needle cricothyroidotomy in the management of the 'can't intubate, can't oxygenate' scenario. Difficult airway equipment should be readily accessible during emergency airway management and hospitals should conduct regular training in how to perform scalpel cricothyroidotomy, to increase familiarity with the technique. The DAS has introduced a four-step approach to emergency front of neck airways. The equipment required is a scalpel, bougie, and size 6.0 cuffed tracheal tube. Using a 'laryngeal handshake', the cricothyroid membrane is first identified. Standing on the patient's left side (for right-handed operators), a horizontal stab incision is made at the cricothyroid membrane, after which the scalpel is rotated through 90°. A bougie is then inserted into the trachea and scalpel removed. The tracheal tube is then railroaded over the bougie. In patients with a high body mass index, where front of neck anatomy may not be easily palpated, a vertical skin incision should first be made in order to facilitate identification of the cricothyroid membrane. Additionally, in non-emergency situations, ultrasound may be used to assess and mark the cricothyroid membrane prior to intravenous anaesthetic induction, as part of 'planning for failure'.[29]

Anaesthetic management of maxillofacial trauma

Preoperative assessment and planning

Timely and thorough anaesthetic assessment should be undertaken to identify patients with actual or potential airway compromise. Factors to consider include indicators of potentially difficult bag mask ventilation, difficult tracheal intubation, and difficult mechanical ventilation, as well as the requirements for impending surgery.

Conscious level

As per ATLS guidelines, a patient with a GCS of ≤8 warrants securing and protection of the airway, as they have lost their airway protective reflexes and may also be at risk of hypoventilation. In the context of major maxillofacial trauma, and significantly reduced conscious level, it is also likely that traumatic brain injury has occurred. Tracheal intubation to facilitate controlled ventilation and optimization of oxygenation and carbon dioxide clearance will also help to minimize secondary brain injury.

Spontaneous ventilation and hypoxia

As described previously, compromised ventilation in the presence of reduced conscious level should be identified. Thoracic injuries such as a flail segment, multiple rib fractures, or haemopneumothoraces can severely compromise ventilation. Patients with dyspnoea, tracheal deviation, or subcutaneous emphysema involving the neck and chest should be identified rapidly.

Extent of facial injuries and markers of difficulty

A standard anaesthetic airway assessment should be undertaken, with mouth opening, Mallampati score, jaw protrusion, and thyromental distance assessed where possible. Airway obstruction may already be apparent and neck mobility may be impaired. The presence of drooling, stridor, odynophagia or dysphagia, tracheal deviation, hoarseness of voice, or airway haemorrhage generally indicates the need for urgent/immediate airway management. Similarly, the presence of significant orofacial burns, gunshot wounds, or unstable facial fractures will expedite the need for definitive airway intervention. General predictors of difficult bag mask ventilation (as seen in the general population, e.g. the presence of a beard or high body mass index) should not be forgotten during the airway assessment. If difficult airway management is anticipated, an examination of the front of neck (including ultrasound assessment, when time permits) should be performed in order to identify the relevant anatomical structures. Experienced help should be sought and, if necessary, marking and local anaesthetic infiltration (in preparation for rescue front of neck access) should be undertaken prior to intravenous anaesthetic induction.

Trismus

Reduced mouth opening may not improve after administration of general anaesthesia (or muscle relaxation) in certain injuries. Delayed presentations with increased swelling will reduce mouth opening, therefore the age of the fracture should be determined. Reduced mouth opening associated with infections, abscesses, or temporomandibular joint pathologies (including dislocation; **Fig. 13.4**) are unlikely to improve after anaesthetic induction. A fractured zygoma that interrupts the coronoid process of the mandible will also result in a fixed restricted mouth opening. Options for management include consideration of a regional anaesthetic technique, flexible fibreoptic tracheal intubation, supraglottic airway insertion as a conduit for tracheal intubation, tracheal intubation with a rigid fibrescope (e.g. Bonfils),[37] or retrograde tracheal intubation. Mouth opening <2.5 cm is unlikely to result in successful direct laryngoscopy. In patients presenting with a degree of restricted mouth opening relating to pain alone, this is almost always overcome following induction of general anaesthesia.

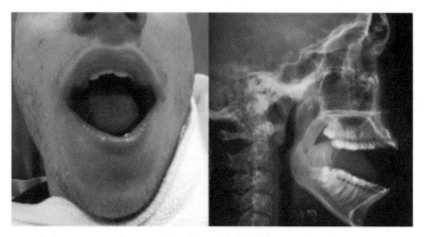

Fig. 13.4 Characteristic open-mouthed appearance of an anteriorly dislocated mandible.

Deangelis AF, Barrowman RA, Harrod R, Nastri AL. Maxillofacial injuries: Dentoalveolar and temporomandibular joint trauma. *Emergency Medicine Australasia*. 2014;26:439–445.

Haemorrhage

Life-threatening haemorrhage associated with maxillofacial trauma is rare, although the polytrauma patient may present with haemodynamic instability through other injuries. Stabilization of the patient should occur prior to induction of anaesthesia. Specific techniques used to manage bleeding associated with maxillofacial trauma include posterior packing[13] or arterial embolization,[14] as discussed previously. Basic management strategies include the timely cross-matching of blood products, correction of coagulopathy, treatment of acidosis, and prevention or correction of hypothermia.

Preparation for surgery

The type of tracheal tube used can impact upon surgical access. South-facing oral Ring–Adair–Elwyn (RAE) tubes are usually used for zygomatic or orbital fractures. Nasotracheal tubes are used for fractures involving the mandible, most Le Fort fractures, and those causing malocclusion. Alternatives to oral or nasotracheal intubation include tracheostomy or submental intubation. The choice of airway management should be discussed with the surgical team prior to induction of anaesthesia, along with the requirement for a throat pack, intermaxillary fixation, or the need for facial nerve monitoring.

Intraoperative management

The shared airway

As with all oromaxillofacial surgery, appreciation of the 'shared airway' is vital for safe anaesthetic management of the patient. Appropriate communication and teamwork are invaluable. Tracheal tubes and circuits should be thoroughly checked and secured prior to preparation of the surgical field and application of surgical drapes, with similar care taken on removal of drapes at the end of surgery to avoid inadvertent tube dislodging or circuit disconnections.

Oral tracheal tubes

Orotracheal intubation via direct laryngoscopy remains the most common technique used to secure the airway in maxillofacial trauma.[10] This can be utilized if the patient is considered appropriate for tracheal extubation at the end of surgery and the orotracheal tube is not interfering with surgical access intraoperatively. Options generally include RAE tubes or reinforced tracheal tubes that can be safely secured away from the operative field or side of surgery.

Nasotracheal tubes

Operations requiring maxillomandibular fixation generally require nasotracheal tubes.[10] Preformed curved nasotracheal tubes can be placed away from the operative field. Specific contraindications to nasotracheal intubation include fractures to the midface and base of skull fractures. Awake nasotracheal intubation techniques can be particularly challenging in the maxillofacial trauma patient. Cooperation is often impaired due to concomitant confusion, and foreign bodies and obstructions can result in inadequate local anaesthetic topicalization, as well as potentially obscuring the glottic view.

Tracheostomies

Patients may come to theatre for surgery with a tracheostomy or surgical cricothyroidotomy already created (either pre-hospital, or in the emergency department—having been involved in major trauma with significant orofacial injuries or impending airway compromise). Formation of an intraoperative tracheostomy should also be considered for patients undergoing maxillofacial trauma surgery whose trachea has been difficult to intubate prior to surgery or in those with previously failed tracheal intubation attempts (with the expectation that, in the context of increased oedema after surgery, the trachea may be impossible to reintubate in the event of airway or respiratory compromise). A tracheostomy may also be indicated if a period of prolonged postoperative ventilation is expected, as this will facilitate respiratory weaning and aid with suctioning of secretions. A tracheostomy may also be necessitated in patients with extensive panfacial fractures, where alternative means of securing the airway that allows surgery to proceed are precluded (e.g. comminuted mandibular fractures or fractures that preclude the use of nasal intubation).[42] Complications of tracheostomy formation include haemorrhage, and damage to airway structures including the trachea (with subsequent stenosis), vocal cords, recurrent laryngeal nerves, or oesophagus.[43]

Throat packs

A throat pack may be required. This requirement should be established during the theatre team brief, including specifically identifying who is responsible for its insertion and removal. The processes surrounding safe throat pack management are discussed in detail in Chapter 10.

Postoperative fixation devices

Postoperative intermaxillary fixation may be required. This has a significant impact upon the decision-making surrounding suitability for tracheal extubation and the chosen extubation strategy at the end of surgery. Tracheal extubation may be more challenging, and the presence of a fixation device is also likely to affect the ease of reintubation if difficulties are encountered. Sometimes, the risk of tracheal extubation immediately following surgery is deemed too great, and continued invasive ventilation in the critical care unit is necessitated. In some cases, for example, severe oedema associated with panfacial trauma, a tracheostomy may be performed in order to create a safe stable airway, regardless of the presence of fixation devices. The development of rigid surgical plating techniques has superseded the requirement for postoperative rigid fixation devices in many cases.[4]

Nerve monitoring

The requirement for facial nerve monitoring will impact the use of neuromuscular blocking agents. In this context, tracheal intubation can often be achieved without the use of any muscle relaxant (e.g. by judicious use of a potent opioid); however, this should not impact safe airway management. Should airway management difficulties arise in the absence of muscle relaxation, a neuromuscular blocking agent should be administered. Of course, an appropriate dose of a short-acting muscle relaxant would be preferable in these circumstances, and repeat dosing should be avoided. Close communication with the surgical team is advised.

Intraoperative tube changes

Intraoperative tracheal tube changes may be necessary in the surgical correction of panfacial fractures (involving the naso-orbitoethmoidal complex and mandibular structures), as nasotracheal tubes can interfere with the surgical correction. Clear communication between team members is essential, and distractions in the operating theatre must be minimized prior to undertaking a tube exchange. Preoxygenation on 100% oxygen and the administration of a neuromuscular blocking agent prior to tube exchange are also advocated. The formation of a surgical tracheostomy may be preferred in order to avoid the risks associated with tube exchanges, particularly when bleeding and oedema may lead to the loss of a previously secure airway.[4]

Submental and retromolar intubation

Tracheal tube exchanges can be minimized by employing a retromolar or more commonly a submental technique for tracheal intubation, as these can enable surgical access to both the oral and nasal cavities.[10] Submental intubation (Fig. 13.5) can be used in patients with comminuted fractures of the midface or the nose, where nasal intubation is contraindicated, and where tracheal extubation is expected to be possible at the end of surgery.[38] Like tracheostomies, submental intubation provides an unobstructed surgical field, but the surgical scar is generally aesthetically superior[43,44] and there may be fewer long-term complications, such as subglottic stenosis. It is, however, contraindicated in the presence of comminuted mandibular fractures, and is not without complication, for example, bleeding, skin infections,[10] salivary fistulae,[39] or damage to the lingual nerve, the marginal mandibular branch of the facial nerve, or the submandibular gland. Conversely, retromolar intubation is considered the technique with the least associated morbidity when compared with submental intubation or tracheostomy formation, but it relies upon the presence of sufficient retromolar space and sometimes may not enable full dental occlusion (and therefore is not always possible).[10,40]

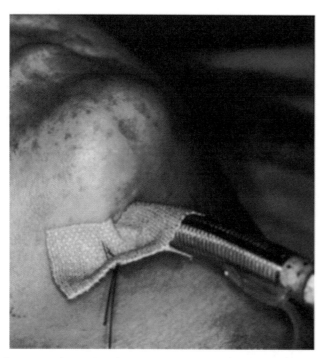

Fig. 13.5 Submental intubation—tracheal tube secured submentally with sutures and tape.
Amin M, Dill-Russell P, Manisali M, Lee R, Sinton I. Facial fractures and submental intubation. *Anaesthesia*. 2002;57:1195–1212.

Other intraoperative considerations

High-dose steroids (such as 8 mg dexamethasone) can be used to minimize postoperative oedema and is administered at the start of surgery and often continued postoperatively in the short term. Prophylactic antibiotic administration of variable duration is also likely to be required. Eye protection using eye tapes and pads are often used. Awareness of the oculocardiac reflex (profound vagal stimulation produced via a reflex arc involving the trigeminal and vagus nerves and the brainstem) is important. This can be associated with orbital and maxillofacial injury, producing severe hypotension and bradycardia.[41]

Surgical factors

Maxillofacial surgery may be very prolonged, and a period of postoperative invasive ventilation may be required due to the duration of anaesthesia alone. Airway oedema, relating to the initial traumatic injuries or the resultant surgery, is likely to worsen immediately postoperatively and may precipitate airway obstruction, therefore continued tracheal intubation and postoperative lung ventilation may be required to allow some of this oedema to subside, enabling safe tracheal extubation further down the line. It is critical that a multidisciplinary discussion occurs between surgeon and anaesthetist that specifically addresses the potential risk of postoperative airway-related complications. In the polytrauma patient, there may also be ongoing surgical requirements, with further staged operative procedures necessitated. Clear communication of the ongoing surgical plan should be relayed before the end of surgery so that this can inform decisions on the most appropriate postoperative destination for the patient.

Anaesthetic factors

Acute postoperative pain can be particularly challenging to manage in the polytrauma patient, and a level two postoperative care facility can often provide better and safer acute pain management for these patients initially. Major perioperative haemorrhage, associated with the initial traumatic injuries or surgical correction, may also warrant critical care admission for further stabilization, cardiovascular support, ongoing blood product administration, and correction of the metabolic derangement.

Patient factors

Other traumatic injuries, in addition to the maxillofacial pathology, may require ongoing airway protection and invasive ventilation, for example, patients with traumatic brain injury or severe thoracic injuries. In this respect, attention to patients' GCS prior to induction of general anaesthesia is crucial as a reduced GCS may well preclude safe tracheal extubation at the end of surgery. Patient comorbidities may also be important, as pre-existing respiratory, cardiovascular, or endocrine disease may be exacerbated in the context of major trauma, requiring additional invasive support postoperatively.

Tracheal extubation

If it is deemed clinically appropriate to wake the patient up at the end of surgery, general considerations to optimize conditions for smooth emergence and tracheal extubation should be employed.[29] Anaesthetic skill mix and level of seniority and experience must be considered when undertaking tracheal extubation in patients with complex airway pathology, and appropriate assistance should be sought if required (especially if there are other confounding factors, such as high body mass index). Difficult airway equipment must be immediately available, along with emergency drugs and drugs for reintubation of the trachea.

Patients should be placed in an upright sitting position (where possible), with neuromuscular blocking agents fully reversed. Prior to tracheal extubation, the anaesthetist should inspect the oropharynx and suction the upper airway under direct vision. A 'check-laryngoscopy' can also be performed, as the grade of laryngoscopy is now likely to be higher than at initial intubation due to the presence of oedema, blood, and secretions. Patients should be fully awake and following commands before extubation of the trachea in maxillofacial trauma. If there are specific surgical concerns regarding bleeding and haematoma development, or suture disruption (applicable to flap surgery), smooth tracheal extubation can be facilitated using a low-dose remifentanil target-controlled infusion.

A bite block may be used to prevent biting and occlusion of the tracheal tube during emergence. Other airway adjuncts such as specially designed 'staged extubation' flexible wires and paediatric airway exchange catheters can be used—these are well tolerated by awake patients, and can provide a conduit for tracheal reintubation if required. Suction catheters have also been used for this purpose, particularly in the paediatric population.

Following tracheal extubation, if there are concerns regarding adequacy of oxygenation postoperatively (despite provision of standard nasal or face mask supplementary oxygen), continuous positive airway pressure masks should generally be avoided as they cause direct pressure on suture lines, potentially causing disruption or bleeding. Instead, high-flow humidified nasal oxygenation (Optiflow™; Fisher & Paykel Healthcare, Auckland, New Zealand) can be considered. Some positive effects on oxygenation, airway patency, and carbon dioxide clearance have been demonstrated using this technique in apnoeic patients at induction of anaesthesia, so-called 'THRIVE' (transnasal humidified rapid-insufflation ventilatory exchange),[45,46] and similar advantages may be conferred in the spontaneously breathing patient postoperatively. For patients suitable for discharge to a postoperative ward rather than critical care facility, a minimum monitoring requirement of continuous pulse oximetry is advocated in order to identify ventilatory insufficiency as quickly as possible.

Postoperative considerations

Planning and preparation for potential airway emergencies is vital ('preparing to fail'). In the event of a failed tracheal extubation, emergency reintubation can be very challenging in these patients. Attention should focus upon a structured escalation plan, with appropriate airway equipment and personnel to deal with anticipated emergencies. Use of an airway exchange device may be considered to facilitate reintubation of the trachea. A senior maxillofacial surgeon should also remain present in the operating theatre during emergence from anaesthesia to assist in the event of any airway compromise.

Delayed airway or respiratory compromise can also occur, often due to worsening oedema or bleeding. Regular postoperative steroids can reduce some of this oedema. However, stitch cutters must be immediately available in the postoperative care unit and beside the patient on the ward/critical care unit, so that sutures can be released in the event of an expanding haematoma causing acute airway

obstruction. In these circumstances, it is important to consider the site of the haematoma and its anatomical relations, as this will affect the subsequent management. For example, mandibular surgery is most likely to cause sublingual, submandibular, and submental haematomas, causing airway obstruction by displacing the tongue upwards and backwards. In this context, if an emergency front of neck airway is required, the trachea is still likely to be in the midline, as the haematoma is superior to the hyoid, and a standard approach to emergency front of neck airway formation can be utilized.

Conclusion

Maxillofacial trauma can result in complex injuries that require urgent anaesthetic involvement and stabilization. A thorough approach to assessment, an awareness of the potential for other significant injuries, and early multidisciplinary involvement are key. A systematic approach to emergency airway management, with a clear airway strategy, a plan for failure, and familiarity with advanced airway techniques (for both tracheal intubation and extubation) will result in safe and effective care of these high-risk patients.

REFERENCES

1. Shahim FN, Cameron P, McNeil JJ. Maxillofacial trauma in major trauma patients. *Aust Dent J*. 2006;**51**(3):225–230.
2. Al Khawalde M. Maxillofacial fractures in Jordan; a 5 year retrospective review. *Oral Surg*. 2011;**4**(4):161–165.
3. Kirkpatrick N. Facial and orbital injuries. *Surgery*. 2004;**22**(8): 186–190.
4. Gassner R, Tuli T, Hachl O, Ulmer H. Cranio-maxillofacial trauma: a 10 year review of 9543 cases with 21 067 injuries. *J Craniomaxillofac Surg*. 2003;**31**(1):51–61.
5. Hutchinson IL, Magennis P, Shepherd JP, Brown AE. The BAOMS United Kingdom survey of facial injuries. Part 1: aetiology and the association with alcohol consumption. *Br J Oral Maxillofac Surg*. 1998;**36**(1):3–13.
6. Fama F, Cicciu M, Sindoni A, Nastro-Siniscalchi E, Falzea R, Cervino G, et al. Maxillofacial and concomitant serious injuries: an eight-year single center experience. *Chin J Traumatol*. 2017;**20**(4):4–8.
7. Scherbaum Eidt JM, De Conto F, De Bortoli MM, Engelmann JL, Rocha FD. Associated injuries in patients with maxillofacial trauma at the Hospital Sao Vincent de Paulo, Passo Fundo, Brazil. *J Oral Maxillofac Res*. 2013;**4**(3):e1.
8. Morosan M, Parbhoo A, Curry N. Anaesthesia and common oral and maxilla-facial emergencies. *Cont Educ Anaesth Crit Care Pain*. 2012;**12**(5):257–262.
9. Hutchinson I, Lawlor M, Skinner D. ABC of major trauma. Major maxillofacial injuries. *BMJ*. 1990;**301**(6752):595–599.
10. Kellman RM, Losquadro WD. Comprehensive airway management of patients with maxillofacial trauma. *Craniomaxillofac Trauma Reconstr*. 2008;**1**(1):39–48.
11. Houghton D, Sidebottom AJ. Pneumomediastinum following zygomatic fracture—an uncommon but potentially life-threatening complication. *Oral Surg*. 2012;**5**(4):198–200.
12. Mittal G, Mittal RK, Katyal S, Uppal S, Mittal V. Airway management in maxillofacial trauma: do we really need tracheostomy/submental intubation. *J Clin Diagn Res*. 2014;**8**(3):77–79.

13. Cogbill TH, Cothren CC, Ahern MK, Cullinane DC, Kaups KL, Scalea TM, et al. Management of maxillofacial injuries with severe oronasal haemorrhage: a multicentre perspective. *J Trauma*. 2008;**65**(5):994–999.

14. Noy D, Rachmiel A, Emodi O, Amsalem Y, Israel Y, Nagler RM. Transarterial embolization in maxillofacial intractable potentially life-threatening haemorrhage. *J Oral Maxillofac Surg*. 2017;**75**(6):1223–1231.

15. Ibraheem K, Kyan M, Rhee P, Azim A, O'Keeffe T, Tang A, et al. "No zone" approach in penetrating neck trauma reduces unnecessary computerised tomography angiography and negative explorations. *J Surg Res*. 2018;**221**:113–120.

16. Zhou H-H, Liu Q, Yang R-T, Li Z, Li ZB. Traumatic head injuries in patients with maxillofacial fractures: a retrospective case-control study. *Dent Traumatol*. 2015;**31**(3):209–214.

17. Adams CD, Januszkiewicz JS, Judson J. Changing patterns of severe craniomaxillofacial trauma in Auckland over eight years. *Aust NZ J Surg*. 2000;**70**(6):401–404.

18. Oh J-W, Kim S-H, Whang K. Traumatic cerebrospinal fluid leak: diagnosis and management. *Korean J Neurotrauma*. 2017;**13**(2):63–67.

19. Bell RB, Dierks EJ, Homer L, Potter BE. Management of cerebrospinal fluid leak associated with craniomaxillofacial trauma. *J Oral Maxillofac Surg*. 2004;**62**(6):676–684.

20. Lynham AJ, Hirst JP, Cosson JA, Chapman PJ, McEniery P. Emergency department management of maxillofacial trauma. *Emerg Med Australas*. 2004;**16**(1):7–12.

21. Abdulrahman H, Ajaj A, Shunni A, El-Menyar A, Chaikhouni A, Al-Thani H, et al. Blunt traumatic esophageal injury: unusual presentation and approach. *Int J Surg Case Rep*. 2014;**5**(1):16–18.

22. Graciano AJ, Stockler Schner AM, Fischer CA. Esophageal perforation in closed neck trauma. *Braz J Otorhinolaryngol*. 2013;**79**(1):121.

23. Tuckett JW, Lynham A, Lee GA, Perry M, Harrington U. Maxillofacial trauma in the emergency department: a review. *Surgeon*. 2014;**12**(2):106–114.

24. Deangelis AF, Barrowman RA, Harrod R, Nastri AL. Maxillofacial injuries: dentoalveolar and temporomandibular joint trauma. *Emerg Med Australas*. 2014;**26**(5):439–445.

25. Aiello G, Metcalf I. Anaesthetic implications of temporomandibular joint disease. *Can J Anaesth*. 1992;**39**(6):610–616.

26. Krausz AA, Abu el-Naaj I, Barak M. Maxillofacial trauma patient: coping with the difficult airway. *World J Emerg Surg*. 2009;**4**:21.

27. Krausz AA, Krausz MM, Picetti E. Maxillofacial and neck trauma: a damage control approach. *World J Emerg Surg*. 2015;**10**:31.

28. Royal College of Anaesthetists. *4th National Audit Project: Major Complications of Airway Management in the UK*. London: Royal College of Anaesthetists; 2011. http://www.rcoa.ac.uk/NAP4

29. Frerk C, Mitchell VS, McNarry AF, Mendonca C, Bhagrath R, Patel A, et al. Difficult Airway Society 2015 guidelines for management of unanticipated difficult intubation in adults. *Br J Anaesth*. 2015;**115**(6):827–848.

30. Hall CEJ, Shutt LE. Nasotracheal intubation for head and neck surgery. *Anaesthesia*. 2003;**58**(3):249–256.

31. Paul M, Dueck M, Kampe S, Petzke F, Ladra A. Intracranial placement of a nasotracheal tube after transnasal transsphenoidal surgery. *Br J Anaesth*. 2003;**91**(4):601–604.

32. Sackles JC, Mosier JM, Patanwalab AE, Dicken JM, Kalin L, Javedani PP. The C-MAC® video laryngoscope is superior to the direct laryngoscope for the rescue of failed first-attempt intubations in the emergency department. *J Emerg Med*. 2015;**48**(3):280–286.

33. Aziz MF, Brambrink AM, Healy DW, Willett AW, Shanks A, Tremper T, et al. Success of intubation rescue techniques after failed direct laryngoscopy in adults: a retrospective comparative analysis from the multicentre perioperative outcomes group. *Anaesthesiology*. 2016;**125**(4):656–666.

34. Lewis SR, Butler AR, Parker J, Cook T, Cook TM, Schofield-Robinson OJ, Smith AF. Videolaryngoscopy versus direct laryngoscopy for adult patients requiring tracheal intubation: a Cochrane Systematic Review. *Br J Anaesth*. 2017;**119**(3):369–383.

35. Mihai R, Blair E, Kay H, Cook TM. A quantitative review and meta-analysis of performance of non-standard laryngoscopes and rigid fibreoptic intubation aids. *Anaesthesia*. 2008;**63**(7):745–760.

36. Healy DW, Maties O, Hovord D, Kheterpal S. A systematic review of the role of videolaryngoscopy in successful orotracheal intubation. *BMC Anesthesiol*. 2012;**12**(32):32.

37. Shollik NA, Ibrahim SM, Ismael A, Agnoletti V, Piraccini E, Corso RM. Use of Bonfils Intubation Fiberscope in patients with limited mouth opening. *Case Rep Anaesthesiol*. 2012;**2012**:297306.

38. Kita R, Kikuta T, Takahashi M, Ootani T, Takaoka M, Matsuda M, et al. Efficacy and complications of submental tracheal intubation compared with tracheostomy in maxillofacial trauma patients. *J Oral Sci*. 2016;**58**(1):23–28.

39. Pieters BMA, Maas EHA, Knape JTA, van Zundert AAJ. Videolaryngoscopy vs. direct laryngoscopy use by experienced anaesthetists in patients with known difficult airways: a systematic review and meta-analysis. *Anaesthesia*. 2017;**72**(12):1532.

40. Jaisani MR, Pradhan L, Bhattarai B, Sagtani A. Intubation techniques: preferences of maxillofacial trauma surgeons. *J Maxillofac Oral Surg*. 2015;**14**(2):501–505.

41. Pham CM, Couch SM. Oculocardiac reflex elicited by orbital floor fracture and inferior globe displacement. *Am J Ophthalmol Case Rep*. 2017;**6**:4–6.

42. Barak M, Bahouth H, Leiser Y, Abu El-Naaj I. Airway management of the patient with maxillofacial trauma: review of the literature and suggested clinical approach. *BioMed Res Int*. 2015;**2015**:724032.

43. Amin M, Dill-Russell P, Manisali M, Lee R, Sinton I. Facial fractures and submental intubation. *Anaesthesia*. 2002;**57**(12):1195–1212.

44. Eipe N, McGuire T. Submental intubation: another anaesthetic option for maxillofacial trauma. *Paediatr Anaesth Correspond*. 2012;**22**(5):494–496.

45. Patel A, Nouraei SAR. Transnasal humidified rapid-insufflation ventilatory exchange (THRIVE): a physiological method of increasing apnoea time in patients with difficult airways. *Anaesthesia*. 2015;**70**(3):323–329.

46. Booth AWG, Vidhani K, Lee PK, Thomsett C-M. SponTaneous Respiration using IntraVEnous anaesthesia and Hi-flow nasal oxygen (STRIVE-Hi) maintains oxygenation and airway patency during management of the obstructed airway: an observational study. *Br J Anaesthesia*. 2017;**118**(3):444–451.

14

Burns and inhalational injury

Caroline A. R. Nicholas and Tim N. Vorster

Introduction

This chapter focuses on the anaesthetic management of oral and facial burns, thermal airway burns, and inhalation injury. It provides a brief overview of general burns management and the principles of burns resuscitation; however, there are alternative resources[1] and courses available for a more generalized perspective of severe burns management.[2]

The surgical aims of treating oral and facial burns are identical to the treatment of burns elsewhere on the body—to excise non-viable tissue, to allow viable tissue to heal in a time frame that reduces scarring, and to cover debrided areas with skin grafts or skin substitutes in order to improve cosmetic and functional results. Conversely, the anaesthetic challenges are quite unique. Oral and facial burns are seldom an isolated injury and are often associated with other immediately life-threatening injuries. Acute thermal airway burns are usually encountered with a facial burn and other aspects of the 'smoke inhalation complex' are commonly involved, requiring rapid assessment and appropriate treatment prior to transfer to a specialist burns unit.

Epidemiology

Although minor cutaneous burns are extremely common, deaths from burns are rare in the UK.[3] In the US, with a population of 300 million, the American Burn Association estimated that 500,000 burns patients were seen in their emergency departments each year, of whom 40,000 were admitted as inpatients and 25,000 went to specialized burn centres. Approximately 2500 of these patients had burns >30% of total body surface area (TBSA), and there were 4000 deaths, with 75% of deaths occurring prior to hospital arrival.[4]

Inhalation injury occurs in approximately 10–20% of patients admitted to burn centres, increasing in frequency as the size of burn increases. Inhalation injury, age, and burns size are the three most cited predictive factors for prolonged ventilator dependence, hospital stay, and death.[5–8] Though not all patients with facial burns will have an associated inhalation burn, the vast majority of patients with inhalation injury will have a facial burn. The presence of a full-thickness facial burn has been shown to be an independent prognostic indicator for significantly increased risk of death, when compared with similar size burns elsewhere on the body.[9] It is proposed that this is due to the close association between this type of burn and an inhalation injury. Facial burns are often just a fraction of the overall burn seen in patients with massive thermal injuries—a significant number of burn victims will have other injuries and coexisting pathologies that will need to be appropriately treated. Isolated inhalation injury, or inhalation injury with a minor cutaneous burn, has a mortality rate of 0.3–5%.[10,11] However, the American Burn Association National Burn Repository database shows that the presence of an inhalation injury increases the risk of death in patients <60 years of age with burns <20% TBSA by 15 times.[12] With increasing age and burn size, the mortality increases dramatically, such that a patient aged >60 years with a burn >40% TBSA and an inhalation injury has a predicted mortality of 90%.[10] This compares with a predicted mortality of 30% in the absence of an inhalation element.

Burns occurring at the extremes of age are more likely a 'symptom' of other pathologies. Toddlers with colds are more likely to be seen with scalds than well children. Burns in the elderly may be caused by underlying cardiac or neurological events. The burn in these patients, especially if minor, may be the least important factor in their prognosis.

Chemical burns represent 3–5% of burns injuries but have a high mortality rate, particularly if there is associated ingestion of the agent.

The emergency department acute major burn admission

The acute major burn patient can be exceptionally emotive for the receiving hospital staff involved. Their injuries may be visually dramatic, overwhelming to the olfactory senses, and the severe pain experienced by the patient can be particularly distressing to witness. Regardless of seniority and experience, it is easy to be distracted by these aspects and fail to manage the patient in the systematic way we would approach other trauma victims. Injuries seldom overlooked in other trauma situations such as cervical spine instability, thoracic emergencies, abdominal crises, long bone fractures, myocardial ischaemia, or concurrent drug overdose, have all anecdotally been missed.

Cutaneous burns are left to the secondary survey of any major burn assessment. Obtaining a quick history from the patient (where possible), relatives, or ambulance staff, and ensuring the team complete a full Advanced Trauma Life Support trauma survey in a stepwise manner are paramount. The presence of immediate life-threatening injuries, in addition to the burn, must be sought and excluded before treating a patient as an isolated burn, as 7% of all burns admissions are reported to have associated polytrauma.[13] Though uncommon, some suicide attempts may involve self-immolation, therefore this should also be considered. Paracetamol and salicylate levels should be taken routinely. An initially overlooked drug overdose in a burn patient can still have the same outcome if detected and treated promptly.

Resuscitation

Airway (and cervical spine protection)

Apnoeic patients and those with decreased consciousness are unable to maintain their own airway safely and, therefore, require tracheal intubation. Impending airway compromise due to inhalation injury must be considered and re-evaluated regularly. All burns patients should initially receive 100% oxygen via a non-rebreathing mask. Cervical spine protection is mandatory until a neck injury has been formally excluded. The presence of hypoxia, hypercapnia, deep facial burns, circumferential neck burns, and/or oropharyngeal oedema warrants tracheal intubation. Early tracheal intubation is advisable where the progression of significant oedema is anticipated. The use of suxamethonium is safe in the first 24 hours following a burn injury; thereafter, the risk of precipitating hyperkalaemic cardiac arrest (due to uncontrolled potassium release from extra-junctional acetylcholine receptors) precludes its subsequent use for up to 2 years. Air flow through a tracheal tube or tracheostomy is mainly laminar (Fig. 14.1) and, therefore, regulated by the Hagen–Poiseuille equation[14]:

$$\text{Flow}\,(Q) = \text{pressure}\,(P) \times \text{radius}^4\,(r) \times \pi\,/ \\ \text{length of the tube}\,(l) \times \text{viscosity}\,(\eta) \times 8$$

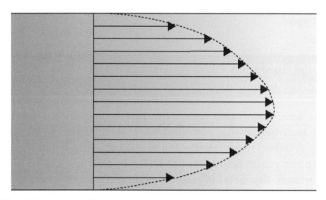

Fig. 14.1 Laminar flow in the airways.

Reproduced with permission from Gilbert-Kawai, E., & Wittenberg, M. (2014). Reynold's number (and turbulent flow). In *Essential Equations for Anaesthesia: Key Clinical Concepts for the FRCA and EDA* (pp. 21–23). Cambridge: Cambridge University Press. doi:10.1017/CBO9781139565387.013

The radius of the tracheal tube has a significant impact on gas flow and lung ventilation. The larger the tracheal tube diameter, the greater the gas flow that can be delivered (reducing work of breathing), as well as facilitating airway toileting and suctioning, and enabling the frequently performed bronchoscopy and bronchiolar lavage to be undertaken with greater ease. In patients with a thermal insult, the direct and indirect chemical injury to the respiratory tract can lead to profound mucus membrane disturbance, and activation of the inflammatory cascade, resulting in increased capillary permeability, loss of intrinsic cilia, and diffuse exudative production. Secretion load can be heavy, potentiating bronchospasm, hypoxia, atelectasis, loss of hypoxic vasoconstriction, airway obstruction, and infection.

Breathing

Full exposure of the chest and neck are required for examination. A history of a blast injury or other trauma will make intrathoracic damage more likely. Inhalation injury may show limited early clinical signs but may exacerbate existing pulmonary pathology. A high respiratory rate is concerning and pulse oximetry should be undertaken and corroborated later with an arterial blood gas sample. Full-thickness burns to the torso will cause the skin to lose its elasticity and the ability to expand, impacting significantly on breathing. Oedema formation around the injury site may also lead to compression of the structures within the neck, causing airway obstruction. This is of particular relevance in children, who have smaller diameter airways. Compliance, and subsequently pulmonary ventilation, may be reduced with circumferential burns of the chest. In children, (predominantly abdominal breathers), this can occur with just isolated anterior burns of the chest and upper abdomen. An urgent escharotomy may be required to avoid airway obstruction, alleviate respiratory distress/failure, or prevent iatrogenic barotrauma secondary to mechanical ventilation.

Circulation

Tachycardia, delayed capillary refill, or tachypnoea may be early signs of cardiovascular impairment. Hypotension is a late sign. Circulatory impairment may be secondary to the burn but other causes must be excluded.

Disability

Alcohol and/or drug intoxication are common causes of accidents leading to burns. Carbon monoxide poisoning, shock due to other causes, and head injuries must be excluded in all obtunded patients.

Exposure

All patients must be fully exposed and examined (Fig. 14.2). However, burns victims lose heat rapidly and, therefore, all means possible should be employed to maintain normothermia.

Fluid resuscitation

Fluid resuscitation is recommended in adult burns >15% TBSA, and in children with burns >10% TBSA. Burn size can be calculated from the 'Rule of Nines' or from a burn body chart. In the acute burn, fluids should be started at the time of the primary survey and formally calculated when appropriate. The subsequent fluid requirements can appear excessive, especially in children, and these should be reviewed and agreed by the regional specialist burns unit, confirming the percentage of the burn involved and the fluid resuscitation volumes

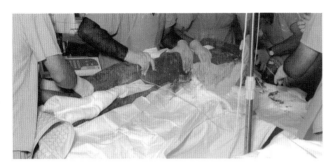

Fig. 14.2 A patient with major burns being fully exposed to ensure all injuries are identified and assessed.
Courtesy of Dr Ali Diba, Consultant Anaesthetist, Queen Victoria Hospital, East Grinstead.

required. Ideally, two large-bore intravenous cannulae should be sited through unburnt skin. In very large burns, this may be difficult, and central venous access via the groin (often spared) is a useful alternative. Depending upon the site of the burn, vascular access via the subclavian or internal jugular veins may be possible. Vascular access devices are known to be a major cause of hospital-associated infections and bloodstream bacteraemias so adhering to all aspects of safe insertion and maintenance of these devices, in addition to timely removal when no longer required, greatly reduce the risk of infection. The UK National Institute for Health and Care Excellence provides comprehensive guidelines on real-time ultrasound-guided central venous access,[15] and the benefits of ultrasonography for peripheral venous access should also be recognized. If peripheral or central intravenous access is not achievable, surgical venous cut down, though rare, remains an alternative when other methods have failed,[16] with intraosseous access also providing another life-saving option in such situations.[17] Both would be considered 'bridging methods' until formal intravenous access can be achieved.

The standard intravenous fluid regimen in the UK is based on the Parkland formula. Fluid resuscitation is calculated as 3–4 mL/kg/% TBSA of burn. The first half of the calculated volume is administered in the first 8 hours (from the time of injury) and the second half is given over the next 16 hours. Children weighing <25 kg, with a greater surface area to mass ratio, should receive additional maintenance fluid (e.g. Parkland plus maintenance fluid for the first 8 hours, then 50% of Parkland plus normal maintenance fluids for the following 16 hours). Any additional fluid requirements may be met with judicious use of colloids. The efficacy of fluid resuscitation should be monitored clinically, principally by observing urine output. Urinary catheterization is, therefore, mandatory in large burns, with the aim of achieving a urine output of 0.5 mL/kg/hr in adults and 1 mL/kg/hr in children. The exception to this is patients with haemoglobinuria or myoglobinuria, where the aim should be to achieve 1–2 mL/kg/hr urine output (utilizing sodium bicarbonate and mannitol).

Inhalation injury, in addition to a cutaneous burn, is associated with an increased fluid resuscitation requirement. However, further fluid should be given cautiously as concerns exist with over-resuscitation resulting in lung and tissue oedema.

Pain management

Pain should be treated with titrated intravenous opioids. The intramuscular route should not be used, as the peripheral circulatory changes associated with burns render this route of absorption unpredictable.

Radiology/imaging

A 'trauma series' including cervical spine, chest, and pelvis should be undertaken.

Secondary survey

History

An 'AMPLE' history (Allergies, Medical history, Past illnesses, Last meal, Events/Environment relating to the injury) should be obtained from the patient (where possible). The burn history should also include duration of exposure, type of clothing worn, temperature and nature of fluid if scalded, and adequacy of first aid measures. An inhalation history should also be taken, as well as any other relevant history of blast, ejection, assault, or other trauma.

Examination

A full body examination is required, including the eyes, ears, and back (commonly overlooked). All limbs need to be evaluated for escharotomy requirement, looking for circumferential burns and any signs of reduced limb perfusion—pain, paraesthesia, pulselessness, and paralysis.

Monitoring

Continuous pulse oximetry, electrocardiography, blood pressure monitoring, fluid balance recording and assessment, and temperature monitoring are minimum standards. Invasive vascular monitoring and cardiac output monitoring are common, and routinely used in the burns critical care unit.

Temperature regulation

Normothermia is desirable but is often difficult to achieve and is also often overlooked. A burns victim may have had cooling first aid, or had their clothes removed or burned off, and undergone significant exposure. Loss of skin integrity and evaporation of exudate also causes heat loss. Core temperature may be further reduced by the vasodilatory effects of any general anaesthetic agents required. Hypothermia has significant deleterious effects, including increased risk of infection and cardiovascular impairment, as well as negative effects more specific to the burn, such as vasoconstriction and reduced blood supply. Patients should be actively warmed where necessary and methods to reduce heat loss should be employed.

Burn wounds

Burns are initially sterile, but ultimately provide an ideal medium for bacterial colonization and growth. Initially, they should be wrapped in a plastic cling film layer until advice is sought from the regional burns unit. Tetanus prophylaxis should be given routinely to patients not fully immunized.

Referral to a specialist burns unit

The National Burn Care Group and British Burn Association have identified the following injuries as those requiring referral to a specialist unit[18]:

- Burn >10% TBSA in adults.
- Burn >5% TBSA in children.
- Burns of special areas—face, hands, feet, genitalia, perineum, and major joints.
- Full-thickness burns >5% TBSA.
- Electrical burns.
- Chemical burns.
- Burns with associated inhalation injury.
- Circumferential burns of the limbs or chest.
- Burns at the extremes of ages.
- Burn injury in patients with pre-existing medical disorders which could complicate management, prolong recovery, or affect mortality.
- Any burn patient with associated trauma.

Transfer of unstable patients can be hazardous, should be planned carefully, and undertaken by adequately trained personnel with appropriate patient monitoring, emergency drugs, and equipment available. The main concern is maintenance of a protected airway, which should be secured prior to transfer if there is any doubt of deterioration during transfer. Intravenous access should be *in situ* and secured thoroughly.

Inhalation injury

Inhalation injury is caused by either direct thermal damage to the airway, the effects of the products of combustion, or both. The products of combustion can be categorized into those due to toxic non-particulate gases, and those due to particulate smoke. These give rise to the 'smoke inhalation complex', a triad consisting of direct thermal injury, injury above the cords, and injury below the cords. While some patients may only suffer one aspect, others will have a range of symptoms and signs involving at least two of these elements.

Diagnosis of inhalation injury

Mechanism of the burn

A flame, blast, or steam injury may lead to an inhalation injury. Conversely, a scald is very unlikely to have an inhalation element, unless associated with a significant steam injury. Nonetheless, a full-thickness scald to the neck can still precipitate airway obstruction, due to loss of skin elasticity and oedema, particularly in children.

Burn environment

A history of fire or smoke in an enclosed space should raise suspicion of an inhalational injury. The longer the duration of entrapment in such an environment, the stronger the suspicion should be. Petrol immolation and prolonged burning of clothing may also increase the risk.

Level of consciousness at the scene

Unconsciousness should raise suspicion that the patient may have suffered a significant inhalation injury. An unconscious patient loses the protective ability to breath-hold, and is also, obviously, unable to extricate themselves quickly from the toxic environment.

Signs of inhalation injury

Burns around the face and mouth, and singed nasal hairs indicate proximity to a heat source and are strongly associated with a thermal airway inhalation injury. They also have the potential to increase the difficulty of tracheal intubation. The oedema associated with facial burns can be significant in the initial phase and if tracheal intubation is warranted, it should be done expeditiously. Exceptions include, facial scalds (without a significant steam injury, or oral ingestion of burning liquids) and 'flash flame' burns—if the patient provides a satisfactory history of these and there is sparing of the 'smile lines' and nasolabial folds, an associated airway injury is unlikely.

The presence of soot in the mouth and/or nose are suggestive of smoke inhalation. Blistering, oedema, or burns within the oral cavity should be taken extremely seriously. A 'brassy' cough, wheeze, tachypnoea, altered/hoarse voice, or dysphagia are all signs indicative of an inhalation injury. A conscious patient complaining of an altered voice, especially when subjectively describing deterioration in voice quality, should be taken seriously. Carbonaceous secretions should be regarded as sign of exposure, but nothing more. Dyspnoea, wheeze, cyanosis, inspiratory stridor, and increased respiratory rate are rare presenting signs, but must be acted upon quickly. Confusion and restlessness, may indicate hypoxia necessitating urgent treatment.

An arterial blood gas sample and carboxyhaemoglobin levels are mandatory to evaluate any degree of carbon monoxide poisoning and can be extrapolated to the time of injury using a nomogram. A chest X-ray should also be taken.

Systemic gaseous toxins

At the scene of a fire, it is unlikely that victims are killed directly by the smoke, but instead die of hypoxia. The hypoxia is due to a decreased availability of oxygen that occurs during a fire, with oxygen concentrations decreasing to 10–15%[19,20] of normal levels. In addition, gaseous systemic toxins (principally carbon monoxide and hydrogen cyanide) lead to histotoxic hypoxia.

Carbon monoxide

Carbon monoxide poisoning causes up to 80% of smoke-related deaths.[21,22] It has an affinity with haemoglobin 210 times that of oxygen, reducing oxygen carriage and delivery[23] and shifting the oxygen dissociation curve to the left. The affinity of carbon monoxide for myoglobin causes myocardial depression, hypotension, and arrhythmias.[24] It also binds to hepatic and other cytochrome enzymes causing peroxidation of cerebral lipids.[23] Neurological signs include confusion, disorientation, visual changes, syncope, seizures, and coma. Arrhythmias and myocardial infarction may be provoked in those with coronary heart disease. The extent of injury is dependent on the concentration of carbon monoxide, the duration of exposure, and pre-existing comorbidities. Neuropsychiatric impairment is a serious long-term complication for survivors.[19]

Normal carboxyhaemoglobin levels are <5% (up to 9% in a smoker). Serious toxicity is often associated with levels >25%, and the risk of death is high at >70%. However, no consistent dose–response effect has been found between measured levels and clinical effects,[25] such that carboxyhaemoglobin levels provide an indicator of level of exposure rather than reliably predicting clinical course or outcome.[26] Normal pulse oximeters cannot distinguish between oxyhaemoglobin and carboxyhaemoglobin and should not be relied upon until carboxyhaemoglobin levels have been restored to the normal range.

The half-life of carboxyhaemoglobin is 320 minutes breathing room air at sea level. This is reduced to 80 minutes with the administration of 100% oxygen.[27] Therefore, all suspected or confirmed cases of carbon monoxide poisoning should have high-flow (humidified) oxygen via a tight-fitting non-rebreathing mask. Tracheal intubation is required in those with thermal damage to the upper airway or in those unable to maintain their own airway safely.

Hyperbaric oxygen therapy has been used to treat carbon monoxide poisoning and may result in even faster displacement of carbon monoxide from the blood. At three atmospheres of oxygen, the half-life of carboxyhaemoglobin is 23 minutes. If commenced >6 hours after exposure, however, it is likely to be ineffective.[28] Currently, six randomized control trials of hyperbaric oxygen therapy for carbon monoxide poisoning exist. A Cochrane review showed that four of these did not demonstrate an improved long-term benefit and there was no evidence of reduction in neurological sequelae.[29] Nevertheless, hyperbaric oxygen may have a place in the management of severe carbon monoxide poisoning, and it should be considered for patients with a carboxyhaemoglobin level >40% (or 20% in pregnant women).

Supportive therapy may be required to manage the sequelae of carbon monoxide poisoning, and long-term neuropsychiatric problems may occur in up to 30% of these patients.[30]

Hydrogen cyanide

Oral cyanide poisoning leads rapidly to coma, apnoea, cardiac dysfunction, and severe lactic acidosis and is associated with a high mixed venous oxygen and low arteriovenous oxygen content difference.[31] There is controversy surrounding whether cyanide toxicity has any role in the morbidity and mortality of fire victims.[32] Those opposing the cyanide poisoning theory of smoke inhalation allude to low cyanide levels obtained in simulated fires,[33] the presence of cyanide as a physiological metabolite,[34,35] its release by many organs after death,[35] and the great variability in data on the levels causing death.[36,37] Proponents highlight the presence of cyanide in smoke and in the blood of fire victims,[38–42] and that oral cyanide poisoning replicates the metabolic acidosis seen in some fire victims. In any event, cyanide poisoning would be synergistic with concurrent carbon monoxide poisoning and the hypoxic gas mixture breathed during a fire, which may explain why sublethal levels of carbon monoxide and cyanide are found in some victims.

Blood levels can be measured, but unfortunately there is no rapid test available, such that it serves only to inform at postmortem and for research purposes. A severe metabolic acidosis, high venous oxygen saturation, and a narrow arteriovenous oxygen gradient may be signs of potential poisoning. Importantly, a burn patient with a metabolic acidosis should first be assumed to be under-fluid resuscitated, to have carbon monoxide poisoning, or have unrecognized concomitant trauma, and these must be excluded before considering the possibility of cyanide poisoning.

Supportive therapy is the mainstay of treatment. 'Antidotes' are available, but they are not without their own, occasionally fatal, side effects. Administration of these agents in an inhalation injury should only be undertaken on the advice of the regional burns unit. Hydroxocobalamin is now being used in the UK in circumstances where initial resuscitation does not immediately correct metabolic imbalances.

Thermal injury to the airway

The thermal injury element of the smoke inhalation triad has the potential to develop into a 'can't intubate, can't oxygenate' event. It is caused by direct heat injury from hot air, gases, or vapours to the oropharynx and upper airway. Because the heat exchange capabilities of the upper airway are so efficient, even super-heated air is rapidly cooled before reaching the lower respiratory tract, such that this is often referred to as injury above the vocal cords. The extent of thermal damage to the airway depends upon the heat capacity characteristics of the gas or vapour and the duration of exposure. Dry gases cause less damage than saturated vapours at the same temperature. Burns below the glottis are extremely rare, and only occur if super-heated soot particles or steam are inhaled. Thermal injury produces immediate damage to the mucosa, causing oedema, erythema, and ulceration. Oedema forms rapidly due to a combination of altered hydrostatic pressures, increased vascular permeability, and release of cytokines and free radicals.[43–50] Though oedema will form spontaneously, it may be accelerated by fluid resuscitation. Anecdotal evidence from un-intubated patients received at the Royal Darwin Hospital (Darwin, Australia) >24 hours following the Bali bombings of 2002, suggested that suboptimal (under-) fluid resuscitation may have been advantageous in maintaining the airway patency in several patients with airway burns. Once more aggressive fluid resuscitation was implemented, there was an increase in associated airway oedema, and the requirement for airway intervention.[51] Nevertheless, intravenous fluids should not be withheld, as delayed fluid resuscitation has been shown to increase the rates of sepsis, renal failure, cardiac arrest, multiorgan failure, and death.[52]

Airway oedema may not be maximal until 24 hours but will usually manifest itself within 2–6 hours of injury. Airway obstruction caused by intraoral and laryngeal oedema is often complicated by anatomical distortion of the face and neck. Oral oedema will also lead to a decreased ability to clear secretions and impaired protection from aspiration.

Signs of impending airway obstruction include erythema and oedema of the mucosa in the mouth, significant facial burns, carbonaceous sputum, singed nasal hairs, and an altered or hoarse voice. Stridor, dyspnoea, laboured breathing, tracheal tug, intercostal recession, paradoxical breathing pattern, or cyanosis are often preterminal indicators.

Potential airway obstruction must be continually considered. High-dose humidified oxygen should be administered in an environment where urgent tracheal intubation can be safely performed. Change in voice quality may be a sign of progressive oedema and should be closely monitored. These patients should have gentle examination of the oropharynx to exclude and assess erythema, oedema, or blistering. Flexible nasendoscopy under topical local anaesthesia allows visualization of the posterior oropharynx and may need repeated assessment depending on the clinical status.

If there are major suspicions or signs of a direct thermal burn, the treatment of choice is early, semi-elective tracheal intubation. A 'wait and see' approach is only justifiable in those where a true airway burn is believed to be unlikely. This is particularly important in patients being transferred to regional burns centres—safe, planned tracheal intubation is preferable prior to transfer if there are any concerns at all regarding the safety of a patient's airway.

Tracheal intubation

A large-diameter uncut tracheal tube should be inserted to secure the airway, facilitate airway toileting, and optimize management of secretions. Where possible, the patient should be allowed a few moments with family members prior to this intervention as the gravity of the situation should not be underestimated.

Videolaryngoscopy is recommended when undertaking anticipated difficult airway management as it allows superior visualization of the supraglottic and glottic structures, for both the operator and the supporting team. It also permits improved documentation of airway damage and images taken at the time of tracheal intubation may well form part of a patient's notes routinely soon. Awake fibreoptic tracheal intubation must always be considered in these situations, although un-swallowed secretions, oedema, and anatomical distortion can make any chosen technique challenging. In such cases, a nasotracheal tube may sometimes be necessitated.

Prognosis of airway burns

Airway oedema, though maximal at 24 hours, will usually take 3–5 days to resolve. During this time, the tracheal tube should be left *in situ*. Tracheal extubation should only be considered when the patient's vital signs and ventilation are stable and satisfactory and after the airway has been evaluated, and an adequate leak is demonstrable around the tracheal tube.[53] Again, videolaryngoscopy is particularly useful for visualizing the glottis and supraglottic structures and can be utilized for serial assessments to inform tracheal extubation planning.

Smoke injury to the lungs

Inhalation of particulate smoke beyond the vocal cords comprises the third element of the inhalation injury complex, also referred to as injury below the cords.

The carbonaceous material present in the smoke particles is not thought to be directly responsible for the damage but rather serves as a carrier for other agents.[54] The exact nature of the associated toxic products depends upon the materials incinerated. Common materials such as cotton and polyvinyl chloride produce multiple toxic compounds,[55,56] which can cause redox reactions, chemical tracheobronchiolitis, and local or systemic cytokine release, resulting in oedematous tracheobronchial mucosa, de-epithelialization, shedding of the epithelial lining, and formation of pseudomembranous casts (Fig. 14.3).[57] These casts are composed of mucous, cellular debris, fibrinous exudates, polymorphonuclear leukocytes, and clumps of bacteria. In these circumstances, pulmonary compliance is markedly decreased[58] and surfactant is inactivated, causing micro-atelectasis and ventilation–perfusion inequality.

Even though pathological changes occur almost immediately following inhalation of smoke, hypoxia, rales, rhonchi, and wheeze are seldom present on admission. Chest radiographs are almost always unremarkable on day 1, although two-thirds of patients develop evidence of diffuse or focal infiltrates, or pulmonary oedema by days 5–10.[59]

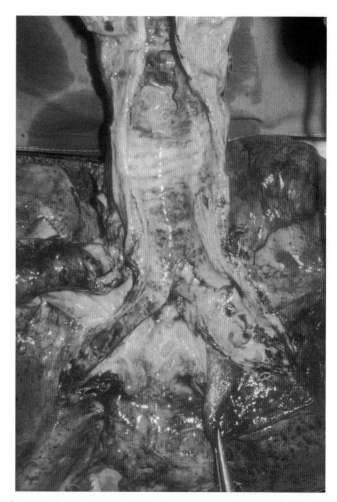

Fig. 14.3 Pathology specimen, showing the larynx, trachea, bronchi, and lungs, from a patient who suffered moderate smoke inhalational injury. There was injury above and below the vocal cords, with soot deposition within the trachea and bronchi. Diffuse pulmonary parenchymal hyperaemia and haemorrhagic changes are visible, as well as cast deposition (particularly in the right main bronchus).
Courtesy of Dr Ali Diba, Consultant Anaesthetist, Queen Victoria Hospital, East Grinstead.

Diagnosis is based upon clinical suspicion, and confirmed predominantly by bronchoscopic findings of soot (Fig. 14.4), mucosal necrosis, airway oedema, and inflammation.[60,61] Xenon scanning can be used to evaluate true parenchymal damage not identified on bronchoscopy.[62]

Supportive therapy including humidified oxygen and nebulizers are the mainstay of treatment. Chest physiotherapy should be instigated early. Despite minimal trial evidence, pharmacological reasoning exists to support the use of nebulizers. Most centres use salbutamol and either heparin, *N*-acetylcysteine, or sodium bicarbonate.[63] Salbutamol relieves the bronchospasm resulting from chemical bronchitis, especially in those with pre-existing reactive airways disease although its role in inhalational injury is not well established, with two large randomized controlled trials showing no benefit.[64,65] Heparin breaks down fibrin, a major component of the cast-like plugs that can obstruct the respiratory bronchioles. Evidence for its use in burns is largely based upon animal models of smoke inhalation.[66] One systematic review demonstrated that inhaled anticoagulants have a positive effect on survival.[67] *N*-acetylcysteine is a

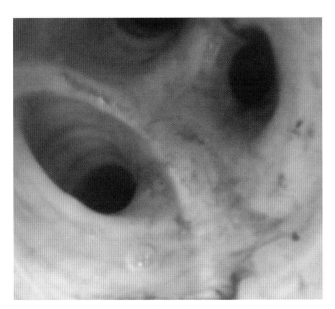

Fig. 14.4 Bronchoscopy image of soot deposition within the bronchial tree.

mucolytic and free radical scavenger. Unfortunately, it is also potentially an irritant to the respiratory tract and may cause bronchospasm. Sodium bicarbonate is also mucolytic but has the additional property that it may buffer some of the toxic compounds within the smoke, decreasing the inflammatory cascade produced by the redox reactions.

Chemical burns

Chemical burns most commonly affect the face and limb extremities and can result from domestic/commercial acids, bleach, ammonia, and chlorination products. Duration of hospital stay is often prolonged, with a delayed and protracted healing process. Severity of the burn depends on a variety of factors, including duration of exposure to the chemical, concomitant inhalation or ingestion of the chemical, location of the insult, and the quantity, strength, and state of the chemical agent (gas/liquid/solid).

Symptoms can be wide ranging, including irritation, redness, burning, discolouration of skin, or numbness of the affected area. Facial swelling and loss of vision can also occur. Some patients may suffer coughing and dyspnoea (which may progress to airway obstruction), difficulty swallowing, headache, dizziness, seizures, cardiac arrhythmias, and loss of consciousness.

Management includes removal of the offending chemical, irrigation of the affected area, assessment of systemic and metabolic disturbances, and thermoregulation. A prompt airway assessment is paramount and tracheal intubation may well be required.

Other considerations in patients with airway burns

Selective decontamination of the digestive tract should be considered in the critically ill patient to reduce hospital-acquired infections. Despite some favourable evidence, there remains considerable apprehension surrounding this intervention.

The most frequent complication following an inhalational injury is pneumonia. Mixed opinion exists in relation to the routine prescribing of prophylactic antimicrobial agents for inhalational injury.[68] Evidence is lacking to support the use of prophylactic antibiotics on admission and there are concerns regarding the global issue of antibiotic resistance.[69,70]

Particulate smoke inhalation victims without any associated upper airway thermal burn and with a normal conscious level, do not need or benefit from immediate tracheal intubation. Non-invasive ventilation options can be considered initially; however, a high level of suspicion for upper airway burn must be maintained. These patients should be closely monitored. Deterioration in serial blood gases and an increasing requirement for supplemental oxygen indicate the need for rapid, semi-elective, tracheal intubation (Box 14.1).

Though often unavoidable, tracheal intubation and prolonged mechanical ventilation have been identified as bad prognostic indicators. There is a vast increase in pneumonia, acute respiratory distress syndrome, septicaemia, and organ failure in those mechanically ventilated for >4 days.[5] While this does not distinguish between cause and effect, it is well known that mechanical ventilation and ventilator-acquired pneumonia are associated with a higher mortality in all patients. Thus, if tracheal intubation can be avoided, it should be. The majority of patients with significant cutaneous burns complicating an inhalation injury will need a prolonged period of mechanical ventilation with lung protective strategies, as described by the Acute Respiratory Distress Syndrome Network multicentre trial.[71] Supplementary strategies such as high-frequency ventilation, administration of nitric oxide and lung surfactant, prone positioning, and extracorporeal membrane oxygenation can also be considered.[72] A ventilator care bundle approach, with 30° head-up nursing, and regular sedation holds should be employed. An early tracheostomy should also be considered as the benefits of improved

---

Box 14.1 Important considerations when undertaking tracheal intubation in the burns patient

- If in doubt, intubate the patient's trachea. Early tracheal extubation is preferable to undertaking an emergency tracheal intubation in an unstable patient, with potentially a very difficult airway.
- Allow the patient time to speak with relatives first, if possible.
- A patient with stridor or other signs of respiratory distress should be considered a difficult airway until proven otherwise.
- Tracheal intubation should be performed quickly, by an appropriately trained anaesthetist, and with the full range of difficult airway equipment available.
- A rapid sequence induction is usually indicated.
- Suxamethonium can be used in the first 24 hours after injury.
- The tracheal tube should never be cut. This is especially important in facial burns, which can swell dramatically, almost obliterating the tracheal tube.
- Always document the grade of tracheal intubation (or ease of videolaryngoscopy), any evidence of soot, oedema, or other airway abnormality. This will be particularly helpful to any receiving hospital in planning further interventions/treatments.
- Tracheal tubes are precious and should be firmly secured with either a tube tie (not impairing venous return) or dental wire.

comfort, reduced sedation, improved communication, earlier mobilization, and reduced airway resistance are well recognized.

Early tracheal extubation should always remain the main goal, but it must be noted that many of the airway burns patients also suffer from significant cutaneous burns. The treatment of the latter vastly complicates the treatment of the inhalation element. The patients often require multiple skin debridement and grafting procedures, and regular dressing changes over a prolonged period, making the timing of tracheal extubation particularly challenging. Prolonged mechanical ventilation, blood transfusion, and sepsis inevitably contribute to the increased mortality seen in these patients with increasing size of burn.

A stepwise approach to tracheal extubation is advisable. The Difficult Airway Society, UK, provides comprehensive extubation guidelines for both the 'low-risk' and 'high-risk' patient. Burns patients may have had prolonged periods of mechanical ventilation, associated with multiple respiratory insults, from infection, inflammation, and/or oedema. Patients should fulfil baseline criteria to be considered suitable for tracheal extubation or decannulation of their tracheostomy:

- Resolution/stabilization of underlying disease process.
- Acceptable gas exchange.
- Minimal ventilatory support.
- Spontaneous respiration.
- Effective cough/gag reflex.
- Haemodynamic stability.
- Conscious and neurologically intact.

A thorough assessment of the predicted ease of oxygenating, bag mask ventilating, and reintubating the trachea must be undertaken. Traditionally, the 'cuff leak test' has provided some useful information in this regard and a videolaryngoscope can also provide an easy means of assessing residual airway oedema.

Prognosis in the airway burns patient

Deaths are invariably due to multiorgan failure, preceded by sepsis.[73] Deaths show a bimodal distribution of early (within a week) and late (weeks to months). The early group of patients often die of rapid overwhelming sepsis or systemic inflammatory response syndrome, and multiorgan failure. The late group of patients show a steadier decline in overall organ function, associated with several septic episodes interspersed with periods of clinical improvement. Survivors can be left with chronic problems secondary to their inhalation injury. Chronic airway disease is relatively rare in adults,[74,75] but children may show decreased pulmonary function for up to 10 years after injury.[76] Subglottic tracheal stenosis can occur in those who required prolonged tracheal intubation but can be reduced by minimizing cuff pressures of the tracheal or tracheostomy tubes.

Critical care therapy

Intensive care treatment of major burns patients is similar to 'normal' intensive care patients, but with a special emphasis on:

- Early nutritional support.
- Stress ulcer prophylaxis, until full enteral feeding is established.

- Micronutrient support.
- Thromboprophylaxis.
- Mandatory patient isolation.
- Increased awareness of infection risk.
- Thermoregulation.
- Early psychological input for patients and relatives.
- Acute and chronic pain management.

Immediate major burn debridement

Early debridement of major burns is now standard practice. The aim is to debride and graft the burn wound as quickly and efficiently as possible, while maintaining a physiologically stable patient. Full-thickness excision of wounds is aimed at decreasing cytokine production, reducing wound infection, and improving overall morbidity and mortality. There is reduced blood loss when compared with late debridement.[77] Blood loss can be rapid and extensive, and must be specifically planned for. The wound is covered with autograft, allograft (cadaveric skin), a synthetic skin substitute, or other dressing. Once healed, skin can be re-harvested from existing donor sites and applied to areas only temporarily dressed. Fine judgement is often required in optimizing the timing of operations and must be tailored to the individual patient.

General considerations in burns anaesthesia

The majority of burn patients have smaller burns that are not complicated by inhalation, thermal, or lung smoke injury. Patients at the extremes of age suffer proportionally more burns than the general population, as do those with pre-existing comorbidities such as epilepsy, alcohol or drug dependence, and/or mental health problems. Some adults with burns (but more commonly children) are the victims of non-accidental injury.

The airway should be evaluated for predictors of difficult mask ventilation and tracheal intubation. Acute burns to the face will cause mask ventilation and, potentially, tracheal intubation to be more challenging. A chronic burn to the face and neck may result in limited mouth opening and reduced neck extension, making tracheal intubation predictably more difficult. Re-evaluating the airway each time long-stay patients present for surgery is important, with some requiring awake tracheal intubation prior to induction of anaesthesia.

Good intravenous access is essential prior to undertaking burns debridement but the usual sites, including central access, are frequently burned, or no longer viable having being obliterated during the resuscitation phase. Femoral access is often possible when other sites are not available.

Standard anaesthetic monitoring of burns patients can be difficult depending on the site and size of the burn. Certain adaptations may be required:

- Electrocardiogram monitoring may require skin staples to be placed through the electrode, or via direct attachment to a staple or wire suture.
- Pulse oximetry can normally be achieved using an ear probe, which can be applied to the cheek or even tongue if necessary.

- Non-invasive blood pressure cuffs can be difficult to place and an arterial line may be needed for relatively small surgical procedures.
- Capnography often assumes greater importance in the face of the above-mentioned difficulties.
- Temperature monitoring is very important.
- Urinary catheters are required in all major cases, and a urometer is essential for continuous accurate fluid balance monitoring.
- Central venous and arterial pressure monitoring are routine for all major burn excisions.
- Cardiac output monitors are a useful adjunct in patients undergoing major debridement where blood loss can be difficult to calculate accurately.

Blood loss can be a significant problem during burns surgery. Predicted blood loss can be very roughly estimated at 100 mL for every 1% TBSA excised. With improved surgical techniques and meticulous thermoregulation, blood transfusion is rare for minor burns debridement. Nevertheless, patients should be cross-matched for all but the smallest excisions and early consideration should be given to the need for platelets, fresh frozen plasma, or factor concentrate when significant bleeding does occur. Thromboelastometry is a useful viscoelastic method for haemostasis testing in whole blood. Despite appropriate planning and intraoperative patient management, major blood loss and/or coagulopathy can still be a problem in major burns debridement and may necessitate suspension of surgery to enable physiological stability to be restored.

Heat loss occurs quickly due to a combination of radiation and evaporation from the wound, compounded by the skin preparation used prior to surgery, the exposure of large surface areas, the prolonged duration of operations, the loss of core–periphery homeostasis caused by anaesthetic agents, and the large volumes of intravenous fluids often required. Hypothermia further increases the high metabolic rate, surgical bleeding, and the risk of wound and pulmonary infection, and impairs cardiac function. Core temperature should be monitored meticulously in all but the shortest operations, and all measures taken to maintain a 'normal' core temperature. The ambient theatre temperature should be maintained at >27°C, and body areas not being operated on should be covered. Forced air warming devices, warming mattresses, overhead radiant heaters, and central venous heat exchangers should be used as appropriate. All intravenous fluids must be administered via a fluid warmer. Prewarming of patients prior to surgery is recommended.

All major surgical debridement procedures should be treated in a high dependency or intensive care setting postoperatively. Good analgesia is essential, and feeding should be resumed as early as possible. For a summary of the key considerations in burns anaesthesia see **Box 14.2**.

Burns pharmacology

Pathophysiological changes following a burn injury alter a patient's normal pharmacokinetics. Absorption, bioavailability, protein binding, volume of distribution, and drug clearance are all affected to a certain degree,[78] dependent on the size and duration since the burn.[79] Initially, hypovolaemia leads to a hypoperfusion state, and

---

Box 14.2 Key considerations in burns anaesthesia

- The burns surgical case mix is not representative of the general population.
- Intravenous access and physiological monitoring can be particularly challenging.
- Difficulty in airway management should be anticipated in patients with facial and neck burns, with a clear airway strategy devised and communicated.
- Blood loss during surgery can be significant and must be planned for accordingly.
- Hypothermia must be avoided, and strategies to minimize heat loss and actively warm patients should be employed.
- Good postoperative care, in an appropriately staffed and equipped environment, is vital.
- There is altered drug pharmacokinetics associated with large burns.

---

absorption of drugs given by any route other than intravenous is impaired and unpredictable.[80] Albumin levels decrease, increasing free fraction of certain drugs.[81] Fluid loss through the burn wound and generalized oedema accumulation can decrease plasma concentrations of many drugs. Most anaesthetic agents are not protein bound and the clinical effect of most agents is largely unaltered.

After this initial phase, a hyperdynamic circulation develops, where there is increased blood flow to the kidneys and liver, and increased drug clearance.[82] Such changes in pharmacokinetics have a wide patient-to-patient variability and may require adjustment in the dosing of various drugs (in particular, antimicrobials) tailored to the individual patient.[83]

Suxamethonium

Suxamethonium is safe to use in the first 24 hours after a major burn, after which it is contraindicated due to the risk of potentiating life-threatening hyperkalaemia, resulting from proliferation of extra-junctional acetylcholine receptors, which also causes resistance to non-depolarizing muscle relaxants.[84] The magnitude of the effect is proportional to the total burns surface area. The greatest risk of hyperkalaemia is from about day 5 to 70 days after injury and may be further prolonged if there is delayed healing due to persistent infection. It is unclear exactly how long suxamethonium should be avoided; however, from 9 months to up to 2 years have been quoted by some sources.

Non-depolarizing muscle relaxants

All non-depolarizing neuromuscular blocking agents have been used successfully in burns patients. The effective dose for 50% of the population is increased proportionally to the size of the burn. If profound muscle paralysis is required for surgery, quantitative neuromuscular monitoring is advocated. A modified 'rapid sequence induction' can be achieved with a dose of 1.5 mg/kg of rocuronium.[85]

General anaesthetic agents

The choice of anaesthetic agents does not appear to influence the outcome from anaesthesia for burn surgery. Sevoflurane is the volatile of choice for inhalational induction. The dose requirements are generally increased due to the hypermetabolism. Minimum alveolar concentration values are raised, and the duration of action is decreased.

Opioids

Opioids, given in conjunction with paracetamol and non-steroidal anti-inflammatory agents (where appropriate), are the mainstay of analgesia. Opioid tolerance can develop quickly and, together with the hypermetabolism associated with large burns, opioid requirements can be huge. Tramadol, with its additional effects on noradrenaline and serotonin, can be a particularly useful adjunct. All critical care patients receiving regular opioids should also be administered regular prophylactic aperients.

Long-term considerations

Patients who have suffered major burns often endure years of corrective surgery and are also just as likely as anyone else to require urgent or elective surgery. Special consideration of any potential difficult airway should be noted. Facial and neck burns can lead to reduced mouth opening and neck contractures. Specifically, assessment of neck extension is vital, with a low threshold for awake intubation. Vascular access may be a significant problem in some patients and may necessitate central venous access.

Conclusion

Orofacial burns patients, especially those with other large burns or associated inhalation injuries, require referral and transfer to a regional burns centre, where they can benefit from the specialist knowledge, skills, experience, and expertise provided by a vast team of multidisciplinary professionals. However, these patients must first rely upon the staff at the receiving hospital to assess and manage them effectively in a logical stepwise approach. Timely, systematic interventions are likely to be critical in those at risk of impending airway obstruction from thermal airway burns.

REFERENCES

1. Herndon DN. *Total Burn Care*, 5th ed. Edinburgh: Elsevier Saunders; 2018.
2. British Burn Association. Homepage. 2020. http://www.british burnassociation.co.uk
3. Goldacre M, Duncan M, Cook-Mozaffari P, Davidson M, McGuiness H, Meddings D. Burns in England 1996 to 2004. Mortality trends. Unit of HealthCare Epidemiology, Oxford University, and South-East England Public Health Observatory. 2006. https://www.uhce.ox.ac.uk/Atlases/Trends/England/Burns_England.pdf
4. American Burn Association. Burn incident fact sheet and national burn repository. 2008. http:// www.ameriburn.org/resources_fa ctsheet.php
5. Smith DL, Cairns BA, Ramadan F, Dalston JS, Fakhry SM, Rutledge R, et al. Effect of inhalation injury, burn size, and age on mortality: a study of 1447 consecutive burn patients. *J Trauma.* 1994;37(4):655–659.
6. Shirani KZ, Pruitt BA Jr, Mason AD Jr. The influence of inhalation injury and pneumonia on burn mortality. *Ann Surg.* 1987;205(1):82–87.
7. Sellersk BJ, Davis BL, Larkin PW, Morris SE, Saffle JR. Early prediction of prolonged ventilator dependence in thermally injured patients. *J Trauma.* 1997;43(6):899–903.
8. Wachtel TL, Frank DH, Frank HA. Management of burns of the head and neck. *Head Neck Surg.* 1981;3(6):458–474.
9. Tredget EE, Shankowshy HA, Taerum TV, Moysa GL, Alton JD. The role of inhalation injury in burn trauma. A Canadian experience. *Ann Surg.* 1990;212(6):720–727.
10. Ryan CM, Schoenfeld DA, Thorpe WP, Sheridan RL, Cassem EH, Tompkins RG. Objective estimates of the probability of death from burn injuries. *N Engl J Med.* 1998;338(6):362–366.
11. Edelman DA, White MT, Tyburski JD, Wilson RF. Factors affecting prognosis of inhalation injury. *J Burn Care Res.* 2006;27(6):848–853.
12. Miller SF, Bessey P, Lentz CW, Jeng JC, Schurr M, MD, Browning S, from the ABA NBR Committee, National Burn Repository 2007 Report: A Synopsis of the 2007 Call for Data. *J Burn Care Res.* 2008;29(6):862–870.
13. Dougherty W, Waxman K. The complexities of managing severe burns with associated trauma. *Surg Clin N Am.* 1996;76(4):923–958.
14. O'Callaghan DJP, Wyncoll D. What size tube doctor? Bigger may be better—at least for weaning. *Crit Care.* 2013;17(2):422.
15. National Institute for Health and Care Excellence. Guidance on the use of ultrasound locating devices for placing central venous catheters. 2002. https://www.nice.org.uk/guidance/ta49/resour ces/guidance-on-the-use-of-ultrasound-locating-devices-for-placing-central-venous-catheters-2294585518021
16. Chappell S, Vilke GM, Chan TC, Harrigan RA, Ufberg JW. Peripheral venous cutdown. *J Emerg Med.* 2006;31(4):411–416.
17. De Caen A. Venous access in the critically ill child: when the peripheral intravenous fails. *Paediatr Emerg Care.* 2007;23(6):422–424.
18. British Burn Association. National Burn Care Group referral guidance. 2012. https://www.britishburnsassociation.org/natio nal-burn-care-referral-guidance
19. Cohen MA, Guzzardi LJ. Inhalation products of combustion. *Ann Emerg Med.* 1983;12(10):628–632.
20. Gill P, Martin RV. Smoke inhalation injury. *BJA Education.* 2015;15(3):143–148.
21. Ernst A, Zibrak JD. Carbon monoxide poisoning. *N Engl J Med.* 1998;339(22):1603–1608.
22. Raub JA, Mathieu-Nolf M, Hampson NB, Thom SR. Carbon monoxide poisoning—a public health perspective. *Toxicology.* 2000;145(1):1–14.
23. Weaver LK. Carbon monoxide poisoning. *Crit Care Clin.* 1999;15(2):297–317.
24. Ganong WF. *Review of Medical Physiology.* East Norwalk, CT: Appleton and Lange; 1995.
25. Hardy KR, Thom SR. Pathophysiology and treatment of carbon monoxide poisoning. *J Toxicol Clin Toxicol.* 1994;32(6):613–629.
26. Scheinkestel CD, Bailey M, Myles PS, Jones K, Cooper DJ, Millar IL, et al. Hyperbaric or normobaric oxygen for acute carbon monoxide poisoning: a randomised controlled clinical trial. *Med J Aust.* 1999;170(5):203–210.
27. Peterson JE, Stewart RD. Absorption and elimination of carbon monoxide in inactive young men. *Arch Environ Health.* 1970;21(2):165–171.
28. Goulon M, Barios A, Rapin M. Carbon monoxide poisoning and acute anoxia due to breathing of hydrocarbons. *Ann Med Interne (Paris).* 1969;120(5):335–349.

29. Juurlink DN, Buckley NA, Stanbrook MB, Isbister GK, Bennett M, McGuigan MA. Hyperbaric oxygen for carbon monoxide poisoning. *Cochrane Database Syst Rev.* 2005;**1**(1):CD002041.

30. Weaver LK, Hopkins RO, Howe S, Larson-Lohr V, Churchill S. Central nervous system oxygen toxicity during hyperbaric treatment of patients with carbon monoxide poisoning. *Undersea Hyperb Med.* 1996;**23**:215–219.

31. Klaassen CD. *Casarett and Doull's Toxicology: The Basic Science of Poisons*, 5th ed. New York: McGraw-Hill; 1996.

32. Barillo DJ. Diagnosis and treatment of cyanide toxicity. *J Burn Care Res.* 2009;**30**(1):148–151.

33. Davies JWL. Toxic chemicals versus lung tissue—an aspect of inhalation injury revisited. *J Burn Care Rehabil.* 1986;**7**(3):213–222.

34. Anderson RA, Harland WA. Fire deaths in the Glasgow area. III. The role of hydrogen cyanide. *Med Sci Law.* 1982;**22**(1):35–40.

35. Symington IS, Anderson RA, Thomson I, Oliver JS, Harland WA, Kerr JW. Cyanide exposure in fires. *Lancet.* 1978;**2**(8080):91–92.

36. Curry AS, Price DE, Rutter ER. The production of cyanide in post mortem material. *Acta Pharmacol Toxicol.* 1967;**25**(3):339–344.

37. Caravati EM, Litovitz TL. Pediatric cyanide intoxication and death from an acetonitrile-containing cosmetic. *JAMA.* 1988;**260**(23):3470–3472.

38. Silverman SH, Purdue GF, Hunt JL, Bost RO. Cyanide toxicity in burned patients. *J Trauma.* 1988;**28**(2):171–176.

39. Clark CJ, Campbell D, Reid WH. Blood carboxyhaemoglobin and cyanide levels in fire survivors. *Lancet.* 1981;**1**(8234):1332–1335.

40. Whetherell HR. The occurrence of cyanide in the blood of fire victims. *J Forensic Sci.* 1966;**11**(2):167–173.

41. Barillo DJ, Goode R, Rush BF, Lin RL, Freda A, Anderson EJ. Lack of correlation between carboxyhemoglobin and cyanide in smoke inhalation injury. *Curr Surg.* 1986;**43**(5):421–423.

42. Barillo DJ, Rush BF, Goode R, Lin RL, Freda A, Anderson EJ. Is ethanol the unknown toxin in smoke inhalation injury? *Am Surg.* 1986;**52**(12):641–645.

43. Lund T, Wiig H, Reed RK. Acute post burn edema: role of strongly negative interstitial fluid pressure. *Am J Physiol.* 1988;**255**(5 Pt 2):H1069–H1074.

44. Arturson G. Microvascular permeability to macromolecules after thermal injury. *Acta Physiol Scand Suppl.* 1979;**2**:111–122.

45. Lund T, Onarkeim H, Reed R. Pathogenesis of edema formation in burn injuries. *World J Surg.* 1992;**16**(1):2–9.

46. Lund T, Reed RK. Microvascular fluid exchange following thermal skin injury in the rat: changes in extravascular colloid osmotic pressure, albumin mass water content. *Circ Shock.* 1986;**20**(2):91–104.

47. Matsuda T, Tanaka H, Reyes HM, Richter HM, Hanumadass MM, Shimazaki S, et al. Antioxidant therapy using high dose vitamin C: reduction of post resuscitation fluid volume requirements. *World J Surg.* 1995;**19**(2):287–291.

48. Yoshioka T, Monafo W, Ayvazian VH, Deeitz F, Flynn D. Cimetidine inhibits burn edema formation. *Am J Surg.* 1978;**136**(6):C81–C85.

49. Nwariaku FE, Sikes PJ, Lightfoot E, Mileski WJ, Baxter C. Effect of a bradykinin antagonist on the local inflammatory response following thermal injury. *Burns.* 1996;**22**(4):324–327.

50. Barrow R, Ranwiez R, Zhang X. Ibuprofen modulates tissue perfusion in partial thickness burns. *Burns.* 2000;**26**(4):341–346.

51. Palmer DJ, Stephens D, Fisher DA, Spain B, Read DJ, Notaras L. The Bali bombing: the Royal Darwin Hospital response. *Med J Aust.* 2003;**179**(7):358–361.

52. Barrow RE, Herndon DN. Early fluid resuscitation improves outcomes in severely burned children. *Resuscitation.* 2000;**45**(2):91–96.

53. Sturgess DJ, Greenland KB, Senthuran S, Ajvadi FA, van Zundert A, Irwin MG. Tracheal extubation of the adult intensive care patient with a predicted difficult airway—a narrative review. *Anaesthesia.* 2017;**72**(2):248–261.

54. Zikria BA, Budd DC, Floch F, Ferrer JM. What is clinical smoke poisoning? *Ann Surg.* 1975;**181**(2):151–156.

55. Dowell AR, Kilburn KH, Pratt PC. Short-term exposure to nitrogen dioxide. Effects on pulmonary ultrastructure, compliance, and the surfactant system. *Arch Intern Med.* 1971;**128**(1):74–80.

56. Einhorn IN. Physiological and toxicological aspects of smoke produced during the combustion of polymeric materials. *Environ Health Perspect.* 1975;**11**:163–189.

57. Walker HL, McLeod CG, McManus WF. Experimental inhalation injury in the goat. *J Trauma.* 1981;**21**(11):962–964.

58. Nieman GF, Clark WR, Wax SD, Webb SR. The effect of smoke inhalation on pulmonary surfactant. *Ann Surg.* 1980;**191**(2):171–181.

59. Putman CE, Loke J, Matthay RA, Ravin CE. Radiographic manifestations of acute smoke inhalation. *Am J Roentgenol.* 1977;**129**(5):865–870.

60. Wanner A, Cutchavaree A. Early recognition of upper airway obstruction following smoke inhalation. *Am Rev Respir Dis.* 1973;**108**(6):1421–1423.

61. Moylan JA, Adib K, Birnbaum M. Fibreoptic bronchoscopy following thermal injury. *Surg Gynecol Obstet.* 1975;**140**(4):541–543.

62. Moylan JA, Wilmore DW, Moulton DE, Pruitt BA. Early diagnosis of inhalation injury using 133 xenon lung scan. *Ann Surg.* 1972;**176**(4):477–484.

63. Prior K, Nordmann G, Sim K, Mahoney P, Thomas R. Management of inhalational injuries in UK burns centers—a questionnaire survey. *J Intens Care Soc.* 2009;**10**(2):141–144.

64. Budinger GRS. β2-agonists in respiratory distress syndrome. *Am J Respir Crit Care Med.* 2014;**189**(6):624–625.

65. Bassford CR, Thickett DR, Perkins GD. The rise and fall of β-agonists in the treatment of ARDS. *Crit Care.* 2012;**16**(2):208.

66. Brown M, Desai M, Traber LD, Herndon DN, Traber DL. Dimethylsulfoxide with heparin in the treatment of smoke inhalation. *J Burn Care Rehabil.* 1988;**9**(1):22–25.

67. Miller AC, Elamin EM, Suffredini AF. Inhaled anticoagulation regimes for the treatment of smoke inhalation-associated acute lung injury: a systematic review. *Crit Care Med.* 2014;**42**(2):413–419.

68. Francis JJ, Duncan EM, Prior ME, Maclennan GS, Dombrowski S, Bellingan GU, et al. Selective decontamination of the digestive tract in critically ill patients treated in intensive care units: a mixed-methods feasibility study (the SuDDICU study). *Health Technol Assess.* 2014;**18**(25):1–170.

69. Avni T, Levcovish A, Ad-El D, Leibovici L, Paul M. Prophylactic antibiotics for burns patients: systematic review and meta-analysis. *BMJ.* 2010;**340**:c241.

70. Liodaki E, Kalousis K, Schopp BE, Mailander P, Stang F. Prophylactic antibiotic therapy after inhalational injury. *Burns.* 2014;**40**(8):1476–1480.

71. The Acute Respiratory Distress Syndrome Network. Ventilation with lower tidal volumes as compared with traditional tidal volumes for acute lung injury and the acute respiratory distress syndrome. *N Eng J Med.* 2000;**342**(18):1301–1308.

72. Asmussen S, Maybauer DM, Fraser JF, Jennings K, George S, Keiralla A, et al. Extracorporeal membrane oxygenation in burn and smoke inhalational injury. *Burns.* 2013;**39**(3):429–435.

73. Saffle, JR, Sullivan JJ, Tuohig GM, Larson CM. Multiple organ failure in patients with thermal injury. *Crit Care Med.* 1993;**21**(11):1673–1683.

74. Demling RH. Smoke inhalation injury. *Postgrad Med.* 1987;**82**(1):63–68.

75. Cahalane M, Demling RH. Early respiratory abnormalities from smoke inhalation. *JAMA.* 1984;**251**(6):771–773.

76. Mlcak R, Desai MH, Robinson E, Herndon DN. Inhalation injury and lung function—a decade later. *J Burn Care Rehabil.* 2000;**21**(1):S156.

77. Desai MH, Herndon DN, Broemeling L, Barrow RE, Nichols RJ, Rutan R. Early burn wound excision significantly reduces blood loss. *Ann Surg.* 1990;**211**(6):753–762.

78. Martyn JA. Clinical pharmacology and drug therapy in the burned patient. *Anesthesiology.* 1986;**65**(1):67–75.

79. Jaehde U, Sorgel F. Clinical pharmacokinetics in patients with burns. *Clin Pharmacokinet.* 1995;**29**(1):15–28.

80. Ziemniak JA, Watson WA, Saffle JR, Russo J Jr, Warden GD, Schentag JJ. Cimetidine kinetics during resuscitation from burn shock. *Clin Pharmacol Ther.* 1984;**36**(2):228–233.

81. Martyn JA, Abernethy DR, Greenblatt DJ. Plasma protein binding of drugs after severe burn injury. *Clin Pharmacol Ther.* 1984;**35**(4):535–539.

82. Bonate PL. Pathophysiology and pharmacokinetics following burn injury. *Clin Pharmacokinet.* 1990;**18**(2):118–130.

83. Boucher BA, Hickerson WL, Kuhl DA, Bombassaro AM, Jaresko GS. Imipenem pharmacokinetics in patients with burns. *Clin Pharmacol Ther.* 1990;**48**(2):130–137.

84. Marathe PH, Dwersteg JF, Pavlin EG, Haschke RH, Heimbach DM, Slattery JT. Effect of thermal injury on the pharmacokinetics and pharmacodynamics of atracurium in humans. *Anesthesiology.* 1989;**70**(5):752–755.

85. Han TH, Martyn JAJ. Onset and effectiveness of rocuronium for rapid onset of paralysis in patients with major burns: priming or large bolus. *Br J Anaesth.* 2009;**102**(1):55–60.

15

Malignancy

Michelle Gerstman, Orla J. Lacey, and Cyrus Kerawala

Introduction

Anaesthesia for oromaxillofacial and head and neck tumour surgery requires particular attention to the location of the tumour and any distortion of airway structures, as well as any previous surgery and radiotherapy. In addition to the routine anaesthetic airway assessment, the anaesthetist needs to assess the mobility and pliability of the tissues affected, review any recent radiological scans of the airway and nasendoscopy findings, and consider the feasibility of front of neck access.

There are >500,000 new cases of head and neck cancer worldwide per annum,[1] with approximately 11,400 being diagnosed in the UK in 2014.[2] This number has increased by nearly 100% over the last 50 years and is expected to continue to grow. Oral cancer is more common in men and older patients. There is, however, an increasing number of younger patients with head and neck cancer largely due to human papillomavirus.

Squamous cell carcinoma accounts for >90% of head and neck cancers with the remaining 10% being made up of a number of rarer tumour types such as sarcoma. The most common locations are the tongue, oropharynx, and larynx. Staging in oromaxillofacial and head and neck tumours uses the TNM classification.

Anatomical distribution of malignancy

The common locations of head and neck cancers include (**Fig. 15.1**)[3]:

- Oral cavity—lips, anterior tongue, floor of mouth, hard palate, and gingiva.
- Nasal cavity and paranasal sinuses.
- Pharynx—nasopharynx, oropharynx, and hypopharynx.
- Larynx—supraglottic, glottis, and subglottic.
- Salivary glands.

Risk factors for malignancy

Smoking tobacco (cigarettes, cigars, and pipe) and smokeless tobacco (chewing tobacco and snuff) are risk factors for malignancy, with a dose–response relationship. Alcohol is also a dose-dependent risk factor, and there is a synergistic effect between tobacco and alcohol. Viral infections, particularly human papillomavirus, account for the increasing number of younger non-smokers and non-drinkers being diagnosed with oropharyngeal cancer. Epstein–Barr virus is also a risk factor for nasopharyngeal cancers. Other predisposing factors include immunodeficiency, betel nut chewing, occupational exposure, radiation, diet, and genetic factors.[1]

Types of surgical procedures

Oromaxillofacial and head and neck cancer patients will require an anaesthetic for a variety of different procedures (each of which pose their own unique challenges):

- Biopsy and tissue diagnosis, including lymph node biopsy, where the primary tumour site may not be known.
- Resection of tumour or locoregional recurrence, and reconstructive surgery, possibly requiring a free flap.
- Neck dissection, either as sole procedure or in combination with resection of a tumour.
- Complications of radiotherapy, including osteoradionecrosis, tissue fibrosis, and tissue breakdown with fistulation or arterial 'blow out'.
- Complications of chemotherapy, including osteonecrosis from bisphosphonates and tyrosine kinase inhibitors.
- Complications of surgery, including voice restoration, vocal cord implants or cordotomy, stenoses, and revision of reconstructive surgery.
- Airway emergencies, often with stridor and impending loss of airway.
- Resection of glandular tissues, including thyroid, parathyroid, and salivary glands.
- Tracheal resection.
- Oral surgery for dental care.

Treatment options

Initially a tissue biopsy will be required, as well as cancer staging to determine the most appropriate treatment. Where possible, fine

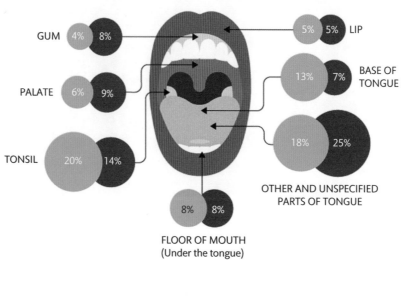

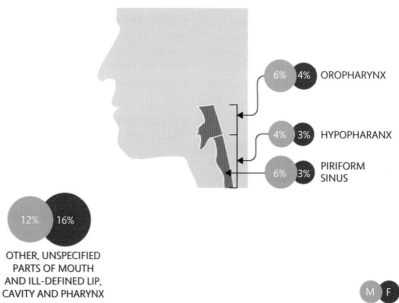

Fig. 15.1 Anatomical site and incidence of oral cancers.
Source: Cancer Research UK, https://www.cancerresearchuk.org/health-professional/cancer-statistics-for-the-uk

needle aspiration cytology or biopsy will be performed, often under ultrasound guidance.

Tissue diagnosis and staging not uncommonly necessitates surgical examination and biopsies under general anaesthesia. Staging is generally completed with computed tomography, magnetic resonance imaging, and/or positron emission tomography scanning. As part of their workup, patients will have undergone outpatient fibre-optic endoscopy, usually nasal.

Depending on the site of the tumour, early-stage disease may be amenable to treatment with simple resection, laser microsurgery, or radiotherapy alone. Larger tumours generally require more extensive surgery and possible tissue reconstruction. Selective neck dissection is often required. In more advanced disease, surgical debulking and chemoradiation may be palliative in nature, rather than curative. Management options should be discussed in a multidisciplinary team meeting. Anaesthetic input into the multidisciplinary team meeting is very useful, especially in the context of significant comorbidities.

Most commonly, patients with oral cavity tumours will be treated primarily with surgery. Postoperative radiotherapy is employed if subsequent pathology confirms close or positive margins, bony involvement, or disease in more than one cervical node. Chemotherapy is not the mainstay of treatment for most oromaxillofacial or head and neck cancers but platinum-based drugs do offer survival benefit in the adjuvant setting for a well-defined group of patients, namely those <70 years of age with positive margins or extracapsular lymph node involvement. Primary radiotherapy is delivered at certain anatomical sites where organ preservation is key, for example, laryngeal disease.[4]

Anaesthetic assessment

Comorbidities and preoperative assessment

Although there is an increasing number of younger patients presenting on oromaxillofacial and head and neck operating lists, the older patient with a history of smoking and alcohol consumption still remains the most typical. These patients are also more likely to have comorbidities, such as chronic airways disease and ischaemic heart disease. It may be necessary to organize investigations such as pulmonary function tests, echocardiography, and stress testing, as well as make referrals to respiratory and cardiology colleagues for their specialist input. These additional investigations and opinions must be balanced against the likely delay associated and the need for expedient surgery. Comorbidities will inevitably have some impact on the surgical techniques employed and may even channel discussions towards non-surgical options. In patients with cancer of the hypopharynx, recurrent aspiration pneumonia must be considered.[4] Oromaxillofacial and head and neck cancer patients are also at risk of malnutrition from both dysphagia and lifestyle factors such as chronic alcohol intake.

Airway examination

When examining any patient, but particularly oromaxillofacial and head and neck cancer patients, the following questions should be considered, with full regard of the 2015 Difficult Airway Society (DAS) unanticipated difficult intubation guidelines[5]:

1. Will face mask ventilation be difficult?
2. Will placing a supraglottic airway device be difficult?
3. Will direct laryngoscopy and tracheal intubation be difficult?
4. Is anterior neck access feasible?

If face mask ventilation is not assured and/or anterior neck access is not feasible, then the tenet of safe oxygenation under general anaesthesia is not assured. In these circumstances, an awake airway intervention should be considered.

Head and neck patients generally have higher rates of difficult tracheal intubation than the general population (7.4–12.6%).[6,7] Of all head and neck patients, the rate of difficult tracheal intubation is much higher in cancer populations than non-cancer populations (12.3–26.3%).[8,9] Thirty-nine per cent of the airway cases reported to the fourth National Audit Project (NAP4) had head and neck pathology.[10]

Risk factors for difficult tracheal intubation in head and neck patients include[6,8]:

- Previous known difficult tracheal intubation.
- Pathology associated with difficult tracheal intubation (particularly a vocal cord mass).
- Interincisor gap <5 cm.
- Poor mandibular or tongue protrusion.
- Short, thick neck.
- Thyromental distance <6.5 cm.
- Limited neck movement.
- Mallampati score of III or IV.

Just as is the case in the general surgical population, each test on its own has limited use but it is the consideration of all measurements together which is particularly valuable.

It is important to also review all available radiological imaging and to liaise with the surgical team about any nasendoscopy findings from the outpatient clinic. Be mindful that these examinations do not specifically assess for any reduced head and neck tissue pliability.

Airway ultrasound is being used increasingly to help identify the difficult airway. It has been found to image structures as reliably as computed tomography scans.[11] Inability to visualize the hyoid bone using sublingual ultrasound predicts difficult intubation with high sensitivity and specificity.[12] The hyomental distance ratio (distance between the hyoid bone and the mentum in the neutral versus hyperextended position), as well as anterior neck thickness, have also been found to help predict difficult tracheal intubation.[13]

Radiotherapy

In some cases, the effects of radiotherapy can be very obvious, with clear signs of non-pliable neck tissues (sometimes described as 'woody'), and a fixed immobile larynx. In the context of radiotherapy, it must be remembered that these patients may be difficult to facemask ventilate, as well as intubate, due to the potential lack of mobility and fixed nature of laryngeal structures, including the epiglottis, base of tongue, and neck tissues.

Other patients, who have also undergone radiotherapy, may not have any classical signs of a predicted difficult tracheal intubation; nevertheless, their history of radiotherapy to the head and neck structures should be treated with a high index of suspicion. Even the placement of a supraglottic airway device may be unsuccessful with a fixed epiglottis. Many experienced anaesthetists have been caught out in these circumstances. In these particular patients, the key to predicting if the airway will be difficult is the quality of the neck structures. The following factors are likely to lead to difficult tracheal intubation:

- Inability to protrude the tongue (fixed, immobile).
- Firm, indurated tissues, 'woody neck'.
- Immobile larynx (identified by palpating the anterior neck), due to the anatomical connection of the epiglottis to the larynx. If the larynx is immobile, the epiglottis is also likely to have reduced mobility, such that it will be difficult to lift the epiglottis when performing direct laryngoscopy.

Tumour location

Distortion, invasion, and compression of tissues is common in airway malignancies and it is essential to review any available radiological imaging. The specific location of the mass is very important. For example, up to 50% of patients with a vocal cord mass may subsequently have a difficult tracheal intubation.[6] In obstructive lesions, it is important to quantify the degree of narrowing as well as the location—oral cavity, base of tongue, supraglottic, glottic, or infraglottic. Figs 15.2 and 15.3 demonstrate two cases which had relatively normal routine external airway examinations, but imaging revealed masses which necessitated awake interventions to secure their airway.

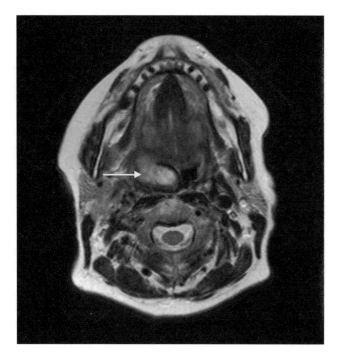

Fig. 15.2 Melanoma deposit filling oropharynx (white arrow).

Previous surgery

Any surgical intervention can make airway management more complicated. Scarring and recent surgery can affect head and neck tissue mobility and pliability making laryngoscopy more difficult. Attention to the nature and position of the previous surgery is paramount. In addition, most patients with local recurrence are also likely to have undergone radiotherapy. In some cases, prior surgery may in fact result in airway management becoming simpler, such as those patients with a tracheostome following laryngectomy.

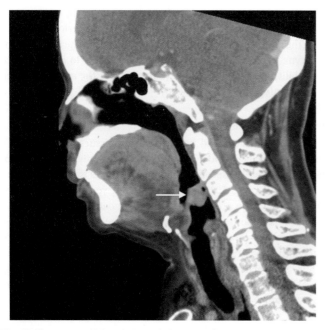

Fig. 15.3 Tumour of the epiglottis (white arrow).

Fourth National Audit Project

Thirty-nine per cent of major airway management complications reported in NAP4 occurred in acute or chronic pathologies of the head, neck, or trachea. Seventy per cent of these cases occurred in patients with obstructive lesions within the airway. Issues with assessment, planning, and communication within teams were identified in one-third of these cases. NAP4 demonstrated that the friable, necrotic, and oedematous nature of head and neck tumours can cause dramatic deterioration in the airway from just a single attempt at laryngoscopy (and even worse after multiple attempts). A large proportion of events were represented by patients who were kept spontaneously ventilated utilizing an inhalational induction technique. It was also noted that awake and asleep fibreoptic techniques are not infallible and a backup plan must be in place. Over half of cannula cricothyroidotomy attempts in NAP4 failed due to misplacement, inability to place, fracture, kinking, blockage, dislodgement, and barotrauma. One-third of all events in NAP4 occurred during emergence or recovery.[14]

Difficult Airway Society 2015 guidelines

In 2015, the DAS released an updated version of the adult difficult tracheal intubation guidelines.[5] One of the major changes was the suggestion of using a scalpel–bougie–tube technique rather than needle cricothyroidotomy (with the caveat that needle techniques remain an option for the anaesthetist who is skilled with this technique). Other important recommendations included:

- Limiting the number of interventions (change something with each attempt).
- Ensuring adequate neuromuscular blockade.
- Using second-generation supraglottic airway devices for airway rescue.
- Avoidance of blind tracheal intubations.
- Planning, education, and training.

Awake airway management techniques

The first decision to be made is whether an awake or asleep technique is required for airway management. Where there is any doubt about the ability to face mask ventilate or the feasibility of anterior neck access, an awake technique is often safer.

Remifentanil target-controlled infusions have increased patient tolerance and comfort of awake techniques. Safe and careful administration of remifentanil can provide adequate patient comfort while still ensuring airway patency, spontaneous ventilation, and an ability to follow commands. The effects may also potentially be reversed using naloxone. Dexmedetomidine is also gaining favour as an effective drug for facilitating awake techniques.

The more recent 'Awake Tracheal Intubation' guidelines, published by DAS (2019), are a very useful resource and set out a safe approach to awake fibreoptic and videolaryngoscopic tracheal intubation, including recommendations for oxygenation, sedation, topicalization, and performance.

Awake flexible fibreoptic tracheal intubation (+/− awake airway wire placement)

Fibreoptic tracheal intubation

It is useful to think about fibreoptic intubation in two main categories. Firstly, the airway with normal oropharyngeal and laryngeal anatomy, but with abnormal tissue mobility (e.g. trismus, cervical spine pathology, and/or radiotherapy). Fibreoptic views and passage through the laryngeal inlet are generally more straightforward. Secondly, the airway with abnormal oropharyngeal or laryngeal anatomy (e.g. due to tumour masses, previous surgery, and/or radiotherapy). In these cases, it is prudent to consider an awake technique and recognize that the passage of the fibreoptic scope through abnormal, bulky, and sometimes friable tissue will be more challenging.

Fibreoptic intubation using an airway wire

This technique is generally reserved for the anatomically abnormal or stenotic airway.

In some cases of severe airway narrowing, a microlaryngoscopy tube may be too large (a size 4.0 mm microlaryngoscopy tube has an external diameter of 5.6 mm). There are a number of potential options in this scenario. In cases of extreme narrowing, a jet ventilation catheter can be used. As the jet ventilation catheter is too narrow to pass over a fibreoptic scope, an airway wire such as that from the Cook® Staged Extubation Set (Cook Medical, Bloomington, IN, USA) (Figs 15.4 and 15.5) can be inserted via

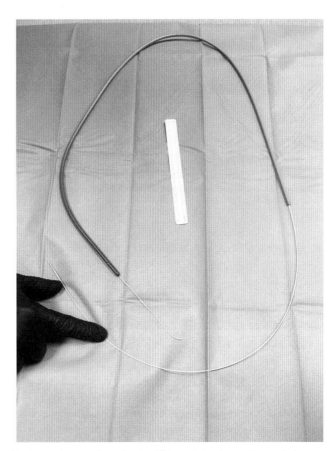

Fig. 15.5 The wire from the Cook® Staged Extubation Set, with the reintubation catheter in place.

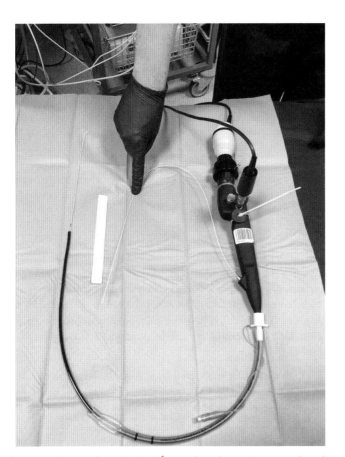

Fig. 15.4 The wire from the Cook® Staged Extubation Set, passed via the working channel of a flexible bronchoscope, to be used as a conduit for tracheal intubation.

the working channel of the bronchoscope, and placed safely in the awake, spontaneously breathing, patient. This can then be used as a conduit for insertion of a larger tube. The Cook® staged reintubation catheter (14 French, 4.7 mm external diameter) can be inserted over the wire in most cases, but in the extremely narrowed airway, a 2 mm jet ventilation catheter can be passed over the airway wire. Oxygenation can then be achieved via jet ventilation, enabling the surgeons to perform airway dilatation procedures. Fig. 15.6 shows severe airway narrowing in a patient with osteochondrosarcoma, which necessitated such a technique. Awake fibreoptic tracheal intubation was performed on several occasions to facilitate balloon dilatation procedures. Depending on the degree of narrowing at presentation, oxygenation was achieved via the bronchoscope itself or via a jet ventilation catheter. An airway wire was then left in place during the dilatations to ensure oxygenation could be maintained after the dilatation was completed. It was not possible to insert an airway transtracheal cannula due to the ossification of the airway tissues.

Awake videolaryngoscopy-assisted tracheal intubation

This technique has gained increasing popularity recently, due to most anaesthetists' greater familiarity and comfort with videolaryngoscopy compared with flexible fibreoptic techniques. When used in patients with a predicted difficult airway, videolaryngoscopy has been shown to result in fewer intubation failures,[21] and the awake technique has been demonstrated safely

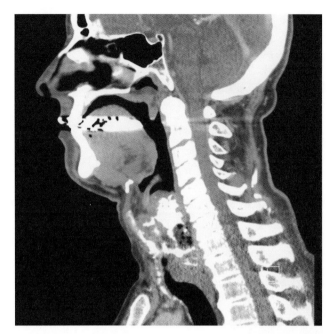

Fig. 15.6 Image demonstrating significant airway narrowing in a patient with osteochondrosarcoma who presented for recurrent dilatation procedures.

in patients with oropharyngeal cancer.[22,23] A meta-analysis of awake videolaryngoscopy versus awake fibreoptic bronchoscopy demonstrated shorter intubation times for videolaryngoscopy, with a similar safety profile.[24] Of course, awake videolaryngoscopy requires a degree of mouth opening, which may limit its use in some oromaxillofacial/head and neck patients.

Awake transtracheal cannula

This technique may be preferred in cases where there is a glottic or supraglottic lesion, or where there is a high risk of airway bleeding from a tumour if a fibreoptic scope is passed. The cannula can be inserted electively under local anaesthetic (as opposed to an emergency needle cricothyroidotomy). This allows the placement to occur in a calm, stress-free environment. Ultrasound has been found to be useful in aiding identification of the cricothyroid membrane and tracheal cartilage.[13] If this technique is to be used, it is important to consider the location of the lesion (ultrasound can also aid with this) and insert the cannula distally, either via the cricothyroid membrane or between the upper tracheal rings. Once the cannula is placed, the position should be checked by both aspirating air and confirming the presence of carbon dioxide with capnography. It is also important to insert the transtracheal cannula all the way to the hilt at the skin to avoid kinking. Once the position has been confirmed, gentle passive oxygenation can be delivered via the transtracheal cannula (apnoeic oxygenation) or jet ventilation can be initiated while a definitive airway is being secured.

Awake tracheostomy

This may be useful in an acute airway emergency where a fibreoptic intubation is likely to be difficult either due to an obstructed or stenotic airway lesion or where there is already soiling or bleeding in the airway.

Oxygenation techniques

Adequate oxygenation of the patient is the priority at all times. Special consideration should be given to optimizing this aspect in all patients, but especially in those with abnormal airways (given the anticipated difficulties and predisposition to airway compromise and hypoxia), so that airway manoeuvres (awake or asleep), induction of anaesthesia, and surgery can be undertaken in the safest manner possible. There have been significant advances in this area in recent times.

Preoxygenation

In its simplest form, preoxygenation can be undertaken via a traditional face mask, with the optional application of continuous positive airway pressure and pressure support. In the predicted difficult airway, adequate preoxygenation should also be combined with per-oxygenation (apnoeic oxygenation) where possible.

Transnasal high-flow humidified oxygenation

This technique can be utilized prior to induction of anaesthesia, during awake airway management techniques, as well as post induction prior to definitive securing of the airway. In the awake, spontaneously ventilating patient, 20–30 L/min of humidified oxygen can be delivered (Optiflow™, Fisher & Paykel Healthcare, Auckland, New Zealand),[15] and up to 70 L/min following induction of anaesthesia (transnasal humidified rapid-insufflation ventilatory exchange, known as 'THRIVE'). Apnoeic oxygenation has been used to increase the safe apnoea time in patients with difficult airways, prolonging the time to desaturation, allowing more time to safely establish a definitive airway.[15] Crucially, the THRIVE technique relies on a patent airway being maintained, and may not be appropriate in circumstances where this is not possible due to collapse of the airway after induction of anaesthesia or secretions blocking an already narrowed airway.[16]

Oxygenation via the fibreoptic scope

Oxygenation can occur via the bronchoscope itself, by delivering oxygen through the working channel, and may be of benefit during an awake fibreoptic intubation.

Jet ventilation

Where high pressure ventilation is necessitated due to the requirement for a narrow diameter tube or during suspension laryngoscopy, jet ventilation can be particularly useful. Jet ventilation causes air to be entrained, in addition to the tidal volume delivered by the high-pressure source. Expiration is then passive and requires a patent airway.[17] Jet ventilation can be supraglottic, transglottic, or infraglottic:

- Supraglottic jetting is achieved via suspension laryngoscopy. This avoids obstruction of the surgical view with a tube. It is also particularly useful in laser surgery as it removes the 'fuel' from the fire triad.
- Transglottic jetting is generally undertaken via a 13-gauge transtracheal needle.
- Infraglottic jetting is achieved via a jet ventilation catheter.

Jet ventilation can be delivered at either a low frequency or high frequency. Low-frequency jet ventilation can be readily achieved using a hand-held device such as a Sanders injector (Manujet III™, VBM Medical, Sulz, Germany). This is usually reserved for short procedures and can also be used for rescue oxygenation via a cricothyroid needle puncture. In low-frequency jet ventilation, the inflation time and the ventilation rate are manually controlled by the operator. It is important to ensure that there is adequate time for expiration. Where a manual jet ventilator is used, the delivered fraction of inspired oxygen (FiO_2) will be approximately 0.8–0.9, due to entrainment of air. The driving pressure is also chosen by the operator.[17] High-frequency jet ventilation requires an automated ventilator machine, for example, the Monsoon III Jet Ventilator (Acutronic®, Hirzel, Switzerland), which comes with advantageous safety features such as high-pressure alarms and a pause pressure facility. The pause pressure is typically set at 15 or 20 millibar such that the ventilator will not deliver the next jetted breath if pressures exceed this preset limit. High-frequency jet ventilation enables finer control of the ventilation parameters. The FiO_2 can be adjusted, although it is generally prudent to leave this at 1.0. Typical settings may include an inspiratory time set at 35–50%, a pause pressure set at 15–20 millibar, and a ventilator frequency in the range of 100–120 per minute. The driving pressure depends on the body dimensions of the patient as well as their pulmonary compliance. Infraglottic jet ventilation will typically require a driving pressure of 0.6–1.2 atmospheres and supraglottic jetting between 1.5 and 2.5 atmospheres.

Carbon dioxide levels are difficult to accurately measure when jetting. The driving pressure has a larger impact on carbon dioxide than ventilator frequency. It is important to allow sufficient expiratory time (determined by both frequency and inspiratory time) for carbon dioxide to be expired and to avoid excessive intrinsic positive end-expiratory pressure. In practical terms, the driving pressure should be approximated to the body mass of the patient and then adjusted by observing diaphragm excursion. It is important to be able to visualize chest movement and to utilize the minimum driving pressure to achieve this.

Jet ventilation equipment should be thoroughly checked prior to use, along with the standard anaesthetic machine and ventilator, which may be required as back-up. Operators should be familiar with the jet ventilation equipment at their particular hospital (and the associated safety features), as well as the potential complications of jet ventilation and how to avoid them.

Airway devices

As in any case with a 'shared airway', it is important to select an appropriate device that optimizes the surgical team's view and access to the surgical field, while not compromising other important patient safety aspects. A good working relationship between anaesthetist and surgeon is essential to achieve this endpoint.

Tracheal tubes

- Reinforced tracheal tubes are often useful as they are more easily secured away from the surgical field without kinking. A smaller diameter tube may be necessary as the reinforcement results in a larger external diameter for the same internal diameter. This is particularly relevant when performing an awake tracheal intubation.
- A microlaryngoscopy tube may be required when the surgical field includes the laryngeal inlet. This smaller diameter tube improves the surgical view, while still providing a seal with an adult trachea due to its relatively larger cuff size. Placing the cuff just below the cricoid enables better surgical views with improved subglottic visualization.
- Laser-compatible tubes may be required for laser airway surgery, and these should be employed along with other standard strategies to reduce the risk of an airway fire.
- North- or South-facing Ring–Adair–Elwyn tracheal tubes are particularly useful in oromaxillofacial and head and neck cancer surgery, but may be more difficult to introduce over a fibreoptic scope due to their preformed nature.

Supraglottic airway devices

The laryngeal mask airway is less bulky and less prominent, therefore potentially more suited to oromaxillofacial and head and neck surgical access requirements than second-generation supraglottic airway devices. However, selection is also based on similar factors affecting the choice of device in any other surgical specialties, such as patient body mass index and duration of intended surgery. For minor, superficial oromaxillofacial or head and neck tumour surgery, however, the reinforced or flexible laryngeal mask airway offers the added advantage of being able to be secured away from the surgical field, optimizing surgical access, which can be particularly useful for some oral cavity and nasal procedures.

Laryngectomy and tracheostomy tubes

Tracheostomes (after laryngectomy) are generally easy to intubate due to the tract being surgically formed. A laryngectomy tube can be used for this purpose. Preoxygenation and ventilation can be achieved with a paediatric face mask or laryngeal mask airway (with cuff slightly inflated) placed over the stoma.

Conversely, if a tracheostomy needs to be reintubated, it is vital to determine how long the tracheostomy has been in place. Long-term tracheostomies are generally easy to reintubate; however, recently formed tracheostomies may be significantly more challenging since the tract may not have formed yet.

Anaesthesia and perioperative care

Induction of anaesthesia

Where an asleep induction of anaesthesia is planned, the choice must be made between an inhalational or intravenous induction technique. Historically, inhalational induction, with a spontaneously ventilating patient, was preferred over intravenous induction for patients with anticipated difficult airway management; however, recent evidence suggests this may not be preferable. Notably, Nouraei et al. compared flow–volume loops in patients with tracheolaryngeal stenosis while spontaneously ventilating prior to induction and after induction with muscle relaxation and positive pressure ventilation.[18] They showed a decrease in inspiratory airway obstruction with positive pressure ventilation. When a patient is spontaneously ventilating, a negative intrathoracic pressure occurs during inspiration. This causes non-rigid components of the trachea to collapse resulting in narrowing of the airway, thus worsening any obstruction. When a patient is face mask hand-ventilated or mechanically ventilated, the ventilation creates a positive intrathoracic pressure for inhalation, which helps to splint the airway open, potentially improving airway flow in a patient with an obstructed airway.[18] Current recommendations for extrathoracic subglottic lesions therefore now recommend intravenous induction with muscle relaxation and positive pressure ventilation.[18] The DAS difficult tracheal intubation guidelines (2015) also promote the use of neuromuscular blocking agents in difficult tracheal intubation situations.[5]

Maintenance of anaesthesia

A total intravenous anaesthesia technique is generally preferred in 'shared airway' cases in order to ensure continuous delivery of anaesthesia, where inhalational techniques may incur interruptions, particularly during unavoidable manipulation of the airway and/or airway device. Retrospective analysis has also shown some positive associations between total intravenous anaesthesia and survival in cancer surgery,[19,20] with further randomized controlled trials expected in this area.

Perioperative emergencies

In oromaxillofacial and head and neck malignancy surgery, significant occult blood loss can occur, with blood pooling in the surgical drapes in particular, therefore constant vigilance is required.

Venous air embolism is a rare, and very serious complication, which these patients are at an increased risk of due to the standard reverse Trendelenburg (elevated head) positioning on the operating table—it requires a high index of suspicion and rapid treatment.

Baroreceptor reflexes and parasympathetic surgical stimulation can cause profound bradycardic responses, including asystole. In most cases, these episodes will resolve within 20–30 seconds following cessation of the surgical stimulus. Where repeated episodes occur with ongoing surgical stimuli in the same site, local anaesthesia can sometimes be used to attenuate the response.

Analgesia

Pain following minor oromaxillofacial malignancy surgery is usually mild to moderate intensity and can generally be controlled with simple analgesia, particularly when combined with generous perioperative local anaesthetic infiltration (some institutions also utilize locoregional blocks to reduce intra- and postoperative analgesic requirements). Non-steroidal anti-inflammatory agents are generally avoided, unless the risk of bleeding is very low. Caution should be taken with excessive opioid administration in this patient cohort, given the prevalence of difficult airways and the potential for respiratory compromise (careful titration is recommended). Nevertheless, in most of the major tumour resection (and/or reconstructive) cases, opioid patient-controlled analgesia is often required. In those patients who have undergone free flap surgery, it is frequently the donor site (particularly if bone is harvested) that is more painful than the reconstruction site. Some oromaxillofacial and head and neck cancers can be associated with pain syndromes, particularly from nerve/muscle tumour infiltration (pain may sometimes be the presenting symptom) —these patients may have complex analgesic

requirements and specialist acute and chronic pain team input is essential.

Tracheal extubation techniques

For all surgery, but particularly for oromaxillofacial and head and neck malignancy surgery, a clear tracheal extubation plan is essential, and should always include a reintubation strategy. Tracheal extubation is a high-risk phase of anaesthesia associated with significant complications in the general population, never mind the oromaxillofacial cancer patient.

Consideration must be given to the optimum timing and best environment for tracheal extubation to be undertaken—at the end of the surgical procedure or in the critical care unit. After major complex cancer resection and reconstruction, the anaesthesia and surgical team must discuss the relative merits and risks of immediate postoperative emergence and tracheal extubation versus delayed extubation and ongoing sedation and ventilation. This discussion needs to take into consideration anaesthetic, patient, and surgical factors. Avoidance of further sedation/anaesthesia may reduce vasopressor requirements and potentially improve flap/tissue perfusion. However, patients with an extensive history of cigarette smoking, alcohol consumption, and/or recreational drug use may benefit from a slower more gradual emergence and delayed tracheal extubation. An airway wire can sometimes be used to facilitate an early tracheal extubation in patients where there is some concern over ease of reintubation. It can be placed prior to tracheal extubation and can be secured to the patient's cheek following extubation (the wire is easily coiled, and can be taped conveniently to the side of the face). They are well tolerated by most patients and can be left *in situ* for several hours (see manufacturer's recommendations). The airway wire can facilitate reintubation of the trachea using the specially designed Cook® reintubation catheter, which can be used for immediate oxygenation, or can be used as a conduit over which a larger diameter reinforced tracheal tube can be passed. While an airway wire can represent part of the contingency plan in some cases, where there is particular concern regarding postoperative airway management (usually relating to the presence of significant airway oedema), an initial period of ongoing sedation and ventilation in the critical care unit may be the safest option (to allow the oedema to subside).

If the decision is made to keep the patient's trachea intubated and to transfer the patient to the critical care unit, a management strategy for the potential loss of the existing secure airway must be formulated, clearly documented, and communicated to the staff responsible for their postoperative care. This must include answers to the same questions posed prior to anaesthesia and surgery—expected ease of bag mask ventilation, insertion of a supraglottic airway device, reintubation of the trachea, or anterior neck access. These elements may have changed significantly since the surgical intervention; therefore, each aspect must be considered carefully.

Following oromaxillofacial and head and neck cancer reconstructive surgery, patients may or may not require a tracheostomy— a decision that should be jointly made by the anaesthesia and surgical teams. A tracheostomy may be necessary due to the specific location of the resection, the extent of the surgery, or patient factors such as underlying respiratory disease (or a combination of factors). Scoring systems have been developed specifically to help determine this requirement, and include tumour location (such as the oropharynx), bilateral neck dissection, particularly if the internal jugular veins are sacrificed, and the need for reconstruction.[35–37]

In patients not requiring a tracheostomy, but requiring ongoing sedation and ventilation, a tube exchange may be necessary at the end of surgery. Flexible reinforced tracheal tubes are often used intraoperatively, and these should ideally be exchanged for a traditional non-reinforced tracheal tube. Many reinforced tubes lack a Murphy's eye and are therefore at an increased risk of becoming obstructed by secretions. A reinforced tube is also potentially at risk of obstruction in the event of the patient biting down on it at tracheal extubation/under light sedation (due to the reinforcing wires becoming compressed). These advantages of changing the tracheal tube must be weighed up against the problems of undertaking a tube exchange immediately after surgery, potential loss of a secure airway, and risk of failure to reintubate. The decision to perform a tube exchange should be discussed with the surgical team, and they should remain in the operating theatre while the tube is being changed.

The DAS extubation guidelines provide a very good resource, comprising simple algorithms for aiding tracheal extubation, with consideration of the important factors involved in the decision-making process.[38]

Range of procedures

Laser surgery

The main concern with the use of lasers is patient safety, and the safety of staff members. Prevention of an airway fire is of paramount importance. A fire requires three essential components—a fuel (such as a tracheal tube), oxygen, and an ignition source (such as the laser). A laser-compatible tracheal tube should be selected (there are a number of laser-safe tracheal tube designs available, either composed of laser-resistant material or requiring specialist foil wrapping [25]), or supraglottic jet ventilation can be employed to obviate the fuel component of the fire triad entirely. The FiO_2 should be reduced to the minimum required for adequate oxygenation. Hospitals where laser surgery is undertaken should have laser surgery protocols in place, which will include the use of wavelength-specific laser protective eyewear, laser-in-use signs, and the appropriate equipment to extinguish a fire if it occurs (sterile water immediately available on the scrub trolley, and carbon dioxide fire extinguishers). In the event of an airway fire, any airway device should be removed immediately, delivery of oxygen ceased, and the fire extinguished with water, after which airway management should be re-established (laser safety is also discussed extensively in Chapter 9).

Selective neck dissection

In addition to resection of the primary tumour, sentinel lymph node biopsy and resection of lymph nodes may be required. Cervical lymph nodes are divided into six levels. The greater the number of levels needing to be explored/removed, the longer the duration of the operation and the higher the risk of damage to underlying structures. Due to the proximity of large blood vessels, major haemorrhage may occur during neck dissection, in particular dissection at levels 2, 3, and 4, therefore large-bore intravenous access should always be placed. Breach of the internal jugular vein may also result

in air embolism, and stimulation of local structures such as carotid bodies can cause profound bradycardia. The recurrent laryngeal nerve is also at risk of damage during a level 6 dissection, such that nerve monitoring is generally required.

Laryngectomy surgery

Tracheal intubation for patients requiring a laryngectomy can be challenging. The principles discussed in the anaesthesia assessment section are crucial in this group of patients. Where tumour size allows, a reinforced tracheal tube is often used. The tracheal tube must be withdrawn when the trachea is resected from the larynx and the tracheostome is formed. A laryngectomy tube is then inserted via the tracheostome for the remainder of the surgery. Generally, a tracheostomy tube is then inserted postoperatively (for the first 24 hours) to allow for easier suctioning and prevention of aspiration of blood.[26]

Tracheal resection

Evaluation of the tumour generally occurs using fibreoptic or rigid laryngoscopy. A reinforced tracheal tube should then be inserted, with the aim of it sitting just above the carina. The larynx will need to be mobilized, the extent of which will depend on the size of the lesion. Postoperatively, the trachea may need to be kept intubated and the patient sedated with their neck in a flexed position for 2–3 days. When tracheal extubation is undertaken, a staged extubation strategy is often appropriate utilizing an exchange catheter or airway wire.

Robotic and endoscopic surgery

Robotic and endoscopic surgery is becoming more common across all surgical specialities, and oromaxillofacial surgery is no exception. One of the major advantages in this particular area is avoidance of the need to 'split' the mandible. However, the robot certainly adds an additional level of complexity to the 'shared airway'. A tracheal tube is placed orally or nasally, depending on tumour site and surgical preference, and then a retractor is used to allow access for the robot arms, which precludes easy access to the airway and necessitates meticulous securing of the tube. In the event of an airway emergency, the robot must un-dock before being able to be removed, therefore this process should be practised regularly by the relevant team members. A continuous infusion of a neuromuscular blocking agent may be used to help avoid any coughing or any other unintentional motor responses while the robot is in place.

Resection of rarer tumours

There are a number of rare tumours which can occur in the oromaxillofacial and head and neck region, each with their own specific issues. Sarcomas, for example, are associated with massive haemorrhage, and neuroendocrine tumours may cause marked intraoperative cardiovascular instability. Consequently, such tumours should be managed in specialist centres.

Reconstructive surgery following resection

Reconstruction aims to restore appearance, form, and functions such as speech, mastication, swallowing, airway protection, nutrition, and protection of local structures (e.g. carotid tree/internal jugular vein).[27,28] Plastic surgeons should follow the 'reconstructive ladder' in order to decide on the most appropriate reconstructive modality for a particular defect, with the aim of minimizing donor site morbidity. Options for surgical closure of a defect or wound post resection include[27,28]:

- Primary closure (or delayed primary closure).
- Skin graft (split thickness or full thickness).
- Tissue expansion.
- Local flap (e.g. nasolabial advancement flap).
- Pedicled flap (e.g. pectoralis major flap).
- Free flaps.
- Prosthetic reconstruction (e.g. obturators used for maxillectomy defects).

Primary closure, skin grafts, and local flaps may be appropriate for smaller lesions. Skin grafts are at risk of forming contractures. Free flaps will give better functional outcomes for larger lesions; however, the duration of surgery is considerably longer. Prosthetic devices have the inconvenience of daily cleaning and periodic adjustment, but may be appropriate for patients with limited defects and significant comorbidities, which have cause to limit the duration of anaesthesia and surgery. The pectoralis major pedicled flap was once the most commonly used flap, but it is now mainly reserved for patients whose comorbidities preclude free tissue transfer. Pedicle flap procedures tend to be shorter procedures as there is no need for microvascular surgery; however, the functional/cosmetic results may be inferior to a free flap reconstruction.

Free flap reconstruction

Free flap procedures can be considered as a separate entity, given the complexities of the surgery and anaesthesia, and the intricacies of perioperative management. There are three main groups of free flap[28]:

- Fasciocutaneous—skin, subcutaneous tissue, and supportive fascia (e.g. radial forearm, anterolateral thigh).
- Myocutaneous—muscle, subcutaneous tissue, and skin (e.g. rectus abdominis, latissimus dorsi).
- Osteocutaneous (e.g. fibular, deep circumflex iliac artery).

The choice of reconstructive technique depends on tumour-related factors (size and location of the defect), patient factors (fitness for long operations, anatomy of the planned flap donor site), and surgical factors (surgical experience and preference). The most commonly performed free flaps are radial, fibular, anterolateral thigh, and deep circumflex iliac artery,[29,30] and the specifics of each are discussed in **Table 15.1**. Jejunal free flaps were more common previously, but have fallen out of favour due to their relatively high failure rate.

Bone flaps can either be non-vascularized or vascularized depending on the indication. Non-vascularized bone, such as from the rib or iliac crest, may be suitable for defects <5 cm but cannot be used when pre- or postoperative radiotherapy is required. Vascularized flaps are the gold standard for oncological reconstruction.[27] Where a bone flap has been used, a supportive cast will generally be placed over the donor site postoperatively (fibular and radial).

Anaesthesia for free flap surgery is based on the general principles of avoidance of hypothermia, avoidance of vasoconstriction, avoidance of acidosis, and a neutral fluid balance. In addition to standard anaesthetic monitoring, an arterial catheter should be inserted to enable meticulous blood pressure monitoring and control, as well as for regular blood gas sampling. Central venous access is advised where vasopressor use is expected. The proposed site of any arterial and venous cannulae should be discussed with the surgical team; for example, a radial forearm flap will commonly preclude cannula placement in the non-dominant arm. Central venous access is generally placed in the femoral vein. Cardiac output monitoring may also be of use in oromaxillofacial and head and neck flap surgery—oesophageal Doppler is rarely possible due to the proximity to the surgical field and the restricted access to adjust the probe placement, therefore other haemodynamic monitoring systems such as LiDCOrapid™ (LiDCO, London, UK) are more commonly used.

There are three distinct phases to free flap surgery: the dissection stage/elevation of the flap, often incorporating tourniquet control; the period of ischaemia following flap division; and the anastomosis of the blood vessels (+/– nerves). During the dissection stage, controlled hypotension may be requested to decrease blood loss and improve the surgical field.[31] This needs to be balanced against the risk of ischaemia in other organ systems, and, generally, it is therefore recommended to keep the blood pressure in the low normal range for the patient. A tourniquet will be used during the dissection stage for certain donor sites (radial, fibula). Tourniquet occlusion time should be limited to 90–120 minutes, and where ongoing dissection is still required, the tourniquet should be released to allow reperfusion of the limb prior to reinflation. Extended tourniquet times

Table 15.1 Specifics relating to common free flap procedures

Type of free flap	Indications and details of harvest	Advantages and disadvantages
Radial forearm (RFFF)	Used for soft tissue reconstructions, such as for intraoral lesions (thin, pliable skin). The long reliable pedicle allows anastomoses to be performed on the ipsilateral or contralateral neck	Bone stock is poor, and the harvest can be associated with morbidity (prophylactic plating of residual radial bone is advised)
Fibular (FFF)	Used for total/subtotal mandibular reconstructions, where up to 25 cm of bone can be harvested	Preoperative imaging (such as computed tomography angiography) is necessary to determine if there is anatomically appropriate vascular supply (three-vessel run off)
Anterolateral thigh (ALT)	This is a reliable soft tissue flap. Large paddles of skin can be harvested with little need for subsequent grafting of the donor site	The flap can be precluded by body habitus (high body mass index). This flap permits two teams to be operating simultaneously, and no preoperative flap investigations are necessary
Deep circumflex iliac artery (DCIA)	This provides good-quality bone that can be subsequently implanted	Bone stock can be tailored to the recipient site. The flap can be transferred with the internal oblique muscle to provide mucosal reconstruction

can result in significant hypertension and tachycardia (which can be impossible to ameliorate), and may also result in significant undesirable sequelae on tourniquet deflation as anaerobic metabolites enter the systemic circulation.

The use of vasopressors in flap surgery has been controversial. Systemic blood pressure should be maintained at such a level that there is adequate perfusion pressure/blood supply to the flap; however, opinions as to the best method of achieving this vary. Historically, there has been some concern regarding the use of vasopressors and the potential for peripheral vasoconstriction to negatively affect blood supply to the flap. An intensive care study investigating the effects of catecholamines on postoperative free flap blood flow found norepinephrine and dobutamine to increase flap blood flow compared with epinephrine and dopexamine which decreased flap flow (norepinephrine provided the greatest increase in flow).[32]

There are several potential causes of free flap failure. Although ischaemic time is kept to a minimum after reperfusion, an inflammatory cascade does occur,[33] resulting in a reduction in blood flow for the first 8–12 hours. Flaps are particularly vulnerable to interstitial oedema, due to the lack of a lymphatic drainage system. The transplanted blood vessels do not have sympathetic innervation, but they are vulnerable to physical stimuli such as cold and physical handling, which may cause vasospasm. Nevertheless, flap failure is most commonly due to thrombus formation. Postoperative flap monitoring is essential, although the exact technique varies depending on surgeon preference and available equipment (implantable Doppler probes are commonly used).[34]

Conclusion

As part of the preoperative evaluation of patients undergoing surgery for oromaxillofacial malignancy, it is essential to review recent radiology and/or views on nasendoscopy as part of the airway assessment. A high index of suspicion of potential airway issues should be retained in any patients who have had radiotherapy, even with an apparently normal airway examination. The airway management strategy must be discussed thoroughly and agreed by the anaesthetist and surgeon prior to the onset of the case. Planning for failure is essential. A clear strategy for rescue oxygenation must be in place, and where there is any doubt over the feasibility of bag mask ventilation or front of neck access, an awake airway management technique should be considered.

REFERENCES

1. Stenson K. Epidemiology and risk factors in head and neck cancer. UpToDate. 2021. https://www.uptodate.com/contents/epidemiology-and-risk-factors-for-head-and-neck-cancer

2. Cancer Research UK. Head and neck cancer statistics. 2021. https://www.cancerresearchuk.org/health-professional/cancer-statistics/statistics-by-cancer-type/head-and-neck-cancers/incidence-qdlbbseomM4PkOxD.99

3. Poon S. Overview of the diagnosis and staging of head and neck cancer. UpToDate. 2021. http://www.uptodate.com/contents/overview-of-the-diagnosis-and-staging-of-head-and-neck-cancer

4. National Institute for Health and Care Excellence. Cancer of the upper aerodigestive tract: assessment and management in people aged 16 and over. NICE guideline NG36. 2016. https://www.nice.org.uk/guidance/ng36

5. Frerk C, Mitchell VS, McNarry AF, Mendonca C, Bhagrath R, Patel A, et al. Difficult Airway Society 2015 guidelines for management of unanticipated difficult intubation in adults. *Br J Anaesth*. 2015;**115**(6):827–848.

6. Karakus O, Kaya C, Ustun FE, Koksal E, Ustun YB. Predictive value of preoperative tests in estimating difficult intubation in patients who underwent direct laryngoscopy in ear, nose, and throat surgery. *Rev Bras Anestesiol*. 2015;**65**(2):85–91.

7. Wong P, Iqbal R, Light KP, Williams E, Hayward J. Head and neck surgery in a tertiary centre: predictors of difficult airway and anaesthetic management. *Proc Singapore Healthc*. 2015;**25**(1):1–8.

8. Arne J, Descoins P, Fusciardi J, Ingrand P, Ferrier B, Boudigues D. Preoperative assessment for difficult intubation in general and ENT surgery: predictive value of a clinical multivariate risk index. *Br J Anaesth*. 1998;**80**(2):140–146.

9. Bhatnagar S, Mishra S, Jha RR, Singhal AK. Predicting difficult laryngoscopy in oral cancer patients: a prospective study. *Indian J Anaesth*. 2005;**49**(5):413–416.

10. Cook TM, Woodall N, Frerk C. *The NAP4 Report: Major Complications of Airway Management in the United Kingdom*. London: Royal College of Anaesthetists; 2011. https://www.niaa.org.uk/NAP4_home

11. Prasad A, Yu E, Wong DT, Karkhanis R, Gullane P, Chan VW. Comparison of sonography and computed tomography as imaging tools for assessment of airway structures. *J Ultrasound Med*. 2011;**30**(7):965–972.

12. Hui CM, Tsui BC. Sublingual ultrasound as an assessment method for predicting difficult intubation: a pilot study. *Anaesthesia*. 2014;**69**(4):314–319.

13. Osman A, Sum KM. Role of upper airway ultrasound in airway management. *J Intensive Care*. 2016;**4**:52.

14. Cook TM, Woodall N, Frerk C; Fourth National Audit Project. Major complications of airway management in the UK: results of the Fourth National Audit Project of the Royal College of Anaesthetists and the Difficult Airway Society. Part 1: anaesthesia. *Br J Anaesth*. 2011;**106**(5):617–631.

15. Patel A, Nouraei SA. Transnasal humidified rapid-insufflation ventilatory exchange (THRIVE): a physiological method of increasing apnoea time in patients with difficult airways. *Anaesthesia*. 2015;**70**(3):323–329.

16. Rummens N, Ball DR. Failure to thrive. *Anaesthesia*. 2015;**70**(6):752–753.

17. Evans E, Biro P, Bedforth N. Jet ventilation. *Cont Educ Anaesth Crit Care Pain*. 2007;**7**(1):2–5.

18. Nouraei SA, Giussani DA, Howard DJ, Sandhu GS, Ferguson C, Patel A. Physiological comparison of spontaneous and positive-pressure ventilation in laryngotracheal stenosis. *Br J Anaesth*. 2008;**101**(3):419–423.

19. Wigmore TJ, Mohammed K, Jhanji S. Long-term survival for patients undergoing volatile versus IV anesthesia for cancer surgery: a retrospective analysis. *Anesthesiology*. 2016;**124**(1):69–79.

20. Soltanizadeh S, Degett TH, Gögenur I. Outcomes of cancer surgery after inhalational and intravenous anesthesia: a systematic review. *J Clin Anesth*. 2017;**42**:19–25.

21. Lewis SR, Butler AR, Parker J, Cook TM, Schofield-Robinson OJ, Smith AF. Videolaryngoscopy versus direct laryngoscopy

for adult patients requiring tracheal intubation: a Cochrane Systematic Review. *Br J Anaesth.* 2017;**119**(3):369–383.

22. Mahran EA, Hassan ME. Comparative randomised study of GlideScope. *Indian J Anaesth.* 2016;**60**(12):936–938.

23. Gaszyński T. The use of the C-MAC videolaryngoscope for awake intubation in patients with a predicted extremely difficult airway: case series. *Ther Clin Risk Manag.* 2018;**14**:539–542.

24. Alhomary M, Ramadan E, Curran E, Walsh SR. Videolaryngoscopy vs. fibreoptic bronchoscopy for awake tracheal intubation: a systematic review and meta-analysis. *Anaesthesia.* 2018;**73**(9):1151–1161.

25. Kitching E. Lasers and surgery. *BJA CEPD Rev.* 2003;**8**(5):143–146.

26. Stephens M, Montgomery J, Urquhart CS. Management of elective laryngectomy. *BJA Educ.* 2017;**17**(9):306–311.

27. Hanasono MM. Reconstructive surgery for head and neck cancer patients. *Adv Med.* 2014;**2014**:795483.

28. Ng W. Reconstructive options in head and neck surgery. *H K Med Diary.* 2007;**12**(7):14–16.

29. Kerawala C, Newlands C. *Oxford Specialist Handbooks in Oral and Maxillofacial Surgery*, 2nd ed. Oxford: Oxford University Press; 2014.

30. Chim H, Salgado CJ, Seselgyte R, Wei FC, Mardini S. Principles of head and neck reconstruction: an algorithm to guide flap selection. *Semin Plast Surg.* 2010;**24**(2):148–154.

31. Adams C, Charlton P. Anaesthesia for microvascular free tissue transfer. *BJA CEPD Rev.* 2003;**3**(2):33–37.

32. Eley KA, Young JD, Watt-Smith SR. Epinephrine, norepinephrine, dobutamine, and dopamine effects on free flap skin blood flow. *Plast Reconstr Surg.* 2012;**130**(3):564–570.

33. Siemionow M, Arslan E. Ischemia/reperfusion injury: a review in relation to free tissue transfers. *Microsurgery.* 2004;**24**(6):468–475.

34. Carroll WR, Esclamado RM. Ischemia/reperfusion injury in microvascular surgery. *Head Neck.* 2000;**22**(7):700–713.

35. Lee HJ, Kim JW, Choi SY, Kim CS, Kwon TG, Paeng JY. The evaluation of a scoring system in airway management after oral cancer surgery. *Maxillofac Plast Reconstr Surg.* 2015;**37**(1):19.

36. Cameron M, Corner A, Diba A, Hankins M. Development of a tracheostomy scoring system to guide airway management after major head and neck surgery. *Int J Oral Maxillofac Surg.* 2009;**38**(8):846–849.

37. Coyle MJ, Shrimpton A, Perkins C, Fasanmade A, Godden D. First do no harm: should routine tracheostomy after oral and maxillofacial oncological operations be abandoned? *Br J Oral Maxillofac Surg.* 2012;**50**(8):732–735.

38. Difficult Airway Society Extubation Guidelines Group, Popat M, Mitchell V, Dravid R, Patel A, Swampillai C, et al. Difficult Airway Society Guidelines for the management of tracheal extubation. *Anaesthesia.* 2012;**67**(3):318–340.

16

Postoperative care and planning

Joshua H. Atkins, Christopher H. Rassekh, and Andrew Herlich

Introduction

With all surgical procedures, postoperative management starts with a carefully prepared set of postoperative measures. This should begin with establishing clear patient expectations for trajectory of recovery, the likelihood and severity of potential complications (including oedema, oozing, nausea, haematoma, and ecchymosis), and the potential need for post-procedure mechanical ventilation or intensive care unit (ICU) monitoring. There are specific guidelines and order sets for many of the oromaxillofacial surgical (OMFS) procedures undertaken. This chapter discusses the general principles underlying postoperative management of OMFS patients, as well as outlining procedure-specific strategies. It is crucial to acknowledge the multidisciplinary nature of postoperative care and recognize the importance of team education and communication for the successful implementation of protocols, process improvements, and other care measures.

Enhanced Recovery After Surgery

The focus of the postoperative period is rapid patient recovery with the goal to return to baseline function and activities of daily living at the earliest possible time. Current realities in healthcare are focused on decreasing cost, increasing access to care, and improving quality as measured through the dual lenses of the qualitative patient experience and quantifiable metrics such as frequency and cost of complications, functional outcome, and length of stay. This defines the 'patient-centred' care model. Decreased length of stay in most cases pleases patients, families, and payers alike. It also frees up scarce inpatient resources for other patients. In the perioperative realm, Enhanced Recovery After Surgery (ERAS) is a focus of evidence-based quality improvement initiatives. ERAS programmes began with colorectal surgery and have rapidly expanded across most surgical specialities.[1] Interventions to date have been broad, and the relative contribution of any single element or bundle of elements to the outcome improvement remains poorly characterized. ERAS pathways focus heavily on multimodal analgesia, early mobilization, and optimization of volume status with goal-directed fluid resuscitation. Literature guidance is limited on how to approach ERAS for OMFS procedures. A recent meta-analysis of ERAS in head and neck free flap surgery included up to 17 potential ERAS pathway interventions and described great variation in application across a variety of surgical procedures. Preoperative carbohydrate loading, pharmacological thromboprophylaxis, perioperative antibiotics in clean-contaminated procedures, postoperative nausea and vomiting (PONV) prophylaxis, goal-directed fluid management, opioid-sparing multimodal analgesia, frequent flap monitoring, early mobilization, and the minimization of preoperative fasting may all contribute in various ways.[2] Overall, clinical data generally support a decreased length of stay resulting from well-implemented ERAS protocols, but data on the long-term goals of improved functional outcomes are lacking.[3] These would include earlier return to work or primary activities of daily living, higher satisfaction with care, and decreased postoperative cognitive dysfunction or impairment. ERAS is an area that catalyses the anaesthetist to assume the role of perioperative physician and coordinator with the goal of integrating multiple disciplines and potential care approaches into a unified pathway. Where possible, careful consideration of new evidence for the development of procedure-specific and resource-appropriate ERAS protocols should be considered. The ERAS Society (https://erassociety.org) and Evidence Based Perioperative Medicine (https://ebpom.org) are two multidisciplinary organizations working to evaluate, distil, and apply evidence regarding perioperative optimization interventions and maintain updated resources on the subject.

A critical aspect of ERAS is the identification of anaemia and its optimization for surgery. Postoperative morbidity and mortality are increased in the face of intraoperative transfusion. A consensus statement published in 2017 made several important and practical suggestions with respect to anaemia and avoidance of transfusion. A best practice care plan of nine points is simply and practically identified.[4] Other work reaffirmed the recommended approach to diagnosis, treatment, and its conclusions.[5] Anaemia is defined as a haemoglobin level <130 g/L and the aetiology should be investigated. The mean corpuscular volume can be used to categorize the type of anaemia as either normocytic, microcytic, or megaloblastic anaemia. A normocytic anaemia indicates chronic disease or acute haemorrhage. A megaloblastic anaemia is likely related to vitamin B_{12} deficiency or folate deficiency (a rather less frequent cause of anaemia). However, the most common form of anaemia is a microcytic anaemia and is generally due to iron deficiency (although other causes do exist). Iron deficiency may be specifically identified by measuring serum ferritin and transferrin levels. If an inflammatory cause of this type of anaemia is suspected, a C-reactive protein level will assist in the diagnostic process. Investigation (and treatment) should be initiated immediately upon the decision to operate, and elective surgery should be postponed until treatment with oral iron has corrected the problem (which may take up to 6–8 weeks). Patients who are intolerant of oral iron, or in whom faster correction is warranted, may also receive intravenous iron. Correction of anaemia prior to urgent or emergency surgery may not be possible, such that intraoperative transfusion may be required. Transfusion should usually not take place unless there is a haemoglobin level of <70 g/L. In the case of minimally invasive cranial base surgery, this surgical approach has reduced the requirement for blood transfusion. However, the benefit of preoperative treatment of anaemia is less clear in patients with squamous cell carcinoma of the head and neck—where overall survival has been shown to be worse in patients where anaemia was corrected preoperatively (including with blood transfusion).[6]

Postoperative levels of care and monitoring

The provision of appropriate levels of postoperative nursing care and monitoring are important considerations in postoperative planning. In general, it is preferable for patients to receive postoperative care on a ward dedicated to OMFS and head and neck patients. Experienced clinical staff are more likely to recognize specialty-specific complications early, are more comfortable with critical tasks such as tracheostomy care, drain management, and neurological and vascular flap checks, and are more likely to escalate care at the appropriate time. They may also be more familiar with and adherent to procedure-specific and emergency rescue protocols. Standard electronic order sets can be generated and modified to individual patients, while still adhering to generally agreed care pathways (Fig. 16.1). Procedure- or patient-specific alerts can also be incorporated into order sets as reminders to enter or adjust specific orders.

The decision on the most appropriate level of postoperative care facility (including ICU) should always be based on multidisciplinary discussion between the anaesthetist and surgical team.[7] The availability of necessary skills and resources outside the ICU, including step-down units, must be considered. Failure to rescue (due to *failure to recognize*) can have an important contribution to morbidity, and may directly relate to the lack of familiarity of clinical staff in the post-procedure unit with the type, signs and symptoms, and trajectory of potential complications—even when the patient is in the ICU; for example, a cardiothoracic ICU team may be less likely to

identify incipient uncal herniation than an experienced neurosurgical ward team.

There is little evidence to support a default critical care pathway for major OMFS patients—a retrospective analysis revealed low utilization of critical care services by patients undergoing head and neck cancer surgery, and did not identify any causes of complications leading to the use of critical care services.[8] Risk factors for complications include bilateral neck dissection, an Acute Physiology And Chronic Health Evaluation II (APACHE II) score >10, massive blood transfusion, early postoperative complications requiring further surgery under general anaesthesia, history of smoking, and perioperative antibiotic choice. In addition, obstructive sleep apnoea syndrome (OSAS) is a common comorbid condition in OMFS patients and requires careful planning. When OSAS is moderate to severe, surgery on the airway or mandibular advancement has been performed, or when use of significant postoperative opioid analgesia is planned, careful consideration should be given to enhanced respiratory monitoring in a high-acuity setting.[9]

Anaesthetic considerations

Postoperative normothermia is important for wound healing, haemostasis, patient comfort, and to reduce metabolic demands.[10] This may be especially relevant after free-flap reconstruction and in patients with cardiopulmonary comorbidities. A post-anaesthesia care unit (PACU) target temperature of 36.0°C has been established as a quality standard in many countries. Active forced air warming and elevated ambient room temperature are the most effective postoperative interventions.

Patients who present with oromaxillofacial and head and neck cancers may have a history of significant, regular alcohol consumption and smoking. Such patients are at substantial risk of acute alcohol withdrawal in the perioperative period. Preoperative assessment should include screening questions about alcohol use and nutritional status. Preoperative alcohol detoxification should be seriously considered and be implemented whenever possible. Attention to this detail should be thought of as part of the overall prehabilitation and optimization of the patient. Perioperative benzodiazepine administration should be considered along with monitoring for signs and symptoms of acute withdrawal. Acute nicotine withdrawal may also contribute to agitation and can be treated with transdermal patches. In either case, intraoperative use of dexmedetomidine can be helpful in attenuating acute withdrawal, as well as ameliorating perioperative agitation. Early removal of urinary catheters will also reduce agitation.

PONV is particularly important to avoid after OMFS and head and neck surgery as repeated Valsalva events can disrupt delicate haemostasis and lead to life-threatening bleeding. Airway

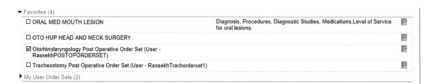

Fig. 16.1 Example of a standard order set menu that can be used for OMFS and head and neck procedures, which can be modified according to the individual patient.

obstruction and pulmonary aspiration is a particular concern in patients with intermaxillary fixation or those who have undergone surgery in the oropharynx that may impair protective reflexes. Multimodal prophylaxis with a serotonin 5-HT$_3$ antagonist with or without dexamethasone (if not contraindicated) should be routine. Total intravenous anaesthesia also reduces PONV. For higher-risk patients (except the elderly), a transdermal hyoscine patch can be added but will result in decreased saliva production. This may exacerbate pre-existing xerostomia and should be avoided in procedures such as sialendoscopy or those involving salivary duct reconstruction where salivary flow should be maintained. For intractable PONV (despite all of the above interventions), oral aprepitant, a neurokinin-1 receptor antagonist, may also be considered. Refractory post-procedure PONV can be treated with haloperidol, prochlorperazine, promethazine, or low-dose propofol depending on the clinical circumstances, the patient's age, and other comorbidities. Where possible, medications with sedative side effects should be avoided in the elderly and those with a history of cognitive impairment.

Oral hygiene

Oral hygiene requires meticulous attention in the postoperative period, and maintenance of oral hygiene in the postoperative period is a hallmark of early recovery. Gentle irrigation with chlorhexidine will help reduce inflammation and possible local infection after maxillary or mandibular surgery. In the case of surgery beyond simple exodontia, brushing of the teeth should be gentle and is easily augmented with oral chlorhexidine 0.014% rinses (several times per day, for the first week). Regimens of benzethonium chloride and hydrogen peroxide have also been described.[11]

Tissue oedema

Irrespective of the type of surgery, postoperative oedema is expected to a lesser or greater extent. The degree of oedema is largely dependent upon the duration of the procedure, the invasiveness of the procedure, and the care by which tissues have been handled. Factors that may be modified by the anaesthetist include volume and type of intravenous fluids administered during surgery (i.e. avoiding large volumes of crystalloid or hypotonic fluids), the incline of the operating table, as well as the timing of intravenous corticosteroid administration. However, postoperatively, the patient should be nursed in the semi-Fowler's position (or more erect if tolerated). Cold packs, facial compression dressings, and care to avoid restriction of venous drainage are additional factors in oedema reduction. Early ambulation is also important in that it promotes peripheral fluid recruitment and excretion.

Cognitive recovery

The American Society of Anesthesiologists launched a Brain Health Initiative (https://www.asahq.org/brainhealthinitiative) to address the growing recognition that a subset of patients have impaired cognition after surgery and anaesthesia. This can present as delirium and/or memory and executive function problems. Although often self-limiting, in some patients this postoperative cognitive dysfunction progresses to long-term cognitive decline.[12] The pathophysiology of this process is poorly understood. Older patients and those with a history of dementia, alcohol abuse, and other neurological disorders (e.g. Parkinson's disease) are at highest risk. At the very least, patients and their families should be counselled regarding this potential complication. Avoiding excessive depth of anaesthesia with processed electroencephalogram monitoring, use of total intravenous anaesthesia, and avoidance of known associative agents such as benzodiazepines may be important. Interdisciplinary communication and shared decision-making as to appropriate interventions for sedation, analgesia, and anxiolysis should be emphasized. Providers are urged to monitor the scientific literature for new recommendations and to consider development of multidisciplinary clinical pathways for patients at risk.

Difficult airway identification

Many health systems have adopted a difficult airway identification system. In most instances, the system involves placement of a difficult airway identity bracelet and an electronic alert in the medical record system on any admitted patient with a known difficult airway, provision of an algorithm or specialized rescue system with equipment[13] for airway emergencies, and a mechanism to communicate the successful initial airway approach that is readily accessible in an emergency. Most centres have a difficult airway trolley, and some have a difficult airway response team with surgical airway equipment for management of any patient with a difficult airway status. Factors such as airway mass, friable airway tissue, intermaxillary fixation, previous radiation therapy to the head and neck, trismus, and risk of haematoma impacting the airway are all common in OMFS patients. In settings where high-risk airways are routine (e.g. transoral robotic surgery, TORS), clear protocols should be in place for emergency surgical airway, and teamwork drills should be regularly conducted to refresh crisis management skills and protocol familiarity.

Consideration should be given to designating select OMFS patients as having difficult airways in the postoperative period. This is particularly true for procedures involving the jaw or airway. Extubation guidelines are just as important as intubation.[13] Even if prior airway management at induction of anaesthesia was straightforward, postsurgical reintubation in the ward may be challenging or impossible due to oedema, bleeding, or surgery-related anatomical changes. After some surgical procedures, tracheal extubation is delayed for airway protection in order to allow oedema to subside. Occasionally, a temporary tracheostomy may be used. We recommend a system to identify 'high-risk extubation' patients, minimizing the risk of inadvertent early extubation, and facilitating appropriate planning and intervention should unplanned extubation occur. This might include a red 'high-risk extubation' sticker placed on the pilot balloon of the tracheal tube or more formal documentation of an extubation and reintubation plan and banner warning alerts in the medical records. Examples of such procedures would be when a patient's trachea remains intubated after a transoral (robotic or laser) posterior hemiglossectomy or supraglottic laryngectomy.

Analgesia

Analgesic needs vary depending upon the procedure undertaken. The analgesic regimen must take into consideration the surgical site, patient expectations, medical history (including chronic use of opioids or chronic pain), sleep-disordered breathing, concomitant use of synergistic medications such as benzodiazepines, and liver and kidney disease that may influence drug bioavailability, metabolism, and excretion. Chronic postsurgical pain is a common, yet underdiagnosed syndrome, which may be lessened by appropriate preventive and multimodal analgesia in the immediate perioperative period.[14] The increase in chronic prescription opioid use and dependence, particularly in the UK and North America, is an evolving challenge to optimal perioperative pain control. Patients with chronic pain and concurrent use of high-dose opioids may benefit from preoperative counselling and assessment by a pain specialist in conjunction with the surgeon and anaesthesia team. Unrealistic patient expectations may contribute significantly to patient dissatisfaction and may cause clinicians to be overly aggressive with analgesic dosing, thereby increasing the risks. The American Pain Society has published consensus guidelines for the management of surgical pain.[15] Consideration may be given to tapering of opioid medications in the preoperative period if this is feasible. Otherwise, the usual dose of opioid medication should be maintained up to the beginning of surgery, including the doses on the day of the procedure. The involvement of the pain specialist in perioperative planning may facilitate patient-controlled analgesia dose titration and conversion of intravenous opioid medications to an oral analgesic regimen suited to outpatient use in preparation for discharge. In most situations, due to the risks of opioid-related respiratory depression, a basal infusion on the patient-controlled analgesia is not recommended.

Multimodal analgesia is currently the standard approach for many surgical procedures, with the emphasis on patients' recovery profile, reduced opioid use, and reduced opioid-related side effects.[16] This is especially true in patients with a complex history of chronic pain, opioid use, morbid obesity, or OSAS for whom the risks of opioid-related complications are high (especially for outpatient procedures and procedures involving the airway). Despite some supporting evidence, there continues to be contradictory data suggesting that multimodal approaches, at least in spinal surgery, have minimal benefit on analgesia specifically.[17] A major concern in many OMFS procedures is postoperative bleeding and haematoma formation. The surgical site is often highly vascular, and small volumes of bleeding can result in substantial morbidity—particularly if the haematoma causes airway compromise. For this reason, there is a reluctance to use non-steroidal anti-inflammatory medications in the immediate perioperative period, even though the absolute risk of bleeding is small.[18] COX-2 selective non-steroidal anti-inflammatory drugs (coxibs) are a popular alternative as they have similar analgesic efficacy with no inhibition of platelet function. Paracetamol has a good safety profile in normal dosing and is available in oral, rectal, and intravenous formulations.[19] Paracetamol exerts its analgesic effects via multiple mechanisms

and can be co-administered with coxibs.[20,21] Oral bioavailability is high and the oral or nasogastric route is preferred if possible.[22] Perioperative infusions of adjuvant medications such as lidocaine, ketamine, and dexmedetomidine have been studied for a variety of surgical procedures. Dexmedetomidine can augment analgesia, facilitate maintenance of blood pressure at lower levels (to reduce haematoma formation and oedema), and reduce risk of withdrawal or agitation in alcohol-dependent patients. Protocols for the continuation of these medications in the PACU, ward, or ICU can be considered. The use of continuous infusions of lidocaine in the immediate perioperative period for reduction in acute surgical pain is relatively recent and the evidence base is limited. Data from small studies continue to emerge, though significant concerns exist regarding its safety.[23,24] Hypothesized mechanisms include direct blockade of voltage-gated sodium channels, modulation of wide-dynamic nociceptive neurons through glycine receptors, and modulation of proinflammatory signalling pathways.[25,26] Opioid sparing, more rapid recovery of bowel function, decreased nausea and vomiting, and enhanced cognitive recovery have all been reported with lidocaine infusions. However, there has been limited investigation in procedures specific to OMFS. A typical approach is a loading dose of 1.5–2 mg/kg and an infusion of 1–2 mg/kg/hr (with a maximum dose based on ideal body weight). In some institutions, the infusion is continued at a modestly reduced dose for up to 48 hours postoperatively.[26] Plasma levels can demonstrate wide ranges and the use of ideal body weight is therefore preferable to reduce risk.[27] Caution should be exercised if significant infiltration of supplemental local anaesthesia by the surgeons is anticipated or in patients with low albumin levels, reduced ejection fraction, impaired liver function, intrinsic or pharmacological cardiac conduction disorders, and in extremes of age. Ketamine exerts analgesic effects through multiple mechanisms, but mainly via antagonist action at the glutamate N-methyl-D-aspartate (NMDA) receptor. Ketamine may contribute to preventive analgesia by modulating ascending nociceptive signalling pathways when given early. The dissociative side effects appear to be rare at the doses used for adjuvant anaesthesia and, in fact, the drug may have positive effects on mood. Most regimens entail a pre-emptive bolus followed by a continuous infusion that may be continued into the postoperative period. Ketamine may be particularly useful in patients with a history of neuropathic pain or chronic opioid use. Gabapentin and pregabalin are neuromodulatory medications with slightly different side effect profiles which may also improve perioperative analgesia.[28,29] Both drugs are commonly used in the treatment of neuropathic pain. Side effects include dizziness, sedation, blurred vision, and less commonly nausea or vomiting. These effects should be considered in patient selection for perioperative adjuvant use, particularly in vulnerable populations such as the elderly. Perioperative gabapentin has been studied in various head and neck-related surgical procedures with a very modest reduction in 24-hour opioid use demonstrated on meta-analysis.[30] Preoperative doses were large, ranging from 600 mg to 1200 mg in a single dose, that in some cases was continued into the postoperative period.

Regional anaesthesia through targeted nerve blocks and field block infiltration are important components of the multimodal postoperative analgesic plan.[31] Techniques include anterior, superior, and middle alveolar nerve blocks, greater palatine and nasopalatine nerve blocks, and local infiltration of the palate. Availability of ultrasound for targeted blocks is increasing the number and options of regional approaches for OMFS procedures.

Obstructive sleep apnoea syndrome

OSAS is increasingly common in all surgical patients, though still frequently goes undiagnosed. However, of any surgical specialty, oromaxillofacial surgeons are likely to have a higher index of suspicion, arising from a greater exposure and awareness of the disease. New surgical approaches for OSAS have evolved, including TORS, tongue base resection, palatopharyngoplasty, and tonsillectomy, as well as implantation of genioglossus nerve stimulators.[32,33] This has resulted in an increasing number of patients with OSAS presenting for surgery. Growing evidence suggests that patients with undiagnosed OSAS are at the highest risk of perioperative complications.[34] A formal sleep study remains the gold standard for OSAS diagnosis. The STOP-BANG tool is a validated bedside screening tool that should be used preoperatively to assess most OMFS surgical patients.[35] A STOP-BANG score of ≥ 5 correlates with a substantial risk of the patient having moderate to severe OSAS. The threshold for specialist management (and nature of the postoperative care facility) should be adjusted to local resources.

Continuous positive airway pressure (CPAP) is the mainstay in OSAS therapy. Anaesthesia and, especially, opioid medications can have a profound impact on OSAS in the perioperative period, yet perioperative use of CPAP may be restricted due to the nature of the OMFS procedure, for example, after sinusotomy, concern may exist about the potential for pneumocephalus with CPAP use. A survey of practising surgeons demonstrated wide variation in when to restart CPAP, with severity of OSAS and extent of surgery considered to be significant factors.[36] Similarly, after TORS, concern about air tracking into the mediastinum generally favours avoidance of CPAP immediately postoperatively. A perioperative plan for resumption of CPAP should therefore be formally discussed by the multidisciplinary team. For nasal/sinus surgery, intraoperative endoscope-guided placement of a nasopharyngeal airway across the defect (sutured in place) can be considered. This allows positive pressure airway support as needed. In extreme cases, consideration should be given to elective tracheostomy for perioperative management. International guidelines have attempted to address questions related to periprocedural monitoring and the appropriateness of outpatient surgery in patients with OSAS.[37,38] There is no universal consensus, and options for monitoring include continuous pulse oximetry, capnography, step-down or ICU level care, and non-invasive minute ventilation.[38] The disadvantages of additional monitoring—principally cost/resource allocation and false-alarms/alarm fatigue—should be weighed up against the benefits of closer surveillance of patients' physiological status. The decision to use additional monitoring modalities must be tailored to local resources, individual patients' conditions, the nature of the surgery, the planned use of postoperative opioids, and the ability to use post-procedure CPAP. Wherever possible, CPAP should be reinitiated in the PACU. Discharge from the PACU is a similarly complicated issue, with limited evidence to guide decision-making. Patients with diagnosed or suspected (untreated) severe OSAS with poorly characterized or poorly controlled comorbid conditions (hypertension, diabetes, and chronic obstructive pulmonary disease), and those

where CPAP is precluded in the postoperative period, should be considered for in-hospital admission for all but the most minor of procedures (if general anaesthesia has been undertaken and opioids will be necessary for postoperative pain control). An extended stay in the PACU or in-hospital admission should be considered after planned ambulatory surgery if there have been repetitive oxygen desaturations or frequent apnoea events in the PACU. This may be particularly important in cases of sedation/analgesia mismatch.

Venous thromboprophylaxis

Most moderate to major OMFS procedures are associated with a level of risk of venous thromboembolism that necessitates routine thromboprophylaxis.[39] Subcutaneous low-molecular-weight heparin and sequential calf compression devices are standard measures, and should be continued until the patient is ambulatory. Sequential compression devices should not be used in the presence of atherosclerosis of the lower extremities. For most procedures, aspirin can be resumed immediately postoperatively, although caution is required following airway surgery (when there has been no covering tracheostomy) due to concerns that even minor bleeding in an oedematous airway could precipitate an emergency.[40,41] Most patients who have undergone free flap reconstructions are placed on aspirin, but they also often have a tracheostomy. Patients on long-term anticoagulants are increasingly common, presenting a challenge for perioperative management—particularly those with coronary artery disease and cardiac stents requiring dual antiplatelet therapy. In general, there is a trend towards continuing patients on their anticoagulants and accepting the greater likelihood of bleeding, rather than risking life-threatening cardiac stent occlusion—though this depends on the type of stent, how long it has been in place, and the individual surgical risk (cardiac risk assessment and management is discussed in detail in Chapter 1).[42]

Perioperative nutrition

Optimizing nutritional status is a critical element of preparation for surgery and postoperative recovery. Patients with oromaxillofacial and head and neck cancer often have preoperative malnutrition with associated hypoalbuminemia and anaemia. Preoperative dietician consultation and prehabilitation should be considered, along with optimization of anaemia (as previously discussed in the ERAS section). Lesions may impair preoperative oral intake due to pain or dysphagia, and surgery may breach the oropharyngeal mucosa or impair pharyngeal function and airway protective reflexes, increasing the risk of aspiration postoperatively. Enteral nutrition via a post-pyloric nasogastric tube (placed during surgery) is routinely used for patients undergoing laryngectomy and TORS. For patients who are unable to speak or swallow without aspiration risk, placement of a percutaneous endoscopic gastrostomy (PEG) or jejunostomy (J-tube) is necessary for feeding. For patients expected to have delayed recovery of swallowing following major OMFS procedures, or for those who have endoscopy followed by chemoradiation, a PEG is usually the best option and can be done at the time of endoscopy or at the time of surgery (depending on the degree of nutritional impairment). Even in patients with a PEG, it is important to continue with some oral intake if possible, as the long-term success of oral dietary rehabilitation is improved in patients who maintain swallowing function despite requiring supplemental nutrition via a feeding tube. In some cases, a PEG tube is best placed preoperatively, particularly in those undergoing major resections with the risk of pharyngocutaneous fistula or aspiration, as they are unlikely to recommence oral intake for a significant period of time. Evaluation of speech and swallowing should be an early part of routine postoperative care for any such procedures.

Neurological sequelae

Cranial nerve injuries following OMFS procedures can be associated with significant morbidity, but fortunately, are quite rare.[43] Injuries to the cranial nerves II, III, VI, and VII have all been reported (both in isolation and in combination). The majority of injuries resolve, but permanent blindness can occur.[44,45] Certain intraoperative monitoring modalities can be employed to tailor the anaesthetic technique, and to detect/avoid excessive hyperextension or flexion positions—these include somatosensory evoked potentials, electromyography, and brainstem auditory evoked potentials. Electromyography monitoring can be used for cranial nerves that have a motor component, such as cranial nerves III–VII and IX–XII, and is most commonly used for monitoring laryngeal function during thyroid surgery and facial nerve function during parotid surgery.[46] Brainstem auditory evoked potentials have been routinely used during skull base surgery. Such monitoring modalities are now incorporated in the American Academy of Otolaryngology-Head and Neck Surgery recommendations.[47] Unfortunately, neurological complications are not always apparent in the immediate postoperative period, and may only become evident as the patient regains full consciousness several days later.[48]

Perioperative antimicrobials

The use of perioperative antibiotics for orthognathic surgery is quite common. The wounds are classified as clean, but contaminated, in that the oral mucosa has been transected, and the nasal mucosa has also been exposed during nasotracheal intubation. The choice of antibiotic and duration of therapy depends on the individual risk, but generally, antibiotics are discontinued after 24 hours. The presence of active infection, or the need for complex reconstruction involving bone grafts and implants, may elongate any prescribed course. Infected, contaminated wounds clearly require more aggressive intravenous antibiotic therapy, which may entail not only Gram-positive but also anaerobic and Gram-negative cover. Wound cultures are helpful, and the input from a microbiology/infectious disease specialist is advisable. Other influencing factors on antibiotic cover include patient comorbidities such as diabetes and immunosuppression, and the extent of any oromaxillofacial cancer.

Procedure-specific considerations

Tracheostomy

Tracheostomy is often performed in conjunction with other procedures, but sometimes in isolation. There are two major subsets of patients who undergo tracheostomy: those who have an oromaxillofacial or airway-specific problem, and those who have a systemic problem requiring a prolonged period of mechanical ventilation and airway toilet. The guidelines vary slightly for these two groups. It takes approximately 3–5 days for the tract between the skin and the tracheal mucosa to mature. Newly formed tracheostomies should be carefully secured, for example, by a pair of 2-0 Prolene® sutures bilaterally, in addition to a tracheostomy tie or securing device, for at least 3 days. For patients with free flap reconstructions, tracheostomy ties are avoided so as not to compress blood vessels and only sutures are used. For high-risk patients, this period of close fixation may be extended significantly (though for most patients, 5 days is ample). In most settings, a cuffed tracheostomy tube is placed at the time of surgery to facilitate mechanical ventilation and secretion management in the immediate postoperative period. For most adult surgical patients, a size 6.0 mm internal diameter cuffed tracheostomy tube is sufficient, with the cuff being left inflated for the first 24 hours postoperatively. Thereafter, the cuff can be deflated if the patient is suitable (it is advisable to have suction ready for the first time the cuff is deflated as secretions often accumulate above the cuff). On postoperative day 3, if the tracheostomy site is not felt to be high risk, the cuffed tube can usually be exchanged for an uncuffed tube, and in some cases, downsized to a size 4.0 mm tracheostomy tube. Again, depending on the patient, a cap or a Passy–Muir valve may be placed. If the patient requires ongoing mechanical ventilation, the tracheostomy tube change is delayed until the cuff is no longer required. The tracheostomy formed is dependent on local preferences, but a Björk flap (an inverted U-flap of tracheal cartilage sutured to the skin) is useful in facilitating the reinsertion of the tracheostomy tube (in event of dislodgement). A stay (rescue) suture is an alternative measure. For morbidly obese patients or patients with short necks, where access to the trachea is difficult, a Shiley™ XLT (Medtronic, Minneapolis, US) extended-length tracheostomy tube may be used and, in general, a longer period of time is allowed before tube changes. On changing the tracheostomy tube for the first time, the stoma site and tract should be assessed, and if it appears safe for future tube reinsertions to be done by staff other than the surgical team, the sutures can be removed, and the tracheostomy tube secured with soft Velcro™ ties. Where there is a free flap, a decision can be made at this point whether to re-suture the tube or to use ties if the early risk of venous compression is considered to have passed. The relatively straightforward OMFS patient with a tracheostomy may be discharged from hospital at this time, if there are no other ongoing medical requirements (dependent on local policies and practices). Plans for home tracheostomy care and suction appliances must be in place prior to discharge, and additional support/training may be needed. Most patients can eat after tracheostomy. However, while a tracheostomy can facilitate pulmonary toilet if there is aspiration, it can also cause dysphagia (and even aspiration) by one of several mechanisms (Box 16.1). A standard set of postoperative orders for tracheostomy management should be in place and can be modified according to the individual patient circumstances (Fig. 16.2).

During the early postoperative period, inadvertent removal of the tracheostomy tube may result in the inability to reidentify the tracheotomy site and subsequent loss of airway. Dislodgement may occur due to inadequate sedation in an agitated patient, during vigorous suctioning or coughing, or during patient turning (pressure

Box 16.1 Causes of dysphagia related to tracheostomies

- Tethering of the laryngeal rotation and elevation.
- Inadequate subglottic pressure needed to expectorate.
- Pain limiting patient swallowing and cough.
- Compression of the oesophagus by the cuff.
- Reduced vocal cord closure reflex.
- Decreased sensation of pharynx and larynx.
- Weakening of the laryngeal muscles.

area management) by nursing staff, especially if the tracheostomy tube has only been advanced a short distance into the trachea due to excessive tissue between the skin and the trachea. As mentioned previously, a Björk flap can facilitate rescue of a displaced fresh tracheostomy. Similarly, in patients with a large neck circumference due to adipose tissue, surgical debulking of the pretracheal tissue near the tracheotomy site will reduce the distance from skin to trachea. This may reduce both the risk of accidental dislodgement and facilitate surgical re-exploration if necessary. In extreme cases, multiple skin flaps may be required to form a fully epithelialized tract to ensure formation of a safe tracheostomy and facilitate tracheostomy replacement. Loss of airway is the most serious post-tracheostomy complication. Tracheostomy-related airway emergencies are not infrequent and have three main causes: tube dislodgement, mucous plugging, and bleeding. These problems are more frequent in patients whose tracheostomies were performed for systemic conditions (rather than temporary surgical cover), and are more likely to have a worse outcome due to comorbid disease and lack of physiological reserve. The UK National Tracheostomy Safety Project (http://www.tracheostomy.org.uk/) sets out a framework for improving quality and safety of tracheostomy management, which can be adapted to local resources and requirements.[49] The programme focuses on education of providers, covering the fundamentals of tracheostomy care, and the assessment and management of tracheostomy emergencies (including a mobile reference app). It highlights the importance of clear communication of the details of the surgical procedure using bedside signs—including the model of tracheostomy tube, the location and type of stay sutures, and the surgical approach (site and type of tracheostomy), so that it is clearly accessible to all postoperative care providers. The accompanying emergency algorithm for the management of a displaced tracheostomy (acute or chronic) should also be displayed, and staff should undergo frequent training using the algorithm. Similar signs and algorithms also exist for laryngectomies. The standardized bedside signs and algorithms can be modified to local institutions and practices (Figs 16.3 and 16.4). In the event of a suspected displaced or

blocked tracheostomy, assessment of tracheostomy patency should occur as the first step, and always precede any attempt at positive pressure ventilation. Patency is most reliably assessed by checking for end-tidal carbon dioxide followed by passage of a suction catheter or a fibreoptic scope through the lumen of the tube. Listening or feeling for air exchange through or around the tracheostomy (with the cuff up and down) may also assist in assessing adequacy of spontaneous ventilation. Attempted positive pressure ventilation through a dislodged tracheostomy will produce mediastinal air and may result in further patient deterioration.

Humidification of supplemental oxygen in the postoperative period is crucial, to minimize mucous plugging—a frequent problem that can cause an airway emergency by obstructing the tube. Inability to pass a suction catheter can be indicative of dislodgement or a mucous plug (though other causes do exist). In the presence of end-tidal carbon dioxide via the tracheostomy tube, partial obstruction is the more likely cause. To prevent mucus plugging, frequent tracheostomy suctioning is advised—usually at least once every 6 hours, though shorter intervals may be required dependent on the extent of secretions. In addition, saline bullets or nebulizers can reduce drying of secretions and consolidation of plugs. In the event of an adverse respiratory event (e.g. oxygen desaturation) that does not respond to suctioning, an airway rapid response team (Box 16.2) should be immediately activated. Simple removal of the inner cannula of the tracheostomy will alleviate the blockage in many cases. However, sometimes the tracheostomy tube itself must be removed to clear secretions—flexible bronchoscopy can be particularly beneficial in this instance, in preventing creation of a false passage on reinsertion of the tracheostomy tube and loss of airway control. Re-intubation of the trachea from above should always be considered if there is difficulty reinserting the tracheostomy tube during an episode of plugging or failure to ventilate via the tracheostomy. During attempts to restore patency and adequate oxygenation/ventilation, oxygen should be delivered via the upper airway (facemask/supraglottic airway) and via the tracheostomy stoma (unless a laryngectomy, rather than tracheostomy has been performed—laryngectomy patients are 'neck-only breathers').

Bleeding from a tracheostomy can also be an airway emergency—especially in the case of a tracheo-innominate artery fistula (TIF, or TIAF). Immediate management consists of inflating the tracheostomy cuff or the cuff of a tracheal tube at the site in an attempt to tamponade the bleeding, followed by prompt surgical exploration. Patients at risk of TIF can sometimes be identified at the time of surgery or in the immediate postoperative period, evidenced by pulsation of the tube itself or within the tissues immediately surrounding the tube, suggesting the close proximity of a major artery. Surgical teams should indicate clearly if they think the

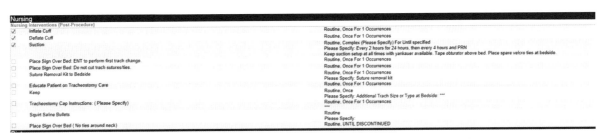

Fig. 16.2 Example of a tracheostomy nursing order set. Default orders can be selected and modified as required.

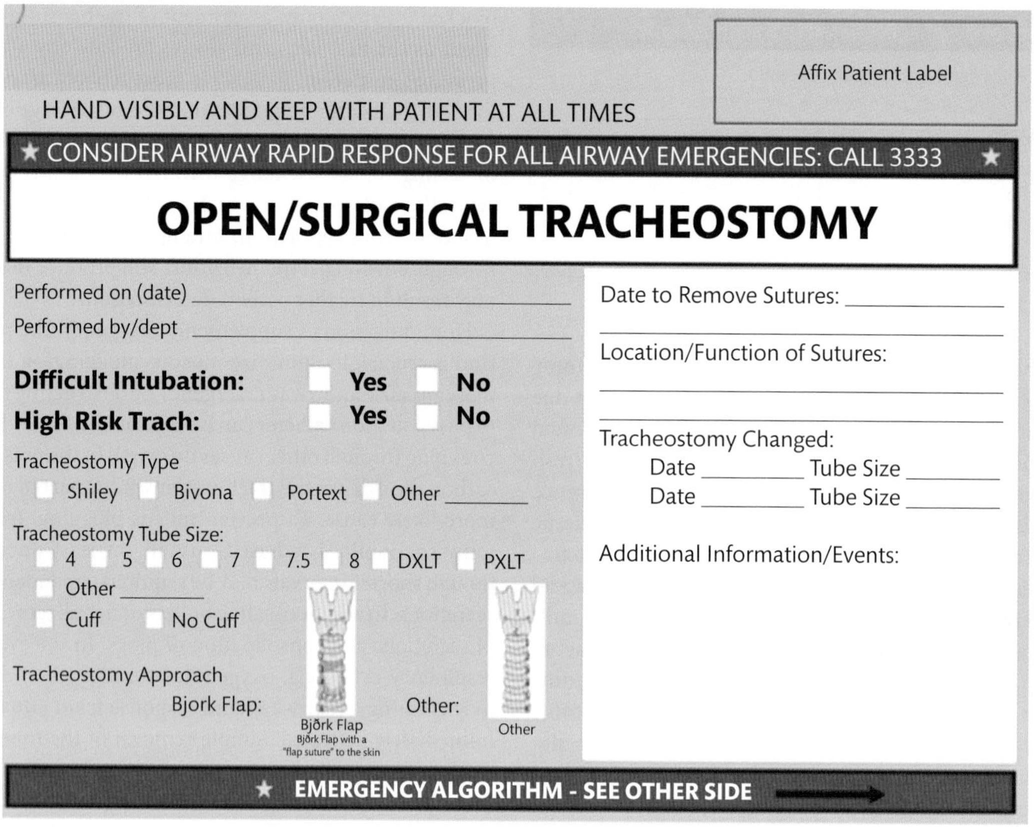

HAND VISIBLY AND KEEP WITH PATIENT AT ALL TIMES

Affix Patient Label

★ CONSIDER AIRWAY RAPID RESPONSE FOR ALL AIRWAY EMERGENCIES: CALL 3333 ★

OPEN/SURGICAL TRACHEOSTOMY

Performed on (date) _____
Performed by/dept _____

Difficult Intubation: ☐ Yes ☐ No
High Risk Trach: ☐ Yes ☐ No

Tracheostomy Type
☐ Shiley ☐ Bivona ☐ Portext ☐ Other _____

Tracheostomy Tube Size:
☐ 4 ☐ 5 ☐ 6 ☐ 7 ☐ 7.5 ☐ 8 ☐ DXLT ☐ PXLT
☐ Other _____
☐ Cuff ☐ No Cuff

Tracheostomy Approach
Bjork Flap: Other:

Björk Flap
Björk Flap with a
"flap suture" to the skin

Other

Date to Remove Sutures: _____

Location/Function of Sutures:
_____
_____

Tracheostomy Changed:
Date _____ Tube Size _____
Date _____ Tube Size _____

Additional Information/Events:

★ EMERGENCY ALGORITHM - SEE OTHER SIDE ➡

Fig. 16.3 Adapted Tracheostomy UK bedside signs used to convey critical information about the type and age of the tracheostomy, model and size of tube, and position of any sutures.

tracheostomy tube is 'low lying', and generally the risk is avoided by formation of tracheostomies between the second and third tracheal rings (occasionally, an even more superiorly placed site is chosen, accepting the higher risk of laryngeal complications). If a TIF is suspected following a controlled 'sentinel' bleed, a computed tomography angiogram can be obtained to confirm the diagnosis. If a TIF presents with massive bleeding, the airway rapid response team should be activated immediately as it may be necessary to intubate the trachea from above, while applying digital pressure to the artery via the tracheostomy site. This digital pressure must be maintained until exploration can be undertaken, and often necessitates the team member's finger to be 'prepped' into the surgical field. A cardiothoracic surgeon is likely to be required for the surgical management, so they must be notified immediately. The blood transfusion laboratory should also be notified, as part of a massive haemorrhage protocol.

An important, delayed, complication of tracheostomies is tracheal stenosis, which is associated with significant morbidity. Stenosis is secondary to chronic inflammation from the presence of the tube and cuff within the trachea. Overinflation of the cuff can also cause ischaemic injury, leading to subsequent stenosis or tracheomalacia. Constant movement of the tube, which commonly results from movement of the patient's head and neck while they remain connected to the ventilator via a breathing circuit, can also contribute to the inflammatory process. Consequently, the breathing circuit should be appropriately supported to minimize the movement of the tracheostomy tube within the trachea.

Transoral robotic surgery

TORS is a treatment utilized for oropharyngeal cancer and for CPAP-resistant OSAS in select patients.[50,51] TORS resection is associated with reduced morbidity, faster recovery, and the avoidance of PEG feeding. Post-TORS airway emergencies usually relate to bleeding or swelling. Patients with a previous history of difficult airway management/difficult laryngeal exposure, prior laryngeal radiation, and/or significant resection of the epiglottis are routinely left intubated for 48–72 hours after surgery, or undergo tracheostomy if especially high risk. Postoperative medical and nursing teams must be prepared for, and well-drilled in, the emergency management of the post-TORS bleed—which necessitates clear communication and rapid and appropriate escalation, in preparation for an emergency bedside surgical airway and immediate return to the operating theatre. Consequently, TORS should only be performed at institutions where the necessary airway and surgical expertise is immediately available. Patients must also be educated in the importance of reporting promptly to the closest emergency department in the event of a suspected airway issue or bleeding.

TORS is typically preceded by a neck dissection during which arterial 'feeders' to the oropharynx can be ligated, and this may reduce the risk of postoperative bleeding. CPAP is generally not reinitiated in the OSAS patients for some time following TORS due to the potential risk of pneumomediastinum if a pharyngo-cervical fistula is present—the first sign of which may be the presence of subcutaneous emphysema. The association between the timing of the neck dissection relative to the TORS procedure and fistula formation is

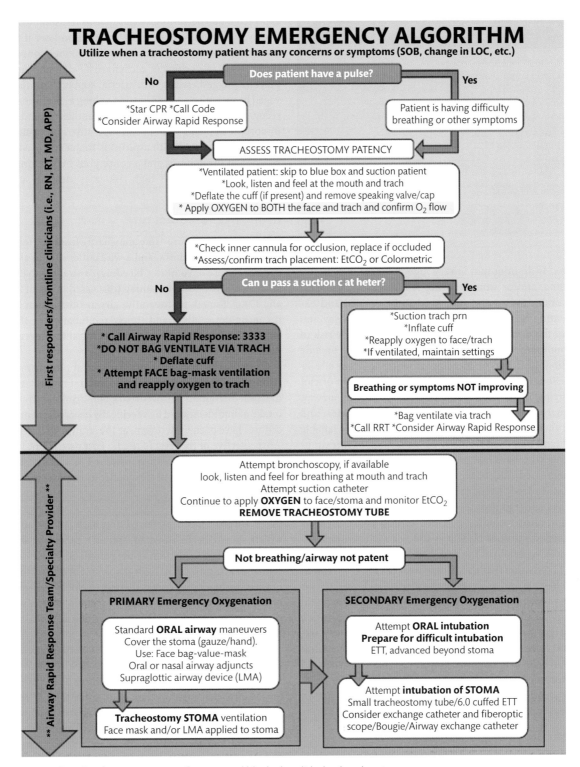

Fig. 16.4 Emergency algorithm for management of a suspected blocked or dislodged tracheostomy.

unclear. Some surgical centres elect to perform a staged procedure, with the neck dissection preceding TORS by up to a week.[50]

Neck dissection

Expanding neck haematoma is a surgical emergency. Consequently, it is routine practice during neck dissection that at least one or two surgical drains are inserted—which should be emptied and recompressed. A common approach is to attach the drains to wall suction for the first 24 hours, after which bulb suction is usually sufficient. Haematoma formation is less likely in those who have undergone neck dissection surgery if drains are left *in situ* and are functional. Mild oozing is not unusual from any neck wound, but active haemorrhage is not! Drains can be passive (Penrose) or active (suction), with drainage output being easier to calculate

Box 16.2 Essential components of an airway rapid response team

- Anaesthetist (consultant level).
- Surgeon (surgical airway experience essential; usually a fellow or consultant level).
- Tracheostomy kit (tracheostomy tubes, skin retractors, etc.).
- Front of neck needle/scalpel kit (depending on local training).
- Rapid response specialist nurse.
- Fibreoptic bronchoscope.
- Videolaryngoscope.
- Difficult airway trolley with additional advanced airway equipment.
- Respiratory/physiotherapist.
- X-ray equipment.
- Established criteria for activation.

from the latter. If drain output is very high, or there is evidence of neck swelling, and/or wound oozing is too great to be managed by the drain, the wound may need to be opened and explored. Expanding neck haematoma can threaten the airway and the viability of the overlying skin, as well as increasing the risk of infection. Symptoms and signs of neck haematoma may include painful swelling, bruising, or bleeding around the drain site or from the incision. Immediate bedside surgical evacuation of clot may be lifesaving if the haematoma is compressing the airway. Multidisciplinary teamwork is critical in such emergencies, and protocols for their management should be immediately available in the PACU (and practised regularly by staff, using *in situ* simulation). Patients who have had previous neck radiotherapy are at particularly increased risk of haemorrhage (along with most other complications). Indeed, haemorrhage in a previously irradiated patient who has undergone oral cavity surgery may signify major vascular compromise, including potential carotid artery haemorrhage (a controlled 'sentinel' bleed may precede a catastrophic carotid 'blow out'), especially if the neck has also been operated on. The triad of (1) radiation (which not only weakens the arterial wall but causes ischaemia and necrosis of the adventitial layer), (2) air (pharyngocutaneous fistula, indicative of wound breakdown and infection), and (3) saliva (the fistula allows direct contact between the carotid artery wall, causing desiccation and digestion by salivary enzymes) is usually required for a carotid bleed to occur, but this process can happen insidiously. Morbidity is high from carotid blow-out syndrome, though both emergency endovascular (embolization or stenting) and open surgical carotid artery ligation (performed less commonly) can be undertaken.

Free flap reconstruction

These patients require frequent assessment of vascular anastomosis patency. This can be accomplished in the ICU, or in other monitored settings—provided that medical and nurse staff numbers and training are appropriate (e.g. a dedicated OMFS/head and neck ward). Reduced blood flow, as detected by Doppler ultrasound, is a surgical emergency, therefore many units use implantable Doppler probes for the first 48–72 hours. For the first postoperative day, *hourly* flap observations are necessary—checking for the colour, texture, and temperature of the flap. Venous congestion or arterial insufficiency can be assessed by a pinprick test, where bleeding with a 1–2 second delay and bright red blood should be

expected if flap perfusion is healthy. This test should be done immediately postoperatively to allow comparison later if there are concerns. Dark blood on pinprick suggests venous congestion, as does the presence of swelling or ecchymosis. Pallor and lack of blood on pinprick suggests issues with arterial supply. Most flaps can be salvaged by prompt revascularization as long as perfusion problems are recognized early. Maintenance of normothermia and euvolemia are important elements of both intraoperative and postoperative care. Antiplatelet therapy (with aspirin) is frequently used to reduce the risk of flap thrombosis, and a continuous heparin infusion may be employed in particularly high-risk cases (dextran solutions are no longer used).

Orthognathic procedures

Patients may require intermaxillary fixation following some orthognathic procedures, and a wire cutter should always be at the bedside in case of vomiting, bleeding, or swelling that compromises airway control and/or breathing (discussed in detail in Chapters 10 and 17). Although postoperative airway obstruction is uncommon, it can be devastating, and timely reintubation of the trachea (or emergency front of neck airway) is crucial in preventing poor patient outcome.

Orthognathic patients require a special postoperative diet, consisting of soft foods (common to most intraoral surgery, where mucosal disruption has occurred), and drinking straws (to aid oral intake of liquids) should be specifically *avoided* if dentoalveolar procedures have been undertaken, as the straw may dislodge any clots.

Irrespective of the level of the Le Fort osteotomy, it is imperative that patients do not blow their nose for 4–6 weeks postoperatively, as this may cause significant subcutaneous emphysema.

Paediatric procedures

Every surgeon has a preferred approach to wound management which should be followed to optimize recovery, and the understanding and collaboration of the patient and their caregivers is essential in achieving this. Early involvement of the child's caregivers in their postoperative care is therefore critical (e.g. gentle cleansing of extraoral wounds). Provision of a liquid, then a soft diet is important in maintaining the child's nutrition as well as the stability of the surgical repair.

Most facial trauma is managed as conservatively as possible in the paediatric population, due to rapid growth and development.[52] Fortunately, patients under the age of 10 years are less likely to sustain facial fractures than adults, due to their relatively larger forehead, increased facial soft tissue/fat, and absence of air in the paranasal sinuses. The frequency of nasal fractures increases with downward and forward growth of the craniofacial matrix as the child develops with age. Non-displaced fractures are usually managed expectantly with appropriate analgesia, soft diet, and surveillance for any changes in fracture position.[53] Subcondylar fractures are repaired with circum-mandibular wires and fixation to the pyriform aperture—required to be in place for only a brief period (7–10 days). Early mobilization is important to prevent temporomandibular joint ankylosis.

Postoperative care of the paediatric OMFS patient requires an additional degree of vigilance due to the relatively narrowed airway and the greater potential for compromise from surgical oedema. Children who have undergone nasotracheal intubation should be expected to have some mild nasal oozing or epistaxis, which may be minimized by nursing in an upright position.

Paediatric tracheostomy formation, especially in the infant or small child, requires specialist expertise and training, and should ideally not be undertaken as an emergency procedure, unless absolutely necessary. In countries where there are insufficient resources to safely perform and manage paediatric tracheostomies, submental intubation may provide a potential alternative. Following surgery, early extubation of the trachea (in the operating theatre, if possible) gives the best opportunity for both the anaesthetic and surgical teams to evaluate the airway together, identify any issues, and address them expeditiously. Any paediatric patient who necessitates the ongoing presence of an oro/nasotracheal tube or tracheostomy tube into the postoperative period must be appropriately sedated to prevent inadvertent displacement of the airway device prior to its planned removal.[54]

Conclusion

Postoperative care should be considered as essential, and delivered in the same meticulous manner as preoperative assessment and intraoperative care. It is a fundamental component of the perioperative journey of the OMFS patient, and complications during this period can lead to significant morbidity and mortality. The postoperative care of each patient should be individualized, and planned carefully, to ensure the appropriate level of physiological monitoring is in place, and so that the patient receives the necessary level of care from the nursing, medical, surgical, and allied health professionals required to achieve the best outcome.

REFERENCES

1. Ljungqvist O, Scott M, Fearon KC. Enhanced recovery after surgery: a review. *JAMA Surg.* 2017;**152**(3):292–298.
2. Dort JC, Farwell DG, Findlay M, Huber GF, Kerr P, Shea-Budgell MA, et al. Optimal perioperative care in major head and neck cancer surgery with free flap reconstruction: a consensus review and recommendations from the Enhanced Recovery After Surgery Society. *JAMA Otolaryngol Head Neck Surg.* 2017;**143**(3):292–303.
3. Jandali DB, Vaughan D, Eggerstedt M, Ganti A, Scheltens H, Ramirez EA, et al. Enhanced recovery after surgery in head and neck surgery: reduced opioid use and length of stay. *Laryngoscope.* 2020;**130**(5):1227–1232.
4. Muñoz M, Acheson AG, Auerbach M, Besser M, Habler O, Kehlet H, et al. International consensus statement on the peri-operative management of anaemia and iron deficiency. *Anaesthesia.* 2017;**72**(2):233–247.
5. Burton BN, A'Court AM, Brovman EY, Scott MJ, Urman RD, Gabriel RA. Optimizing preoperative anemia to improve patient outcomes. *Anesthesiol Clin.* 2018;**36**(4):701–713.
6. Baumeister P, Canis M, Reiter M. Preoperative anemia and perioperative blood transfusion in head and neck squamous cell carcinoma. *PLoS One.* 2018;**13**(10):e0205712.
7. Ghaffar S, Pearse RM, Gillies MA. ICU admission after surgery: who benefits? *Curr Opin Crit Care.* 2017;**23**(5):424–429.
8. de Melo GM, Ribeiro KC, Kowalski LP, Deheinzelin D. Risk factors for postoperative complications in oral cancer and their prognostic implications. *Arch Otolaryngol Head Neck Surg.* 2001;**127**(7):828–833.
9. Chung F, Memtsoudis SG, Ramachandran SK, Nagappa M, Opperer M, Cozowicz C, et al. Society of Anesthesia and Sleep Medicine guidelines on preoperative screening and assessment of adult patients with obstructive sleep apnea. *Anesth Analg.* 2016;**123**(2):452–473.
10. Sessler DI. Perioperative thermoregulation and heat balance. *Lancet.* 2016;**387**(10038):2655–2664.
11. Mizuno H, Mizutani S, Ekuni D, Tabata-Taniguchi A, Maruyama T, Yokoi A, et al. New oral hygiene care regimen reduces postoperative oral bacteria count and number of days with elevated fever in ICU patients with esophageal cancer. *J Oral Sci.* 2018;**60**(4):536–543.
12. Belrose JC, Noppens RR. Anesthesiology and cognitive impairment: a narrative review of current clinical literature. *BMC Anesthesiol.* 2019;**19**(1):241.
13. Mark LJ, Herzer KR, Cover R, Pandian V, Bhatti NI, Berkow LC, et al. Difficult airway response team: a novel quality improvement program for managing hospital-wide airway emergencies. *Anesth Analg.* 2015;**121**(1):127–139.
14. Tawfic Q, Kumar K, Pirani Z, Armstrong K. Prevention of chronic post-surgical pain: the importance of early identification of risk factors. *J Anesth.* 2017;**31**(3):424–431.
15. Chou R, Gordon DB, de Leon-Casasola OA, Rosenberg JM, Bickler S, Brennan T, et al. Management of postoperative pain: a clinical practice guideline from the American Pain Society, the American Society of Regional Anesthesia and Pain Medicine, and the American Society of Anesthesiologists' Committee on Regional Anesthesia, Executive Committee, and Administrative Council. *J Pain.* 2016;**17**(2):131–157.
16. Bruhn J, Scheffer GJ, van Geffen G-J. Clinical application of perioperative multimodal analgesia. *Curr Opin Support Palliat Care.* 2017;**11**(2):106–111.
17. Maheshwari K, Avitsian R, Sessler DI, Makarova N, Tanios M, Raza S, et al. Multimodal analgesic regimen for spine surgery: a randomized placebo-controlled trial. *Anesthesiology.* 2020;**132**(5):992–1002.
18. Stephens DM, Richards BG, Schleicher WF, Zins JE, Langstein HN. Is ketorolac safe to use in plastic surgery? A critical review. *Aesthet Surg J.* 2015;**35**(4):462–466.
19. McNicol ED, Ferguson MC, Haroutounian S, Carr DB, Schumann R. Single dose intravenous paracetamol or intravenous propacetamol for postoperative pain. *Cochrane Database Syst Rev.* 2016;**5**:CD007126.
20. Apfel CC, Souza K, Portillo J, Dalal P, Bergese SD. Patient satisfaction with intravenous acetaminophen: a pooled analysis of five randomized, placebo-controlled studies in the acute postoperative setting. *J Healthc Qual.* 2015;**37**(3):155–162.
21. Shaffer EE, Pham A, Woldman RL, Spiegelman A, Strassels SA, Wan GJ, et al. Estimating the effect of intravenous acetaminophen for postoperative pain management on length of stay and inpatient hospital costs. *Adv Ther.* 2017;**33**(12):2211–2228.
22. Jibril F, Sharaby S, Mohamed A, Wilby KJ. Intravenous versus oral acetaminophen for pain: systematic review of current evidence to support clinical decision-making. *Can J Hosp Pharm.* 2015;**68**(3):238–247.
23. Bailey MA, Toner AJ, Corcoran TB. A survey of perioperative intravenous lidocaine use by anaesthetists in Australia and New Zealand. *Anaesth Intensive Care.* 2020;**48**(1):53–58.
24. Ates İ, Aydin ME, Ahiskalioglu A, Ahiskalioglu EO, Kaya Z, Gozeler MS. Postoperative analgesic efficacy of perioperative

intravenous lidocaine infusion in patients undergoing septorhinoplasty: a prospective, randomized, double-blind study. *Eur Arch Otorhinolaryngol.* 2020;**277**(4):1095–1100.

25. Kościelniak-Merak B, Batko I, Kobylarz K, Sztefko K, Tomasik PJ. Intravenous, perioperatively administered lidocaine regulates serum pain modulators' concentrations in children undergoing spinal surgery. *Pain Med.* 2020;**21**(7):1464–1473.

26. Dunn LK, Durieux ME. Perioperative use of intravenous lidocaine. *Anesthesiology.* 2017;**126**(4):729–737.

27. Greenwood E, Nimmo S, Paterson H, Homer N, Foo I. Intravenous lidocaine infusion as a component of multimodal analgesia for colorectal surgery-measurement of plasma levels. *Perioper Med.* 2019;**8**:1.

28. Kong VKF, Irwin MG. Gabapentin: a multimodal perioperative drug? *Br J Anaesth.* 2007;**99**(6):775–786.

29. Bhavaraju SA, Vorrasi JS, Talluri S, Kalladka M, Khan, J. Pre-emptive administration of gabapentinoids to reduce postoperative pain and opioid usage following oral and maxillofacial surgical procedures. *Oral Surg.* 2022;**15**:106–115.

30. Sanders JG, Dawes PJD. Gabapentin for perioperative analgesia in otorhinolaryngology-head and neck surgery: systematic review. *Otolaryngol Head Neck Surg.* 2016;**155**(6):893–903.

31. Herlich A. Focused local anesthesia and analgesia for head and neck surgery. *Int Anesthesiol Clin.* 2012;**50**(1):13–25.

32. Baptista PM, Costantino A, Moffa A, Rinaldi V, Casale M. Hypoglossal nerve stimulation in the treatment of obstructive sleep apnea: patient selection and new perspectives. *Nat Sci Sleep.* 2020;**12**:151–159.

33. Bisogni V, Pengo MF, De Vito A, Maiolino G, Rossi GP, Moxham J, et al. Electrical stimulation for the treatment of obstructive sleep apnoea: a review of the evidence. *Expert Rev Respir Med.* 2017;**11**(9):711–720.

34. Fernandez-Bustamante A, Bartels K, Clavijo C, Scott BK, Kacmar R, Bullard K, et al. Preoperatively screened obstructive sleep apnea is associated with worse postoperative outcomes than previously diagnosed obstructive sleep apnea. *Anesth Analg.* 2017;**125**(2):593–602.

35. Nagappa M, Liao P, Wong J, Auckley D, Ramachandran SK, Memtsoudis S, et al. Validation of the STOP-Bang questionnaire as a screening tool for obstructive sleep apnea among different populations: a systematic review and meta-analysis. *PLoS One.* 2015;**10**(12):e0143697.

36. Cohen JC, Larrabee YC, Weinstein AL, Stewart MG. Use of continuous positive airway pressure after rhinoplasty, septoplasty, and sinus surgery: a survey of current practice patterns. *Laryngoscope.* 2015;**125**(11):2612–2616.

37. Corso RM, Gregoretti C, Braghiroli A, Fanfulla F, Insalaco G. Practice guidelines for the perioperative management of patients with obstructive sleep apnea: navigating through uncertainty. *Anesthesiology.* 2014;**121**(3):664–665.

38. Memtsoudis SG, Cozowicz C, Nagappa M, Wong J, Joshi GP, Wong DT, et al. Society of Anesthesia and Sleep Medicine guideline on intraoperative management of adult patients with obstructive sleep apnea. *Anesth Analg.* 2018;**127**(4):967–987.

39. Blatt S, Al-Nawas B. A systematic review of latest evidence for antibiotic prophylaxis and therapy in oral and maxillofacial surgery. *Infection.* 2019;**47**(4):519–555.

40. Yoshimoto Y, Fujikawa T, Tanaka A, Hayashi H, Shimoike N, Kawamoto H, et al. Optimal use of antiplatelet agents, especially aspirin, in the perioperative management of colorectal cancer patients undergoing laparoscopic colorectal resection. *World J Surg Oncol.* 2019;**17**(1):92.

41. Gibb C. The Yin and Yang of perioperative aspirin: a clinician's perspective. *Int J Cardiol.* 2018;**258**:74–75.

42. Lee LKK, Tsai PNW, Ip KY, Irwin MG. Pre-operative cardiac optimisation: a directed review. *Anaesthesia.* 2019;**74** Suppl 1:67–79.

43. Brignardello-Petersen R. Uncertainty regarding risk factors for cranial nerve injury after Le Fort I osteotomy owing to serious methodological limitations of systematic review. *J Am Dent Assoc.* 2019;**150**(6):e103.

44. Hanu-Cernat LM, Hall T. Late onset of abducens palsy after Le Fort I maxillary osteotomy. *Br J Oral Maxillofac Surg.* 2009;**47**(5):414–416.

45. Kim JW, Chin BR, Park HS, Lee SH, Kwon TG. Cranial nerve injury after Le Fort I osteotomy. *Int J Oral Maxillofac Surg.* 2011;**40**(3):327–329.

46. Deng Y, Navarro JC, Markan S. Advances in anesthesia monitoring. *Oral Maxillofac Surg Clin N Am.* 2019;**31**(4):611–619.

47. American Academy of Otolaryngology-Head and Neck Surgery (AAO-HNS/F). Position statement: intraoperative nerve monitoring in otologic surgery. 2017. https://www.entnet.org/content/intraoperative-cranial-nerve-monitoring.

48. Koht A, Sloan TB, Hemmer LB. Neuromonitoring in surgery and anesthesia. UpToDate. 2020. https://www.uptodate.com/contents/neuromonitoring-in-surgery-and-anesthesia?s

49. Wilkinson K, Freeth H, Kelly K. 'On the right trach?' A review of the care received by patients who undergo tracheostomy. *Br J Hosp Med (Lond).* 2015;**76**(3):163–165.

50. Miller SC, Nguyen SA, Ong AA, Gillespie MB. Transoral robotic base of tongue reduction for obstructive sleep apnea: a systematic review and meta-analysis. *Laryngoscope.* 2017;**127**(1):258–265.

51. Tomifuji M, Araki K, Uno K, Kamide D, Tanaka S, Suzuki H, et al. Transoral videolaryngoscopic surgery for laryngeal and hypopharyngeal cancer—technical updates and long-term results. *Auris Nasus Larynx.* 2020;**47**(2):282–290.

52. Ryan ML, Thorson CM, Otero CA, Ogilvie MP, Cheung MC, Saigal GM, et al. Pediatric facial trauma: a review of guidelines for assessment, evaluation, and management in the emergency department. *J Craniofac Surg.* 2011;**22**(4):1183–1189.

53. Cole P, Kaufman Y, Hollier LH. Managing the pediatric facial fracture. *Craniomaxillofac Trauma Reconstr.* 2009;**2**(2):77–83.

54. Taiwo OA, Ibikunle AA, Braimah RO, Suleiman MK. Submental intubation in paediatric oral and maxillofacial surgery: review of the literature and report of four cases. *Afr J Paediatr Surg.* 2015;**12**(4):296–300.

17

Surgical complications

Justin P. Curtin and Gene Lee

Introduction

This chapter aims to familiarize the oral and maxillofacial anaesthetist with perioperative surgical complications, from the perspective of the surgeon. This insight and awareness of operative concerns and potential complications should allow the anaesthetist to anticipate problems, minimize sequelae, and appreciate the requirement for further surgical intervention.

Airway management

Preservation of a patent, secure airway is fundamental to safe management of the oromaxillofacial surgical (OMFS) patient. Challenging airway management may be more frequently encountered, and the essence of 'shared airway' surgery means that the type of airway device and its position may have a considerable impact on the facility of surgery (Box 17.1). Most surgeons have their own preference, and this is a key item to discuss at the 'pre-brief', prior to commencing the operating list.

Distinguishing between airway issues affecting the 'upper airway' from those distal to the larynx is pivotal in airway management decision-making (Box 17.2). Limited mouth opening is the most common upper airway issue and may be related to mechanical causes (e.g. ankylosis of the temporomandibular joint (TMJ) or joint fibrosis following radiotherapy) or functional causes (muscle spasm due to trauma or infection)—most of which are apparent prior to anaesthesia and surgery. Reduced tissue bulk and

sarcopenia is relatively common in patients with head and neck malignancy. Subglottic stenosis resulting from previous tracheostomy may not be recognized on routine examination; however, a tracheostomy scar should raise suspicion. Patients with long-standing limitation of mouth opening or those specifically undergoing TMJ surgery should be considered to have mechanical obstruction that will *not* be improved by anaesthesia or muscle relaxation. TMJ ankylosis, while rare, necessitates advanced airway management. Conversely, limitations of mouth opening related to muscle spasm or TMJ/mandibular pain are often relieved by analgesia or anaesthesia. However, delayed presentation must be treated with caution as prolonged mandibular immobility from pain may cause structural TMJ stiffness, fibrosis, and limited mouth opening not relieved by anaesthesia.

Diligent preoperative assessment and consideration of how the airway may change over time significantly influence the optimal timing of surgery. In instances of trauma, airway swelling may regress and a delay in surgery may be beneficial, while infections may progress and airway management may become increasingly difficult. Consideration of the developmental age in paediatric cases with congenital deformity is essential when deciding on the most appropriate time for corrective surgery.

Tumour extension into the posterior tongue and inflammation of the masticatory muscles requires thorough preoperative airway assessment and special consideration of postoperative management due to the high potential for upper airway obstruction. Inflammatory processes within the neck may cause laryngeal oedema that can rapidly progress to airway obstruction, and any patient with dysphagia, drooling, or requirement to sit forwards

---

Box 17.1 Surgical considerations affecting choice of airway management/device selection

- Optimize surgical access.
- Minimize alteration of anatomy and potential impact on aesthetic assessment (and surgical correction), for example, traction of nasotracheal tubes or tapes impairing assessment of facial symmetry, operative access, or free mandibular movement (precluding intraoperative occlusion checks).
- Protection from potential soiling by blood, tissue, or bone/tooth fragments.
- Permit instrumentation—bite blocks/gags/suspension/osteotomes, etc.

Box 17.2 Pre-existing pathology causing impaired airway access

- TMJ disease and dysfunction.
- Anatomical deformity—infection, congenital malformation, malignancy, or trauma.
- Cleft palate, and other congenital conditions.
- Severe obstructive sleep apnoea and excessive soft tissue.
- Previous surgery or treatments, for example, revision orthognathic surgery such as maxillary advancement following previous cleft palate surgery.

should prompt urgent airway intervention and management of the underlying cause.

In selecting the appropriate airway management device for OMFS procedures, the anaesthetist must consider the requirement to withstand local movements and instrumentation, and the need for protection from potential airway soiling. The type of airway device, and where and how it is secured may be influenced by the location of surgical incisions, therefore this must be specifically discussed prior to anaesthesia. Surgical access to the mandible may be gained via oral incision alone, or in combination with incisions in the neck (submental, submandibular). The TMJ may be accessed endoscopically via oral access, or via temporal, transparotid or retromandibular incisions. Isolated orbital fractures may be accessed via cutaneous or transconjunctival incisions. Zygomatic fractures may require oral, temporal, or brow incisions. Fractures involving the frontal sinus, naso-ethmoid region, or complex zygomatic fractures may require access via a coronal incision (also called bicoronal incision—which extends from ear to ear, allowing the scalp to be reflected anteriorly exposing the facial bones). Rainey clips or haemostats are used to minimize scalp bleeding. Fractures involving much of the facial skeleton and Le Fort III osteotomies require combinations of these incisions to gain access to the facial skeleton.

Surgical gags are often used to hold the mouth open while the surgeon operates, and these may dislodge or compress any airway device. Foreign objects, ranging from bone or teeth fragments to screws, may fall posteriorly into the airway, and may be extremely difficult to locate and retrieve due to their size.

In contrast to many other surgical specialties, procedures involving the mouth, jaws, or neck may disturb a previously stable airway such that it may need replacement or exchange for an alternative device. Tracheal tubes may be inadvertently perforated or the cuff punctured by surgical drills, or during maxillary down-fracture or maxillectomy. Adequate ventilation may not still be possible, and tube exchange is often indicated if inadequate or much of the operation remains. Tube exchange must be undertaken through an active sterile field and is often best undertaken using an exchange catheter, necessitating good cooperation from anaesthesia and surgical teams (**Box 17.3**).

Box 17.3 Considerations for the shared airway

- Airway instrumentation.
- Accidental tracheal extubation, or tracheal tube cuff damage from surgical site manipulation or instrumentation.
- Surgical gags causing tracheal tube occlusion or displacement.
- Nasotracheal tube laceration following lateral nasal osteotomy or laceration from surgical drills or saws.
- Foreign bodies, including retained surgical packs or throat packs.
- Intermaxillary fixation (IMF) application and management.
- Tracheal extubation plans and strategies for early and late reintubation.
- Inspection and suctioning of the airway prior to extubation (remove throat packs, blood, and secretions).
- Intraoperative changes to the airway device (planned, and emergency airway exchanges).
- Airway oedema or haematoma compromising airway patency in the postoperative period (and consideration of delaying extubation).

Extubation planning and postoperative airway compromise

Upper airway oedema and ongoing 'surgical ooze' (bleeding from undefined sources) common to OMFS procedures mean that immediate tracheal extubation following completion of surgery may not always be advisable, and extubation may be delayed by several minutes, extending up to several days (with extubation being undertaken in the intensive care unit) (**Box 17.4**). The decision regarding optimal timing for extubation requires careful consideration of both anaesthetic and surgical factors, and multidisciplinary team discussion (**Box 17.5**). Prolonged mechanical ventilation is not without risk; however, a period of stabilization following prolonged surgery, allowing any temporary airway oedema to reside, may be indicated. It is usually relatively straightforward to distinguish those patients suitable for standard ward care and those requiring intensive care. Prolonged surgery, significant comorbidities, advanced airway management, potential airway issues, and microvascular tissue transfer (and perfusion pressure management) all potentially warrant a higher level of postoperative care.[1]

A potentially fatal triad of compromised airway patency and access, diminished consciousness, and upper airway secretions may exist following major OMFS procedures. Simple manoeuvres that are usually easily instituted to manage airway obstruction (e.g. jaw thrust and oropharyngeal suctioning) may not be possible in the OMFS patient (**Box 17.6**).

Patients *most at risk* of airway complications are those that require IMF, where the maxillary teeth are ligated to the mandibular teeth (with wires or elastics). Placed intraoperatively (after airway inspection, suctioning, and removal of any throat pack), the IMF device may be required to remain *in situ* postoperatively, posing unique challenges to post-anaesthesia care unit (PACU) staff in the short-term and ward nursing staff later on—with responsibility often falling to the anaesthetist where problems arise. Communication with patients can be very challenging and, more importantly, access to the upper airway to undertake suctioning of secretions may be significantly impaired, or impossible. The entire team must be aware when patients are being transferred from theatre to PACU, and they must be reviewed prior to discharge/transfer from PACU. PACU and ward staff must also be trained and familiar with managing these patients and the potential life-threatening complications (**Box 17.7**). The principal risk to the patient relates to the potential for upper airway obstruction from secretions, bleeding, or vomitus (or even a retained throat pack). Jaw thrust is impossible and

---

Box 17.4 Potential indications for delayed tracheal extubation

- Prolonged surgery and anaesthesia, and potential effect on physiological stability, respiratory drive, and airway tone.
- Impaired airway protection and high aspiration risk.
- Upper airway obstruction secondary to oedema, haematoma, or foreign body.
- Concerns over laryngeal oedema, and potential for laryngeal obstruction.
- Direct surgical causes—to facilitate IMF stability or prevent wound breakdown.

Box 17.5 Extubation strategies and airway rescue planning

- An individualized extubation strategy should be agreed for each patient by the surgical and anaesthetic teams; the appropriate equipment and personnel should be present; it should be undertaken in the most appropriate environment, with a back-up plan in case of failure.
- Patients should be risk stratified in order to decide upon immediate or delayed tracheal extubation:
  - Is the airway considered 'safe' for immediate extubation?
  - Is there expected to be significantly worsening oedema/continued bleeding?
  - Should the patient return to theatre for further surgical intervention (usually to arrest ongoing bleeding)?
- Advanced options include a bridging tracheostomy or staged extubation using an airway exchange catheter.
- Smooth emergence is desirable with minimal coughing and straining to reduce bleeding and airway soiling.
- Extubation strategies may need to be adapted to avoid tight-fitting facemasks on midface and mandibular wounds, or nasal airways with vulnerable nasal wounds.

Box 17.7 Concerning postoperative clinical signs in the OMFS patient

- Restlessness—may be caused by hypoxia.
- Confusion—may be caused by hypoxia.
- Stridor—may suggest laryngeal oedema.
- Persistent vomiting—especially after orbital surgery.
- 'Tripod' patient positioning/desire to sit up—may suggest base of tongue or sublingual swelling.
- Bleeding per oral—may warrant urgent return to theatre.

prophylactic tongue suture for anterior traction should obstruction occur. Placement of a nasopharyngeal airway may initiate bleeding from the raw palatal surfaces and should be judiciously performed only after consultation with the surgical team. Having excluded other causes of airway obstruction, application of continuous positive airway pressure is usually sufficient to relieve obstruction until oedema has resided and the infant has mastered mouth breathing.

Return to theatre!

The necessity to 'return to theatre' in the early postoperative period is most commonly related to airway compromise, bleeding, or other surgical issues—all of which may present significant challenges to the anaesthetist. All aspects of airway management may be more difficult. Facemask oxygenation may be impaired by oedema or facial surgical wounds, and excessive positive pressure ventilation may cause unwanted and potentially dangerous tissue insufflation. Insertion of a nasopharyngeal airway in patients who have had midfacial fractures, osteotomies, or other procedures that have disrupted the nasal septum/mucosa requires particular caution to avoid tearing of the nasal mucosa and associated bleeding—nevertheless, it may be a potentially life-saving intervention in patients with IMF. IMF devices should of course be released as soon as possible—either during, or prior to anaesthetic management. An oropharyngeal airway may bypass some upper airway obstruction as well as facilitating airway suctioning in preparation for laryngoscopy. Bleeding from the surgical site and into the upper airway may severely limit laryngoscopy views and adequate lighting and large-bore suction devices are essential. Fragile facial bones (due to fractures or reconstruction) and/or tissue reconstructive flaps (dependent on

suctioning is limited. In the conscious patient, assisting them to sit forwards will facilitate passage of secretions/blood per oral. The unconscious patient should be placed in the lateral position, with suctioning performed immediately inside the mouth between the cheeks and teeth. A nasopharyngeal airway (often placed prior to tracheal extubation and emergence) can provide an additional route for suctioning of the oropharynx, though care must be taken not to cause mucosal injury and precipitate bleeding. Crucially, PACU and ward staff must be shown where the wires (or elastics) that secure the teeth together are located, and how to cut them, and equipment for releasing the IMF must be always immediately available and functional (**Box 17.8**).

Patients who have undergone cleft palate repair also pose a number of unique postoperative challenges. Prolonged bloody ooze is common from the 'raw' superior surface of the transposed palatal flaps; however, nasal suctioning is not advisable given that these form the new nasal floor. Oral suctioning must be performed with great care to protect the surgical repair. Some surgeons place small intraoral packs, and while they are sutured in place, they still constitute a potential aspiration risk. These patients have anatomically smaller airways at baseline, and palatal reconstruction significantly reduces available space for the tongue (which prior to surgery may have protruded into the nasal cavity), which may now obstruct against the newly formed soft palate. Recovery in the supine position puts them at high risk of both aspiration and airway obstruction, and patients are best nursed either in the lateral or prone position (allowing secretions to flow out freely). Some surgeons place a

Box 17.6 Challenges of airway rescue in OMFS patients

- Impaired access to oral airway, by surgical fixation and IMF devices.
- Limitations on available rescue techniques—facemask ventilation impaired by tissue oedema, vulnerable facial wounds, and limited range of movement of condyles and soft tissue; desire to avoid jaw thrust and chin lift manoeuvres in certain OMFS patients.
- Impaired access to nasal airway due to prior surgical involvement.

Box 17.8 Essential equipment for management of patients with IMF

- High-volume suction device with range of flexible-tipped suction catheters.
- Independent light source for aiding in identifying bleeding points and accurate suction catheter placement.
- Wire cutters.
- Scissors (if elastic IMF).
- Cheek retractor.
- Range of appropriately sized and lubricated nasopharyngeal airways.
- Picture board to facilitate communication between patient and staff members.

recently anastomosed blood vessels), mean that laryngoscopy must be performed with the lowest forces necessary. Videolaryngoscopic or fibreoptic techniques may cause less tissue disruption; however, views may be impaired by excessive secretions or blood. The priority should always be to maintain patient oxygenation and restore a secure airway—the surgical team will appreciate that some disruption/manipulation of tissues may be required to achieve these goals and will make the necessary revisions. In some cases, a surgical front of neck airway may be required, for which the decision largely depends on the underlying aetiology.

Bleeding

Following acute oral and maxillofacial trauma, significant bleeding may necessitate urgent nasal packing or the placement of wire ligatures around grossly mobile fragments of the mandible—in order to regain control while other definitive management can be undertaken. Importantly, anterior mandibular trauma may result in floor of the mouth haematoma which has the potential to threaten airway patency.

Intraoperative bleeding

Haemodynamically significant bleeding is generally uncommon, but may occur intraoperatively or postoperatively. Intraoperative bleeding during OMFS procedures is rarely life-threatening but can significantly accumulate over time. More likely is that bleeding will obscure the surgical field, impacting the facility and length of the procedure, and, ultimately, patient outcome. Certain anatomical regions are prone to significant blood loss and knowledge of when these areas are involved in certain procedures permits the anaesthetic team greater planning and preparation. These areas include the pterygoid plexus, palatine vessels, nasal floor and septum, and great vessels in the neck—named arteries, and internal jugular vein (IJV; also note the attendant issue of air embolism) (**Box 17.9**).

Bleeding into the floor of the mouth is a rare yet recognized complication following insertion of mandibular implants (**Box 17.10**).[2]

Due to the rich blood supply of the head and neck regions, even small intraoperative bleeding points can result in postoperative haematoma formation that may compromise airway patency or threaten perfusion of free flap reconstructions. There are numerous pharmacological and non-pharmacological strategies for reducing bleeding, each with relative advantages and disadvantages, and these are discussed extensively in Chapters 7, 9, and 10.

Box 17.9 Vascular complications of maxillary surgery

- The maxillary artery, major palatine or sphenopalatine artery, and nasoethmoidal arteries can be injured with the osteotome (surgical chisel) and during down-fracture of the maxilla. These include Le Fort osteotomies and midface fracture surgical procedures.[3]
- The pterygomaxillary venous plexus is a potential source of persistent venous blood loss, requiring cauterization and use of surgical haemostatic agents.
- Direct visualization of the lacerated vessels by the surgeon is required for ligation and control.
- In rare cases of severe bleeding, angiography and embolization may be required; ligation of the external carotid artery may also be necessary.

Box 17.10 Vascular complications of mandibular surgery

- Haemodynamically significant bleeding is generally uncommon, but may occur intraoperatively or postoperatively.[4]
- Retromandibular vein, inferior alveolar artery, and facial artery are at risk.
- Laceration of masseter or pterygoid muscles may also lead to surgical bleeding.
- Surgical control is achieved with packing, ligation, and diathermy as required.

Infection

Surgical wound infections

Postoperative infections following elective OMFS procedures are relatively infrequent, are typically caused by the abundant oropharyngeal flora, and can usually be managed by local debridement and intravenous antibiotics. In common with other surgery specialties, contributory factors include prolonged surgery, patient comorbidities, pre-existing methicillin-resistant *Staphylococcus aureus* colonization/infection, and perioperative hypothermia. Optimally positioned surgical drains will reduce fluid re-accumulation (and its sequelae) post surgical drainage.

Deep neck space infections

Deep neck space infections that spread along fascial planes within potential spaces of the head and neck can be life-threatening, potentially causing airway obstruction, mediastinitis, severe sepsis, and other catastrophic complications. Most frequently caused by necrotic teeth, infection spreads through the cortical plate, into adjacent soft tissues, and beyond. The pathophysiology, microbiology, range of clinical presentations (depending on direction of spread), and the management priorities are discussed in detail in Chapter 12, including management of impending airway obstruction. Postoperative infection following dental extractions can also spread into the soft tissues of the face, base of skull, and/or neck.

Early intervention by an experienced multidisciplinary team is critical. Firmness of the floor of the mouth, dysphagia, and adoption of the tripod position are very concerning signs. Trismus may be present when infection involves either the masticatory space (medial to the mandibular ramus and the medial pterygoid muscle) or submasseteric space. It should be noted that, while masticatory space infections often result in very obvious facial swelling, submasseteric infections have virtually none. A relatively insubstantial submasseteric collection on computed tomography imaging may limit mouth opening to just a few millimetres, which, importantly for anaesthesia, will not improve with muscle relaxation, necessitating advanced airway management. Removal of the cause of infection, and drainage of pus are the cornerstones of management. Crucially, oedema (including laryngeal oedema) may worsen postoperatively and decisions regarding optimum timing of extubation and/or bridging tracheostomy must be discussed and agreed by the multidisciplinary team (also discussed in detail in Chapter 12).

Other perioperative complications

Other perioperative surgical complications are discussed in **Table 17.1**.

Table 17.1 Additional perioperative surgical complications

Intraoperative arrhythmia	Bradyarrhythmias (including asystole) resulting from the trigeminocardiac reflex occasionally occur during down-fracture of the midface or from manipulation of midface bones Similarly, midfacial osteotomies may illicit bradyarrhythmias[5]
Dental injury	Inadvertent damage/fracture of teeth or artificial dentition may occur, and may also be lost into the airway
Flap perfusion issues	Flap ischaemia or aseptic necrosis of the maxilla or mandibular segments may occur due to impaired vascular support of the segment or flap
Ophthalmic complications	The eyes are at risk of injury given the shared airway and proximity of the oral and maxillofacial procedure and equipment. Eyes should be protected with a water-based lubricant, tapes, steri-strips, or corneal shields where appropriate Blindness following Le Fort osteotomies has been reported, with proposed mechanisms including propagation of fractures to involve orbital fissure structures[6]
Base of skull complications	Though generally rare, extended fracture lines (from Le Fort osteotomies) may transmit injury to base of skull structures. Complications of this include cavernous sinus thrombosis, pseudoaneurysms, and arteriovenous fistula formation[7,8]
Soft tissue injury	The lip is at risk of pressure injuries, as well as the nasal tip from excessive traction caused by the nasotracheal tube Pressure injuries may occur during prolonged procedures (especially if hypotensive anaesthesia techniques are employed), and particular attention must be paid to protecting pressure areas
Nasolacrimal complications	Laceration of the lacrimal duct or facial oedema (causing obstruction) may cause epiphora and recurrent dacryocystitis—necessitating return to theatre for dacryocystorhinostomy
Thrombotic complications	A perioperative strategy for thromboprophylaxis must be specifically agreed by the surgical and anaesthesia teams, particularly when microvascular procedures are being undertaken Prolonged procedures, a protracted period of immobility after major surgery, and underlying malignancy may also contribute to risk of venous thrombosis
Major circulatory complications	During neck dissection, manipulation of the internal carotid artery may dislodge atherosclerotic plaque compromising cerebral perfusion Dissection of lymphatics around the internal jugular vein may cause significant blood loss. Perioperative 'head-up' patient positioning aids in reducing distension of neck veins. Air embolism can also rarely occur if neck veins are opened Brisk bleeding may also occur during maxillary osteotomies or maxillectomy, following cleavage of the maxilla from the pterygoid plates (arterial and/or venous sources)—usually managed with cautery, packing, and ligation[3]
Delayed bleeding	This typically occurs within the first 2 weeks, presenting with epistaxis from a recanalized blood vessel, wound breakdown, or a pseudoaneurysm (which requires packing, surgical intervention or angiography, and embolization)[9,10]
Unsatisfactory surgical outcome	Unfavourable surgical correction, relapse, and/or instability of fractures or osteotomies may necessitate further surgical intervention/revision procedures
Neurological injury	Postoperative neurological injury is relatively common following OMFS procedures[11] Branches of the trigeminal or facial nerve may be compressed during dissection or retraction/protection from the operative field.[12] Most of these neuropraxia will recover, although not all, with some developing into chronic pain syndromes.[13] Central hypersensitization measures (e.g. nociceptive blockade, anti-inflammatory agents, and gabapentin) have shown some reduction in postoperative neuropathies.[14] Melatonin has also shown some initial promise, though larger trials are needed[15] Third molar extraction bears special mention here, due to the frequency with which these procedures are performed, and the risk to both the inferior alveolar and lingual nerves, which may proximate to the surgical site resulting in subsequent altered sensory function. Despite these risks, removal is still warranted as third molar teeth may cause localized infections (pericoronitis) that spread into the deep spaces of the floor of mouth and neck Impaired sensation of the lips and chin may occur following bilateral sagittal split osteotomies[16] The prolonged nature of major OMFS procedures carries the risk of peripheral nerve compression injuries

Procedure-specific complications

Oral surgery

Oral surgery largely refers to procedures involving the alveolus and adjacent structures, including removal of teeth, mucosal procedures, and insertion of dental implants. Complications mostly relate to infection and bleeding. Wound breakdown, tissue loss, and/or localized infections following oral surgical procedures are uncommon but may require management under general anaesthesia. While also rare, postoperative bleeding can cause airway compromise.[17] Crucially, swelling of the floor of the mouth can occur following relatively minor surgery and is a potentially life-threatening complication. Foreign objects (e.g. surgical screws) may also fall into the oropharynx, warranting consideration of a throat pack (though, as discussed in Chapter 10, throat packs carry their own risks).

Oral and maxillofacial trauma

All patients presenting with facial trauma should be assumed to have sustained significant head and/or cervical trauma until excluded, and warrant a 'trauma survey' (discussed in Chapter 13). The restoration of a functional dental occlusion following fractures of the jaw(s) requires the teeth to be 'fixed' in place while the bones either heal (conservatively) or while fixation plates are placed surgically. Once the plates have been inserted intraoperatively, the maxillomandibular fixation can usually be released prior to undertaking tracheal extubation. It is relatively rare for patients to leave the operating theatre with their jaws still wired closed (IMF), though elastics may remain *in situ* (specific IMF precautions were discussed earlier in this chapter). Postoperative identification of functional discrepancies in dental occlusion may necessitate return to theatre. Postoperative infection, failure of bony fixation, or non-union of facial fractures are uncommon outcomes following open reduction and internal fixation; nevertheless, management entails fracture revision and free bone grafting (if bony continuity has been lost).

Mandibular trauma

Mandibular fractures often present with trismus (limited mouth opening due to muscle spasm) that may or may not be relieved by neuromuscular blocking agents. Most mandibular fractures require nasotracheal intubation so that the teeth can be brought together for functional reduction, and most do not require advanced airway techniques. Direct laryngoscopy is less likely to be impeded by fractures involving the mandibular body or passing through the third molar tooth socket, as the upward and forward movements of the laryngoscope will usually lift the entire glossal apparatus anteriorly, allowing visualization of the glottis. In contrast, fractures beneath the ascending ramus of the mandible (i.e. under the masseter and medial pterygoid muscles) can be more problematic as spasm of these muscles (causing trismus) can limit the anterior movement of the mandible during laryngoscopy. Secondary displacement of fractures can occur during laryngoscopy, and while clearly not desirable, tracheal intubation must always take precedence, with any unavoidable displacement addressed by the surgical team during fracture reduction.

Midfacial trauma

Fractures of the midface tend to occur in patterns, classified according to the level at which the fractures cross the facial skeleton (discussed in detail in Chapter 13). Le Fort I fractures separate the dental-bearing portion of the maxilla from above, extending from the level of the lateral nose to the pterygoid plates posteriorly. Le Fort II fractures extend from the nasal rim, along the orbital floor to beneath the zygomas, to the pterygoid plates posteriorly. Le Fort III fractures cleave the entire facial skeleton from the cranial base, and signify significant cranial and cervical impact (with their concomitant risks). Naso-ethmoidal fractures tend to be localized, but are significant due to the potential for haemorrhage and intracranial involvement. 'Panfacial' fractures involve most of the facial skeleton, requiring multiple incisions, that are subsequently joined subperiosteally to provide access to the facial skeleton beneath the facial soft tissues.

Orbital trauma

Orbital trauma deserves special mention due to the risk of blindness following surgical repair. The visual status of the affected eye must be established prior to commencement of surgery. If the eye cannot be fully examined due to lid swelling, a bright light can be used to at least confirm light perception and the integrity of the optic nerve. Blindness may be caused by the initial trauma causing damage to the optic nerve, or increased perioperative intraocular pressure resulting in retinal ischaemia and blindness postoperatively. Measures should be taken to avoid/minimize increases in intraocular pressure. Repair of orbital floor fractures requires the globe to be elevated which may compress the globe and raise intraocular pressure. The oculocardiac reflex (associated with profound bradycardia) can be precipitated as the surgeon accesses the orbital floor, though release of the applied retraction usually leads to spontaneous resolution.[18] Anything that might increase the risk of venous bleeding within the orbit postoperatively must also be prevented, for example, coughing

at tracheal extubation, and vomiting in the recovery period. Signs of retrobulbar haematoma include severe pain behind the eye, proptosis, and reduced vision/reaction to light in the affected eye. Patients should be closely monitoring for these signs, and the surgical team must be notified *immediately* if there is any concern, with acetazolamide and dexamethasone administered, and an immediate return to theatre for surgical release via lateral canthotomy. Retrobulbar haemorrhage (and blindness) can also occur following indirect elevation of zygomatic fractures (due to involvement of the lateral orbital wall) therefore these patients require the same degree of vigilance.

Facial osteotomies

Facial osteotomies (discussed in detail in Chapter 10) are performed for functional and aesthetic reasons. These procedures require significant collaboration between the orthodontist (who plans the desired dental occlusion preoperatively) and the surgeons (who move the bony segments bearing the teeth into the pre-planned positions). In a similar manner to the reduction of jaw fractures, the occlusion of the teeth is used to guide the bony segments into position. A satisfactory functional result requires fixation accurate to within one or two millimetres (on dental occlusion); however, functional reproducibility of osteotomies can be affected by the presence of multiple bony segments, TMJ ligament laxity, and variations in muscle tone. A discrepancy of >2 mm detected postoperatively may require subsequent (non-urgent) return to theatre—which is usually undertaken within the first 10 days, when airway management may be complicated by incomplete resolution of surgical oedema and the presence of early fibrosis throughout the local musculature. Voluntary mouth opening may be restricted, but usually improves upon induction of anaesthesia. Extra caution should be taken with the bimaxillary osteotomy patient returning to theatre as the fixation screws used to hold the facial skeleton in place are small (usually 2 mm in diameter) and the bone is generally thin. Fixation can be easily disrupted during tracheal intubation, with the bony fragments displaced. The surgeon will be aware of this possibility and will check the final revised reduction; however, a return to theatre for correction of a 'small discrepancy' can sometimes turn out to be not such a simple undertaking.

Maxillary osteotomies roughly mimic the correspondingly named midfacial (Le Fort) fracture patterns. All involve transection of the nasal septum and disarticulation of the maxilla from the pterygoid plates in some manner, and are therefore always associated with the risk of perioperative haemorrhage.[3] During a Le Fort I osteotomy (the most commonly undertaken maxillary osteotomy), the mucosa of the nasal floor is frequently breached exposing the nasotracheal tube to potential damage. Le Fort II and III procedures involve orbital osteotomies, and therefore pose the same risks mentioned earlier during orbital fracture management. Le Fort III osteotomy involves cleavage of the entire facial skeleton from the cranial base, requiring coronal, orbital, and oral surgical incisions for access. The vitality of the osteotomized facial bones and dental segments is dependent on random diffusion through adherent periosteum. Hypoperfusion, evidenced by decreased bleeding from the osteotomized segments, threatens the viability of the bone segments and dental tissues, therefore maintenance of adequate perfusion is essential. Avascular necrosis of bone and dental tissues following facial osteotomies are relatively uncommon. Management involves waiting for the extent of necrosis to be clearly defined, and then secondary debridement and revision.

Tumour resection and reconstructive surgery

Malignancy can have a significant impact on airway management, relating to distortion of anatomy from the tumour itself, previous surgery, and the presence of scar tissue, or the effects of radiotherapy on tissues (discussed in detail in Chapter 15). Oral and maxillofacial pathology includes epithelial tumours (skin and mucosa), salivary gland tumours (major and minor), tumours relating to the dental apparatus (odontogenic—benign and malignant), and tumours arising from the tissues covering the facial skeleton and within the bony skeleton itself. Resective surgery may require facial osteotomies (as osteoplastic flaps) to disarticulate the facial skeleton, providing access to tumours deep to the facial skeleton (e.g. base of skull).[19] These approaches employ orthognathic surgical techniques, avoiding the need to resect uninvolved tissues, and this ability to reposition large anatomical units following tumour resection allows restoration of facial form and function, while greatly reducing surgical morbidity.

Neck dissection is frequently undertaken as part of the management of malignant tumours, with the aim of removing the regional draining lymph nodes. The superficial lymph nodes of the head and neck drain to the vertical deep chain surrounding the IJV, within the carotid sheath. Neck dissections that extend beyond the superficial lymphatics breach the carotid sheath, exposing the length of the IJV to injury. Damage to the IJV may cause significant rapid bleeding that also obscures the injury site until control can be regained by application of pressure and suturing. Without the application of appropriate pressure, a significant breach in the IJV may also result in air embolism. The 'great vessels' of the neck are replete with arterial and venous branches, and the IJV's multiple feeding veins must be sealed to prevent postoperative haematoma. Hypotensive anaesthesia may assist during neck dissection; however, restoration of 'normal' blood pressure is essential prior to wound closure to ensure any potential sources of bleeding (that may cause postoperative haematoma) are identified and addressed. The carotid sheath also carries the vagus nerve which gives off motor branches to the soft palate, pharynx, and larynx as it travels into the chest and abdomen. In addition, the phrenic nerve, glossopharyngeal nerve, hypoglossal nerve, and ansa cervicalis all traverse the region involved in neck dissection (at various levels) and therefore any of these may also be the source of postoperative dysfunction. Return to theatre for such a patient is likely to be severely complicated by upper airway oedema and relatively fragile bony fixation.

Tumour resection in the oral and maxillofacial region often results in substantial bony and soft tissue defects that, if left uncorrected, would result in poor functional and aesthetic outcomes. Reconstructive efforts are therefore often considerable, entailing the use of local, regional, and distant microvascular flaps carrying bone and soft tissue. While alloplast and xenografts avoid the issues of donor site morbidity, the incidence of postoperative complications and the lack of true biological integration with host tissues, generally favours the use of autogenous grafts. The choice of graft material is largely determined by the size of the defect and the requirement for vascular integration of the graft at the donor site. Regional flaps (e.g. pectoralis major and temporalis muscle flaps) are harvested on a defined anatomical vascular pedicle, which provides relative resilience to fluctuations in systemic blood pressure and fluid status. However, bone is frequently required in oral and maxillofacial reconstruction to restore continuity, with the donor site being determined by the volume of bone needed. Relatively small amounts of bone may be harvested locally, while sites such as the anterior iliac crest are used for larger defects. The size of free bone grafts is limited by their reliance upon ingrowth of a new vascular supply over time. Because blood supply of free flaps is restored intraoperatively, they are often preferred in patients scheduled for radiotherapy.[20] Miniplate fixation of the grafted bone to the resection margins can provide an immediate structure to which soft tissues and musculature can be attached. This enhanced structural integrity has improved functional and aesthetic outcomes, largely obviating the requirement for postoperative IMF, and allowing more effective application of an anaesthetic facemask (if required postoperatively).

Each flap type has its own potential complications. For example, the temporalis muscle flap (frequently used for maxillary reconstruction) may be a source of persistent bleeding in the early postoperative period (usually evident at the anterior nares or within the oropharynx). The exact source of bleeding is rarely identifiable and due to its inaccessibility, is often addressed by local packing via the anterior nares. Conversely, the pectoralis major muscle flap may impair respiratory function in the immediate postoperative period.[21] Bone harvest from distant sites may necessitate additional postoperative analgesia. Patient-controlled analgesia or continuous infusion of local anaesthetic may be safer in patients who have undergone major OMFS procedures, where excessive sedation in the context of oedema and secretions should be avoided.[22] Since flap survival depends upon adequate tissue perfusion, excessive patient movement and physiological disturbance should be avoided in the early postoperative period—especially in the case of free tissue flaps, in which perfusion depends upon anastomotic integrity.[1] Impairment of either arterial supply or venous drainage can jeopardize the flap, and free flap perfusion must be closely and frequently monitored postoperatively. Flaps that are swollen, pale, blue, or cold should prompt urgent physiological optimization of the patient, treatment of any reversible causes, and surgical review—most surgical teams have a low threshold to return to theatre.

Anaesthetic management impacts regional flap integrity to a greater extent than local flaps.[1] Optimizing fluid status, temperature control, and analgesia/sedation are crucial in the success of microvascular tissue transfer (different types of flaps and their management are discussed in detail in Chapter 15).

Cleft lip and palate repair

Thorough preoperative assessment is essential in these patients due to the association with other congenital defects (particularly cardiac and renal) and recognized syndromes (discussed in detail in Chapter 11). There are several different facial cleft classification systems to aid in identification and medical communication, most of which are anatomically or clinically based (rather than developmental).[23] The most frequent facial cleft affects the lip, alveolus (either unilaterally or bilaterally), and both the hard and soft palate. While cleft lip may be more aesthetically distressing, it is the loss of palatal integrity that has the most significant clinical and functional impact—recurrent upper and lower respiratory tracts infections and nutritional deficiencies may affect overall physical development, and the timing of surgery.

Both cleft lip and palatal repairs are undertaken with an oral tracheal tube (usually a south-facing Ring–Adair–Elwyn or flexible reinforced tube) secured carefully to avoid traction on facial soft tissues and positioned in the midline to facilitate optimal repair of the defect. For palatal repair, a mouth gag (e.g. Dingman) is inserted by the surgeon to facilitate access, by widening mouth opening, retracting the cheek, and depressing the tongue. During the application of the mouth gag, tracheal tube position and patency may be affected, and placement of a gauze swab over the lower lip and under the tracheal tube may help prevent tube compression. Following gag insertion (and any necessary tracheal tube optimization), the patient is then placed in a 'head-down' position with considerable head extension—which again may alter tracheal tube position, warranting further confirmation of adequacy of ventilation and potential tube adjustment.

Repair of the palate (closure of the alveolar cleft) requires soft palate muscle dissection and elevation of mucosal flaps, which are then advanced over the defect, covering the bone that has been harvested from a distant site which has been used to fill the bony gap in the alveolus. The volume of intraoperative blood loss is not usually significant; however, any bleeding can severely impede the procedure, in turn leading to further bleeding, and increased surgical time. Closure of the midline palatal defect achieved by medial movement of the mucosal flaps leaves exposed mucosal and bony surfaces which are prone to bleeding—in fact, the entire nasal surface of the reconstructed palate is left to granulate and is, therefore, a potential source of postoperative bleeding. The exposed bone surface is therefore usually covered by a haemostatic pack (resorbable or non-resorbable) that must be sutured in place. As mentioned earlier, nursing and medical staff caring for these patients postoperatively must be aware of these packs and the potential airway hazard they may pose if they become loose. A certain degree of early postoperative bleeding is to be expected; however, persistent bleeding should always warrant urgent review and consideration of re-exploration.

Patients with craniofacial cleft syndromes have an increased incidence of disordered breathing beyond the structural issues of the cleft itself,[24,25] which should be identified at preassessment, and may necessitate a temporary tracheostomy to enable corrective surgery to be safely undertaken. Closure of the palatal defect can result in sudden and significant reduction in volume of the oral airway, which may cause temporary upper airway difficulties—usually addressed by postural measures or traction on a previously placed temporary tongue suture (discussed in the earlier section on extubation planning). Postoperative pain can be significant, impairing the child's ability to feed, and bilateral infraorbital nerve blocks are commonly used as an adjunct.

Conclusion

The shared airway of OMFS dictates that the surgeon and anaesthetist have a mutual understanding of each other's perspectives, needs, and concerns. This can never be truer than when there is a complication during or following surgery as those relating to OMFS procedures, even minor operations, can be potentially life-threatening. Good communication and combined input to the whole perioperative care process will undoubtedly achieve better outcomes.

REFERENCES

1. Kruse AL, Luebbers HT, Grätz KW, Obwegeser JA. Factors influencing survival of free-flap in reconstruction for cancer of the head and neck: a literature review. *Microsurgery.* 2010;**30**(3):242–248.

2. Tomljenovic B, Herrmann S, Filippi A, Kühl S. Life-threatening hemorrhage associated with dental implant surgery: a review of the literature. *Clin Oral Implants Res.* 2016;**27**(9):1079–1084.

3. Lanigan DT, Hey JH, West RA. Major vascular complications of orthognathic surgery: hemorrhage associated with Le Fort I osteotomies. *J Oral Maxillofac Surg.* 1990;**48**(6):561–573.

4. Flanagan D. Important arterial supply of the mandible, control of an arterial hemorrhage, and report of a hemorrhagic incident. *J Oral Implantol.* 2003;**29**(4):165–173.

5. Kiani MT, Tajik G, Ajami M, Fazli H, Kharazifard MJ, Mesgarzadeh A. Trigeminocardiac reflex and haemodynamic changes during Le Fort I osteotomy. *Int J Oral Maxillofac Surg.* 2016;**45**(5):567–570.

6. Cruz AAV, dos Santos AC. Blindness after Le Fort I osteotomy: a possible complication associated with pterygomaxillary separation. *J CranioMaxillofac Surg.* 2006;**34**(4):210–216.

7. Chepla KJ, Totonchi A, Hsu DP, Gosain AK. Maxillary artery pseudoaneurysm after Le Fort I osteotomy: treatment using transcatheter arterial embolization. *J Craniofac Surg.* 2010;**21**(4):1079–1081.

8. Kramer FJ, Baethge C, Swennen G, Teltzrow T, Schulze A, Berten J, Brachvogel P. Intra- and perioperative complications of the LeFort I osteotomy: a prospective evaluation of 1000 patients. *J Craniofac Surg.* 2004;**15**(6):971–977.

9. Hacein-Bey L, Blazun JM, Jackson RF. Carotid artery pseudoaneurysm after orthognathic surgery causing lower cranial nerve palsies: endovascular repair. *J Oral Maxillofac Surg.* 2013;**71**(11):1948–1955.

10. Park B, Jang WH, Lee BK. An idiopathic delayed maxillary hemorrhage after orthognathic surgery with Le Fort I osteotomy: a case report. *J Korean Assoc Oral Maxillofac Surg.* 2019;**45**(6):364–368.

11. Renton T. Chronic orofacial pain. *Oral Dis.* 2017;**23**(5):566–571.

12. Dos Santos Alves JM, de Freitas Alves BW, de Figueiredo Costa AC, Carneiro BGDS, de Sousa LM, Gondim DV. Cranial nerve injuries in Le Fort I osteotomy: a systematic review. *Int J Oral Maxillofac Surg.* 2019;**48**(5):601–611.

13. Devine M, Hirani M, Durham J, Nixdorf DR, Renton T. Identifying criteria for diagnosis of post-traumatic pain and altered sensation of the maxillary and mandibular branches of the trigeminal nerve: a systematic review. *Oral Surg Oral Med Oral Pathol Oral Radiol.* 2018;**125**(6):526–540.

14. Correll D. Chronic postoperative pain: recent findings in understanding and management. *F1000Research.* 2017;**6**:1054.

15. Lee TYC, Curtin JP. The effects of melatonin prophylaxis on sensory recovery and postoperative pain following orthognathic surgery: a triple-blind randomized controlled trial and biochemical analysis. *Int J Oral Maxillofac Surg.* 2020;**49**(4):446–453.

16. Essick GK, Phillips C, Turvey TA, Tucker M. Facial altered sensation and sensory impairment after orthognathic surgery. *Int J Oral Maxillofac Surg.* 2007;**36**(7):577–582.

17. Law C, Alam P, Borumandi F. Floor-of-mouth hematoma following dental implant placement: literature review and case presentation. *J Oral Maxillofac Surg.* 2017;**75**(11): 2340–2346.

18. Lang S, Lanigan DT, van der Wal M. Trigeminocardiac reflexes: maxillary and mandibular variants of the oculocardiac reflex. *Can J Anaesth.* 1991;**38**(6):757–760.

19. Kamalpathey LCK, Sahoo MGNK, Chattopadhyay CPK, Issar MY. Access osteotomy in the maxillofacial skeleton. *Ann Maxillofac Surg.* 2017;**7**(1):98–103.

20. Venkatesulu BP, Mahadevan LS, Aliru ML, Yang X, Bodd MH, Singh PK, Yusuf SW, Abe JI, Krishnan S. Radiation-induced endothelial vascular injury: a review of possible mechanisms. *JACC Basic Transl Sci.* 2018;**3**(4):563–572.

21. Talmi YP, Benzaray S, Peleg M, Eyal A, Bedrin L, Shoshani Y, et al. Pulmonary function after pectoralis major myocutaneous flap harvest. *Laryngoscope.* 2002;**112**(3):467–471.

22. Agochukwu UF, DeVine JG. Evaluating post-operative pain management at the iliac crest bone graft site: an editorial. *J Spine Surg.* 2016;**2**(3):237–239.

23. Tessier P. Anatomical classification of facial, cranio-facial and latero-facial clefts. *J Maxillofac Surg.* 1976;**4**(2):69–92.

24. MacLean JE, Hayward P, Fitzgerald DA, Waters K. Cleft lip and/or palate and breathing during sleep. *Sleep Med Rev.* 2009;**13**(5):345–354.

25. Wynne DM, Justice RE, Russel CJH, Gibson NA, Moores T, Ray AK, et al. Evaluation of changes in sleep breathing patterns after primary palatoplasty in cleft children. *S Eur J Orthod Dentofac Res.* 2014;**1**:10–14.

18

Non-technical skills

Frances Lui

Introduction

It has been estimated that one in ten patients suffer from an adverse event during hospital admission and nearly half are preventable.[1] Medical errors account for a reported 44,000–98,000 deaths annually in the US,[2] and are postulated to be the third leading cause of hospital death.[3] In 2010, the European Board of Anaesthesiology and the European Society of Anaesthesiology established the Helsinki Declaration on Patient Safety in Anaesthesiology. This declaration was universally endorsed, and was a major step forwards in improving patient safety with the World Health Organization (WHO) Surgical Safety Checklist (SSC), and other safety recommendations.[4]

The importance of human factors and system safety have long been recognized within industries such as nuclear energy and aviation—indeed, crisis resource management (CRM) training has been a licensing and revalidation requirement for commercial airline pilots for many years. These high-risk, high-hazard organizations have well-established safety records, based upon intrinsically low absolute error rates and resilient systems designed to minimize sequelae when errors do occur. Conversely, awareness of the importance of human factors has only permeated into healthcare relatively recently. Human factors have often been mislabelled as human errors, with critical incidents attributed to individual carelessness, poor knowledge, or negligence, rather than exploring (and improving) the limitations of the system that contributed. The importance of human factors, ergonomics, and non-technical skills in healthcare are now being recognized—reflected by their overdue inclusion in medical education and postgraduate curricula.

Non-technical skills refer to a set of cognitive and social skills that must be integrated with medical knowledge, clinical skills, and procedural skills, to deliver high-quality, safe, and effective patient care.

Anaesthetic non-technical skills (ANTS) framework

ANTS developed from a list of desirable skills identified for consultant anaesthetist and trainee interviews.[5] Critical incident reports from the Australian Anaesthetic Incident Monitoring System were reviewed to support the concept, and taxonomy and rating systems were derived.

Video clips of simulated anaesthetic crises were filmed at the Scottish Clinical Simulation Centre and consultant anaesthetists, who had been given training on the system, rated observed behaviours of relevant non-technical skills. The scores were analysed and found to have acceptable internal consistency, reliability, validity, and usability.[6] The system has subsequently been modified and translated into many different languages.[5,7] The ANTS framework[8] (Table 18.1) includes four categories and 15 elements, with desirable and less desirable behavioural attributes under each element, with a 4-point rating scale (1, poor; 2, marginal; 3, acceptable; 4, good; N, not observed).

Challenges of oromaxillofacial anaesthesia

In the UK, most procedures are performed in hospitals with anaesthesia provided solely by trained anaesthetists. In other countries, minor oromaxillofacial surgical (OMFS) procedures continue to be performed in outpatient settings—a practice that is accredited by several national bodies, including the Accreditation Association for Ambulatory Health Care and the American Association for Accreditation of Ambulatory Surgery Facilities.[9] In this setting, the operating surgeon often administers sedation (nitrous oxide gas,

Table 18.1 The ANTS framework

Categories	Elements
Task management	Planning and preparing
	Prioritizing
	Providing and maintaining standards
	Identifying and utilizing resources
Team working	Coordinating activities with team members
	Exchanging information
	Using authority and assertiveness
	Assessing capabilities
	Supporting others
Situation awareness	Gathering information
	Recognizing and understanding
	Anticipating
Decision-making	Identifying options
	Balancing risks and selecting options
	Re-evaluating

benzodiazepines, and/or opioids) and there is significant variability in sedation expertise, medical knowledge, and crisis management training. The office environment is rarely equipped with an anaesthetic machine, and resuscitation may be impaired by poor ergonomics, lighting, and electricity supply, as well as restricted access to oxygen sources and monitoring devices. In the US, the 'Office Anesthesia Evaluation' is designed to check for the *presence* of essential equipment, but does not encompass equipment functionality, calibration, or electrical testing. Anaesthetists may be called urgently to assist in the middle of an OMFS procedure, having had no prior patient interaction and without any pre-anaesthetic evaluation. Staff numbers may be reduced, with scrub nurses often fulfilling the role of theatre runner as well, and anaesthetists expected to work completely independently. A post-anaesthesia care unit is usually absent, with patients recovering in the office environment before discharge home the same day. The curriculum of the Association of British Academic Oral and Maxillofacial surgeons incorporates only a small element on medical crisis training.[10] In contrast, dental anaesthesia in Japan is an independent entity and anaesthetists must undergo additional specialist training before being certified to practise. Such disparity in legislation and organizational structures combined with highly variable patient characteristics pose significant challenges to anaesthesia providers.

For some patient groups, only hospital-based anaesthesia is appropriate, even for minor OMFS procedures (e.g. dental extractions). These include most paediatric patients (especially those with complex syndromes and/or congenital heart disease), patients with behavioural/psychosocial disorders (anxiety, phobia, cognitive impairment, and attention deficits), patients with significant comorbidities (heart failure, chronic obstructive pulmonary disease, dementia), patients unable to lie still, and those who require more extensive surgery.[11] Medical errors and complications are poorly tolerated in these vulnerable patient groups due to their limited physiological reserve. Indeed, 44 paediatric dental deaths were identified from a US database between 1980 and 2011.[12] Patients with significant comorbidities may require medical optimization, and treatment courses may be prolonged, involving multiple staged procedures, scheduled around complex social needs. An estimated 40%[13,14] of children with autistic spectrum disorders require multiple dental visits. Arrangements for patient transfer into hospital from their home or institution can be particularly challenging. Emergence delirium is more common in the paediatric and elderly populations, and the incidence of airway complications following OMFS is higher. Consequently, some patients require additional monitoring after anaesthesia, although most still expect rapid recovery and same-day discharge following dental extractions. Turnover of patients is usually high and with constant demand for efficiency, there is increased propensity for medication errors, wrong-site surgery, retained throat packs, and communication gaps.[15] Clearly, not just technical skills are required to meet the complex demands posed by these environmental, organizational, and patient challenges.

Task management

Task management is defined as 'skills for organizing resources and required activities to achieve goals, applied to both individual case plans and longer-term scheduling issues', comprising four skill elements[8]:

Planning and preparing

Strategies for task management must be developed for both primary and contingency pathways, reviewed regularly, and modified as required. This is especially important for minor OMFS procedures, as scheduling issues and ad hoc requests arise frequently. The anaesthetist may be the first physician to assess the patient, reconcile the medication list, and take a relevant history and airway examination. A postoperative discharge plan should also be discussed with patients in the pre-anaesthetic assessment.

Prioritizing

Anaesthetists must allocate varying degrees of attention and importance to different tasks, and avoid being distracted—for example, prioritizing airway control and oxygenation over optimal surgical access during sedation for dental extractions.

Providing and maintaining standards

Guidelines, protocols, and checklists should be adhered to whenever possible. Drugs must be labelled (preferably colour coded) and in standardized dilutions. Equipment, including the anaesthetic machine, must be checked and records kept accurately. Pre-anaesthetic evaluation should be standardized,[16] particularly the airway assessment, given that OMFS patients are more likely to pose airway management difficulties. Anaesthetists practising in office-based environments must be especially aware of potential safety threats, and meticulously check monitoring and resuscitation equipment, as well as oxygen and electricity supplies. Algorithms and emergency manuals are indispensable cognitive aids, and the WHO SSC is especially important in prevention of wrong tooth extraction (where marking of the surgical site is not possible).[17]

Identifying and utilizing resources

Anaesthetists should be able to establish the requirements for task completion with minimal disruption, stress, and overload to the individual or team. Adverse events such as emergence delirium or OMFS crises such as local anaesthetic toxicity require additional resources (personnel, expertise, equipment, and time). The team may not be optimally prepared if simulation drills are not practised regularly. Good anticipation of potential problems and early recruitment of resources is helpful, with task allocation appropriately matched to skill levels.

Situation awareness

Situation awareness is a human performance construct in which an individual understands their current situation, the constantly changing nature of their environment, making correct decisions, and undertaking appropriate actions. Situation awareness can be divided into three levels: perception (level I), comprehension (level II), and projection (level III).[18] In an anaesthesia closed claims analysis, lack of situation awareness contributed to death or brain damage in 74% of claims.[19] Inadequate oxygenation or ventilation, difficult tracheal intubation, and pulmonary aspiration were more common where situation awareness was impaired. In 81.5% of cases reported to the German critical incident reporting system, situation awareness errors occurred most commonly at the levels of perception and comprehension.[18] This is of particular relevance during complex shared airway procedures, or when managing OMFS emergencies; for example, postoperative bleeding, oedema, or vomiting following bimaxillary osteotomy with intermaxillary fixation (where immediate oral access is impaired) can rapidly escalate to critical hypoxaemia if correct decisions and prompt actions are not taken. A number of different methods can assess situation awareness. These include performance measures—either direct (outcomes, time to task completion, error rate) or indirect (self-assessment, observer ratings); mental workload measures (subjective ratings, physiological parameters)[20]; task analytic measures (eye tracking, time and motion, time spent on task components, communication analysis); questionnaires (Situation Awareness Global Assessment Techniques); behavioural indicators (ANTS scale, Ottawa Global Rating Scale)[21]; and psychophysiological measures—heart rate, ocular movements, cerebral blood flow, electroencephalography, and event-related evoked potentials.

Situation awareness depends upon mental workload determinants and the capacity of the human brain to process extra information in evolving situations, which is influenced by exogenous factors (task demands, difficulty, priority, and urgency) and endogenous factors (attention, perception, working memory, expertise). Spatial distribution of visual attention of anaesthetists during simulated induction of anaesthesia with or without critical incidents has shown that more experienced anaesthetists are able to dedicate less time to unrelated tasks, concentrating on manual tasks during critical incidents.[22] This suggests a higher degree of situation awareness allowed them to direct their spare mental capacity to the most relevant tasks, especially in a crisis. Endsley described eight 'demons' of situation awareness[23]:

1. *Attention tunnelling*—for example, an anaesthetist continues to increase the depth of intravenous anaesthesia in response to hypertension, failing to notice drug extravasation.

2. *Requisite memory trap*—especially for auditory information which is not subjected to visual review at a later occasion, for example, an anaesthetist may not remember to remove a throat pack when only verbally, but not visually reminded.

3. *Workload, anxiety, fatigue, and other stressors.*

4. *Data overload*—for example, in a tight schedule with high turnover of patients (common to dental anaesthesia operating lists), the clinical history of different patients may overload the working memory of the anaesthetist.

5. *Misplaced salience*—humans are naturally attracted to environmental features such as the colour red, flashing lights, and moving objects. If these features are overused (e.g. multiple emergency crisis algorithms displayed in operating theatres), their impact will deteriorate.

6. *Complexity creep*—for example, adding too much information will cause cognitive overload and an inability to notice and interpret the information.

7. *Errant mental model*—working with a single mental model and an inability to break out of it.

8. *Out-of-the-loop syndrome*—this problem is created by automation. Automation occurs when a system performs so well that a potential problem with it no longer occurs to the team members—for example, most anaesthetists will not check for signs of hypoxaemia if a pulse oximetry reading is good; however, when the saturation probe reading is low, anaesthetists may repeatedly check for interference rather than for signs of hypoxaemia.

Importantly, there is a relationship between cognitive capacity and established knowledge and understanding. Compared with novices, experts are able to apply their superior domain-specific factual and procedural knowledge to solve problems more quickly. Training in situation awareness (especially using simulation) is therefore designed so that tasks are domain specific for skill acquisition. Visual aids are also encouraged rather than auditory cues, in order to reduce overloading the working memory (cognitive aids are discussed in greater detail later in this chapter).

Situation awareness can be derived at an individual or team level—involving shared requirements, devices, mental models, and processes ('distributed' situation awareness),[24] taking into account the complex interactions that occur within a collaborative system. In this case, the interactions between components of the system become the focus of any root cause analysis in the event of a critical incident.[25]

ANTS applied to situation awareness

Situation awareness in ANTS is defined as 'the skills for developing and maintaining an overall awareness of the work setting, based on observing all relevant aspects of the theatre environment (patient, team, time, displays, equipment); understanding what they mean, and thinking ahead about what could happen in the near future'. It encompasses three skill elements:

Gathering information

Information is collected from all sources including records, drug charts, monitor displays, equipment databases, clinical symptoms, surgical field, theatre settings, and team communication threads. Information gathered is verified, and continuously updated for ongoing interpretation. Good communication between the surgeon and the anaesthetist is essential for accurate data gathering, as the anaesthetist's view of the surgical field can be compromised during OMFS procedures.

Recognizing and understanding

Information is integrated and interpreted to identify any mismatch (a simultaneous diagnostic and management process). Not only the quantity, but also the significance of each information point is analysed to achieve specific goals; for example, if there has been significant bleeding, a patient may become hypotensive, therefore the frequency of non-invasive blood pressure monitoring should be increased. Team members should be alerted and initial management options might include volume expansion, vasopressor administration, upgrading existing intravenous access, point-of-care testing, optimizing anaesthetic depth, and simultaneous actions of the surgeon to achieve haemostasis. Further escalation might include activation of transfusion algorithms, tranexamic acid administration, prevention of hypothermia, and so on.

Anticipating

This involves projection of potential outcomes associated with different actions, and constant review of the evolving situation. In the above example, an anaesthetist may wish to call for extra personnel in anticipation of the increased number of tasks associated with massive bleeding.

Decision-making

How an individual selects a particular course of action depends upon the context, perceived consequences, time permitted, information reliability, and influence of the group (if they are working as part of a team). Perhaps the most significant threat to rational decision-making is a tendency to have preconceived notions and the desire to seek confirmation of these. Several different cognitive models[26] are used to explain the processes involved in decision-making:

Normative model

The optimal decision is made with rationality. A good decision is based on projecting the relevant consequences of different actions, accurate assessment of situations, and making trade-offs in between. An alternative, with the greatest subjective expected utility, is chosen to maximize return and risk aversion.

Behavioural model

This model explains discrepancies in human estimates of probabilities and inference using heuristics, biases, and effects of memory (see later for a list of cognitive biases).

Naturalistic model

This model states that decisions are made in a routine and non-analytical manner, in a dynamic and realistic environment, for example, decisions based on following previous behavioural patterns (especially for manual tasks).

Sometimes, clinical decisions are based upon pattern recognition, and judgements may be made without considering all available options. Decision-making at a group level adds another layer of complexity, as groups are often bounded by social and ethical norms. A 'group' may not necessarily infer 'team' as individuals within the group may not share the same mental model, such that trade-offs must be made and conflicts may arise (large groups are especially prone to arrive at polarized conclusions). Conflict resolution involves discussion, argument, voting, negotiation, arbitration, and third-party intervention. A variety of approaches have been developed to enhance 'group thinking', such as brainstorming, Delphi techniques, attaining consensus, agendas, and computer-based decision support.

Ideally, anaesthetists would make rational decisions in accordance with the normative model; however, human decision-making is influenced by emotion and subconscious processes, such as clinical sense, 'rule of thumb', educational guess, and 'common things are common'. Heuristics are not necessarily incorrect, and represent a means of tackling complex situations in a mentally economical way. Some of these cognitive biases are described below[27]:

1. *Anchoring heuristics*—a tendency to rely on the first piece of information offered, for example, if an anaesthetist chooses to intubate the trachea using a nasal flexible fibreoptic approach, this is an 'anchoring' point for the team to focus on, and alternative options may not be considered.

2. *Availability heuristics*—the ease with which an idea is conceived, for example, an anaesthetist may choose a fibreoptic approach because they have just attended an advanced airway workshop.

3. *Framing effects*—preferences between medical interventions change dramatically depending on whether the outcomes are posed as losses or gains, for example, an anaesthetist may not choose to perform a fibreoptic intubation when they are informed the technique has a 10% failure rate. Conversely, they may select the technique if they are told it has a 90% success rate.

The 'rule of three' has been described as a potential de-biasing strategy[28]: if a treatment for a diagnosed condition is initiated and repeated once without an effect, at least three other possible diagnoses should be considered prior to attempting the same intervention a third time. In addition, explanation for a particular treatment effect should also consider three other possible causes for the effect, for example, a patient's oxygen saturation falls during intermittent positive pressure ventilation, leading to secretions being suctioned. If oxygen desaturation persists on repeat suctioning, three differential diagnoses should be considered. Even if secretions are present upon suctioning, differential diagnoses for oxygen desaturation should still be considered. Cognitive aids and checklists can aid this process of considering differential diagnoses and in avoiding fixation errors.

ANTS applied to decision-making

There are three skill elements in this category[8]:

Identifying options

This requires the anaesthetist to problem-solve—a stepwise approach considering all the alternatives, involving patients in decision-making, and seeking opinion from experts in challenging cases. For example, determining whether a patient's trachea be extubated immediately after elective intermaxillary fixation; if extubation is not appropriate immediately, then when might it be undertaken and how might it be done safely—what will the airway rescue strategy involve; and were all these options discussed with the patient in advance?

Balancing risks and selecting options

This is the ability to consider both advantages and disadvantages before making a choice, specifically tailored to the patient's individual situation, and then judicious implementation of the chosen action. For example, the decision is made to proceed to tracheal extubation; however, if the patient's oxygen saturations fall following extubation, the priority must be rescue oxygenation and a plan for reintubation must be formulated and prepared for.

Re-evaluating

The chosen option must be constantly reassessed and the situation updated. Interventions may take time to take effect, during which the patient may continue to deteriorate, necessitating change in their management. If proven wrong or new information arises, the course of action must be revised. In the previous example, if the oxygen saturations continue to fall despite initial airway rescue techniques, the anaesthetist must transition down the difficult intubation algorithm rather than becoming fixated on reintubation.

Teamwork

In operating theatres, staff from different disciplines, educational backgrounds, and cultures must work together in a complex and dynamic environment. Each team member contributes to patient care and can have an impact on their outcome. The US Institute of Medicine report 'To Err is Human: Building a Safer Health System'[2] emphasized team training in critical care areas to provide safe, effective, efficient, personalized, timely, and equitable medical care. Team Strategies and Tools to Enhance Performance and Patient Safety (TeamSTEPPS™)[29] is an example of such a team training system. The WHO SSC also encourages collaboration between team members, to reduce communication errors and improve safety. The constituents of an effective team vary according to task characteristics, such as task complexity and time pressure. Great teamwork depends on team members' respective competencies in the 'Big Five': leadership, mutual performance monitoring, backup behaviour, adaptability, and team orientation.[30]

ANTS applied to teamwork

Teamwork in ANTS is 'skills for working in a group context, in any role, to ensure effective joint task completion and team member satisfaction'. It involves five skill elements at an individual level[8]:

Coordinating activities with team members

Oromaxillofacial anaesthetists are required to collaborate with many other operating theatre staff members during manual and cognitive tasks, and they must understand the roles and responsibilities of each team member. It is crucial that tasks are allocated according to the best use of labour and resources, and not necessarily assuming that all senior staff members are 'leaders' and all juniors are team 'members' in every task. Everyone (regardless of seniority or training) can contribute positively to any situation, especially in an emergency/crisis. In an evolving situation, the role of each member may need to change, and role allocation should be frequently reviewed. Responsibility and coordination should certainly not be assumed.

Exchanging information

Great teams give and receive knowledge and data, and confirm their understanding for better coordination. For example, in the event of significant intraoperative bleeding, surgical gauze should be regularly weighed and correlated with the volume of irrigation fluid, and the anaesthetist should update the surgeon on the estimated blood loss, so that the entire team is sharing the same mental model towards achieving haemostasis.

Authority and assertiveness

Instructions given by the team leader should be clear, precise, and delivered in a decisive manner. Team leaders should also be able to assume a non-leading role when appropriate. Nevertheless, conflicts may still arise, and a good team should be able to recognize and resolve these effectively. In a patient with impending airway obstruction, the anaesthetist and surgeon may differ on the preferred airway management strategy (e.g. awake fibreoptic intubation versus awake tracheostomy)—an effective, cohesive team must be able to appreciate their colleagues' perspectives, and reach consensus on the best strategy, based upon the available skill mix and individual patient pathology and presentation.

Assessing capabilities

Each team member has their own specific knowledge and skills, and is influenced by factors unique to themselves—previous experience, stress, fatigue, sickness, and so on. Inquiry into the relative experience of team members is essential prior to task delegation. If a team member is not performing to the expected standard, support and assistance (beyond the task) may be required.

Supporting others

Physical, cognitive, and emotional support should be provided to other team members, particularly when a critical incident/untoward incident has occurred. Team members can often be second 'victims' from patient incidents, and even the team leader needs reassurance and appropriate debriefing.

Team communication

Unlike some other surgical specialities, the nature of oromaxillofacial surgery and the 'shared airway' dictate that good communication between operating surgeon and anaesthetist is *essential* to ensuring patient safety and optimizing patient outcome. Numerous strategies exist to improve communication within teams:

Distraction and noise avoidance

In the aviation industry, unnecessary conversation is not permitted in the cockpit when flying below 10,000 feet.[31] Similarly, extraneous noise and interruptions should be minimized in anaesthesia—particularly during time-critical and potentially challenging procedures such as airway management in the oromaxillofacial patient. Notably, the American College of Surgeons has issued a statement addressing the use of smartphones and handheld electronic devices, and the importance of avoiding noise distraction[32] in the operating theatre. Rather unsurprisingly, the frequency of case-irrelevant conversations is lower during more challenging surgical procedures.[33]

Communication techniques and tools

'Read-back' is a technique in which the individual receiving the information repeats it back verbally to the sender, so that the sender knows their message was understood. This technique increases information transfer between anaesthetists and post-anaesthesia care unit nurses, and can be of particular use during patient emergencies.[34]

Weller et al.[35] have also described a structured tool for improved information sharing, 'SNAPPI': Stop, Notify, Assessment, Plan, Priorities, Invite ideas. In simulated scenarios of local anaesthetic toxicity and pulmonary embolus, the SNAPPI tool improved information sharing between anaesthetists and other team members, and verbalization of the diagnosis. The tool also facilitated nursing staff and assistants to speak up (having been invited by the anaesthetists), empowering often-overlooked team members.

To ensure a task is completed, the three Cs of communication—Clear instructions, Closing the loop, and Citing names—have also been shown to be beneficial.[36]

'Speaking up' culture

The two-challenge rule in the aviation industry is an example of a tool to improve communication, and is covered in the TeamSTEPPS™ programme: if a pilot has endangered flight safety by his/her actions, the co-pilot *must* challenge it. If there is no answer after two challenges, or an irrational response is given, the co-pilot is entitled to assume control of the flight. Similarly, United Airlines have promoted the use of provocative words in a crisis, so that junior staff can attract their seniors' attention, C (I am 'concerned'), U (I am 'uncomfortable'), and S (I am 'scared').

Senior medical staff must specifically encourage feedback from junior team members, nursing staff, and assistants, as these individuals may not willingly speak up due to perceived hierarchy, lack of confidence, or in the assumption that the leader already knows the information. Green et al.[37] suggested that phrases such as 'anyone can and should speak up if you have any concerns whatsoever, without fear of retribution' should be repeated throughout the day by senior clinicians to encourage assertive challenges from nursing staff about patient safety concerns. In some languages, particular words and sentence structures can be chosen to emphasize politeness and to highlight the relative hierarchy of the speaker and listener—in crisis situations, the speech pattern should be clear, avoiding overly convoluted language, and should follow a 'horizontal' gradient.[38]

Team performance

Optimal team performance can be affected by a number of external factors.

In a simulation study,[39] it was found that all categories of non-technical skills performance declined during cardiopulmonary resuscitation when there were external stressors present (extraneous noise or a scripted actor playing the role of a family member). However, when the leader possessed superior non-technical skills, the entire team demonstrated improved technical performance, with the authors recommending non-technical skills training specifically for team leaders, in order to benefit overall team performance.

Fatigue may be a particularly important factor in performance. Fatigue can arise not only from sleep deprivation but also boredom, work overload, physical exhaustion, and changes to circadian rhythm. Syringe swaps and wrong drug dosages were identified as the most common medical errors associated with fatigue in the Australian Incident Monitoring Study database from 1987 to 1997.[40] In 2014, the Association of Anaesthetists published guidelines on anticipating and mitigating the effects of fatigue in the workplace. Nevertheless, in a subsequent national survey on the effects of fatigue on UK anaesthetic trainees,[41] fatigue was cited as impairing physical health, psychological well-being, and personal relationships.

Crisis resource management and simulation training

Concepts derived from the aviation industry have been translated to anaesthesia CRM courses to enhance non-technical skills training, focusing on tasks performed by anaesthetists in the operating theatre using simulation-based training.[7]

The principles of anaesthesia CRM include the following key points[42]:

1. Knowing the environment.
2. Anticipating and planning.
3. Calling for help early and identifying who and how to call.
4. Exercising leadership with assertiveness; planning, decision-making, and distribution of tasks with clear instructions.
5. Distribution of workload—the '10-seconds-for-10-minutes rule': at critical moments, when a team 'feels stuck', it should pause for a 10-second time-out to re-evaluate. The leader should identify issues, gather information, and check with team members for their concerns. This 10-second delay is offset by the benefits of aligning rational decision-making and planning.
6. Mobilizing all available resources.
7. Communicating effectively.
8. Using all available information—both primary (patient physiological status, monitor displays) and secondary (patient charts and records, cognitive aids, online resources).
9. Preventing fixation errors—cognitive biases may warrant a second opinion.
10. Cross-checking and double-checking—never assume anything.
11. Using cognitive aids—checklists, handbooks, guidelines, dose calculators, and advice hotlines.
12. Repeated re-evaluation—application of the '10-seconds-for-10-minutes rule'.
13. Implementation of good teamwork—coordination with and support of others.
14. Astute allocation of attention.
15. Dynamic prioritization.

Simulation has been applied to nearly all healthcare domains, to assist with acquisition of technical psychomotor skills for clinical procedures, in evaluation of cognitive and interpersonal skills, and to assess the effects of performance-shaping factors.[43] As well as an educational tool, it has also become a key component of competency-based assessment in many anaesthesia certification programmes. Simulation-based CRM training has demonstrated significant and reproducible improvement in team communication and improved coordination in the management of obstetric,[44] critical care,[45] neonatal,[46] and trauma emergencies/resuscitation.[47] The use of *in situ* high-fidelity simulation in the operating theatre also offers a means of testing the functional aspects of the clinical location during daily activities (surgical procedures) and to assess workplace attitudes.[48] The participants gain intrinsic motivation and positive self-efficacy from their involvement as well.[49] It is more challenging to prove simulation-based CRM training directly improves *patient* outcomes; nevertheless, a few studies have demonstrated such a change, in adult cardiac arrest team responses,[50] neonatal resuscitation,[51] and in-hospital paediatric cardiac arrest survival.[52] High fidelity simulation training has been shown to improve anaesthetists' technical performance and ANTS scores in malignant hyperthermia scenarios,[53] and has been used successfully for medical crisis training of dental practitioners.[54,55]

Cognitive aids

Cognitive aids are tools created to assist an individual or team in reducing errors and omissions, and to increase speed and team fluidity during performance of a task.[56] Examples relevant to OMFS include adult life support algorithms,[57] management of local anaesthetic toxicity protocols,[58] difficult airway algorithms,[59] and SBAR (Situation, Background, Assessment, Recommendations) for structured handover of complex airway patients to recovery nurses.[60] Cognitive aids should be evidence based, context specific, contain only salient information in an easily readable format, and be immediately available in the relevant clinical environment. Linear cognitive aids have been shown to be more effective than branched flow charts,[61] and paper checklists are generally preferable to electronic versions—particularly in emergency situations.[62] Most importantly, education and training using the cognitive aids are essential as part of their implementation.[56] The WHO SSC, introduced in 2009,[63] is one of the most widely adopted checklists internationally, and has successfully reduced postoperative surgical complications including surgical site infections, unplanned reoperations, pneumonia, and overall mortality.[64,65] Of course, adherence to the checklist is essential to influence outcome. Unfortunately, compliance and the quality of the process is highly variable,[66,67] with some staff perceiving it as a 'tick box' exercise rather than recognizing its potential benefits.[68] Its use can be particularly helpful in OMFS, where it may assist in highlighting potentially difficult airway management and/or significant blood loss. Similarly, its application in dental operating theatres and outpatient settings may reduce 'wrong-site surgery' during dental extractions.[69] Interestingly, improved checklist adherence has been observed when the checking process is initiated by surgeons,[67] although successful implementation requires collaborative intention, with engagement of all staff members.[70] At a university hospital in Taiwan, the WHO SSC was used as the basis for an entire educational programme for dental residents, successfully reducing their erroneous dental extraction rate from 0.026–0.046% in 1991 to zero in 2001.[71]

Continued path towards improving patient safety

Patient safety depends upon optimizing hazard control, by limiting safety threats that may result in morbidity, mortality, and/or legal liability. Hazards can be controlled by a three-phase response system: (1) eliminate it, (2) defend against it, and (3) warn about it. Total elimination of potential threats is often impossible, such that patient safety is often reliant upon robust processes and effective warning systems. In OMFS, pre-assessment clinics can be considered such a defence system, identifying potentially high-risk patients who require special planning and management, and patient difficult airway alert bracelets may represent a warning measure.

Of course, like many interventions, these involve behavioural change and compliance, training, and appropriate personnel selection, and none are foolproof. Warnings should never compensate for inadequate or poorly designed defence measures.

Ultimately, the aim should be to establish a *culture* of safety within the workplace, across all settings and environments. This can be exemplified by the effect of simply broadening the WHO SSC into a five-step intervention (pre-list briefing, sign-in, time-out, sign-out, and post-list debriefing)—implementation of which has been shown to have significant improvement in five of the six safety culture domains: working conditions, perceptions of management, job satisfaction, safety climate, and teamwork climate[72] (staff members' perception of stress, the sixth domain, worsened, although this response may have resulted from improvements in the other domains). The climate of safety created not only alerted frontline staff to adverse patient outcome indicators but also encouraged positive domains in the workplace.

Conclusion

Training in anaesthetic non-technical skills has crucially raised awareness of the important contribution of human factors and behavioural learning to patient safety, but should only be considered part of the framework necessary to create a culture of safety. Errors will continue to occur and, while they can be dreadfully damaging to both patients and the staff involved, they serve as the basis for continued improvement. The commitment to achieving a climate of safety must permeate through entire organizations, supported by healthcare policies, organizational structures, and professional regulations, and driven by dedicated leaders and engaged staff.

REFERENCES

1. de Vries EN, Ramrattan MA, Smorenburg SM, Gouma DJ, Boermeester MA. The incidence and nature of in-hospital adverse events: a systematic review. *Qual Saf Health Care.* 2008;**17**(3):216–223.
2. Kohn JT, Corrigan JM, Donaldson MS. *To Err Is Human: Building a Safer Healthcare System.* Washington, DC: National Academies Press; 1999.
3. Makary MA, Daniel M. Medical error-the third leading cause of death in the US. *BMJ.* 2016;**353**:i2139.
4. Mellin-Olsen J, Staender S, Whitaker DK, Smith AF. The Helsinki declaration on patient safety in anaesthesiology. *Eur J Anaesthesiol.* 2010;**27**(7):592–597.
5. Flin R, Patey R. Non-technical skills for anaesthetists: developing and applying ANTS. *Best Pract Res Clin Anaesthesiol.* 2011;**25**(2):215–227.
6. Rutherford JS, Flin R, Irwin A, McFadyen AK. Evaluation of the prototype Anaesthetic Non-technical Skills for Anaesthetic Practitioners (ANTS-AP) system: a behavioural rating system to assess the non-technical skills used by staff assisting the anaesthetist. *Anaesthesia.* 2015;**70**(8):907–914.
7. Flin R, Maran N. Basic concepts for crew resource management and non-technical skills. *Best Pract Res Clin Anaesthesiol.* 2015;**29**(1):27–39.

8. Flin R, Glavin R, Maran N, Patey R. *Anaesthetists' Non-Technical Skills (ANTS) System Handbook v1.0. Framework for Observing and Rating Anaesthetists' non-Technical Skills*. Aberdeen: University of Aberdeen; 2012.

9. Keeley KA. Equipment safety, maintenance and inspection: what the oral surgeon needs to know. *Oral Maxillofac Surg Clin North Am.* 2017;**29**(2):209–221.

10. Macluskey M, Durham J, Cowan G, Cowpe J, Evans A, Freeman C, et al. UK national curriculum for undergraduate oral surgery subgroup for teaching of the Association of British Academic Oral and Maxillofacial Surgeons. *Eur J Dent Educ.* 2008;**12**(1):48–58.

11. Giovannitti JA Jr. Anesthesia for off-floor dental and oral surgery. *Curr Opin Anaesthesiol.* 2016;**29**(4):519–525.

12. Lee HH, Milgrom P, Starks H, Burke W. Trends in death associated with pediatric dental sedation and general anesthesia. *Paediatr Anaesth.* 2013;**23**(8):741–746.

13. Bagattoni S, Sadotti A, D'Alessandro G, Piana G. Dental trauma in Italian children and adolescents with special health care needs. A cross-sectional retrospective study. *Eur J Paediatr Dent.* 2017;**18**(1):23–26.

14. Nelson T, Chim A, Sheller BL, McKinney CM, Scott JM. Predicting successful dental examinations for children with autism spectrum disorder in the context of a dental desensitization program. *J Am Dent Assoc.* 2017;**148**(7):485–492.

15. Todd DW. General concepts of patient safety for the oral and maxillofacial surgeon. *Oral Maxillofac Surg Clin North Am.* 2017;**29**(2):121–129.

16. Lieblich S. Preoperative evaluation and patient selection for office-based oral surgery anesthesia. *Oral Maxillofac Surg Clin North Am.* 2018;**30**(2):137–144.

17. Assael LA. Preventing wrong-site surgery in oral and maxillofacial surgery. *Oral Maxillofac Surg Clin North Am.* 2017;**29**(2):151–157.

18. Schulz CM, Krautheim V, Hackemann A, Kreuzer M, Kochs EF, Wagner KJ. Situation awareness errors in anesthesia and critical care in 200 cases of a critical incident reporting system. *BMC Anesthesiol.* 2016;**16**:4.

19. Schulz CM, Burden A, Posner KL, Mincer SL, Steadman R, Wagner KJ, et al. Frequency and type of situational awareness errors contributing to death and brain damage: a closed claims analysis. *Anesthesiology.* 2017;**127**(2):326–337.

20. Wright MC, Taekman JM, Endsley MR. Objective measures of situation awareness in a simulated medical environment. *Qual Saf Health Care.* 2004;**13** Suppl 1:i65–i71.

21. Schulz CM, Endsley MR, Kochs EF, Gelb AW, Wagner KJ. Situation awareness in anesthesia: concept and research. *Anesthesiology.* 2013;**118**(3):729–742.

22. Schulz CM, Schneider E, Fritz L, Vockeroth J, Hapfelmeier A, Brandt T, et al. Visual attention of anaesthetists during simulated critical incidents. *Br J Anaesth.* 2011;**106**(6):807–813.

23. Endsley MR. Situation awareness. In: Salvendy G (ed) *Handbook of Human Factors and Ergonomics*, pp. 553–568. Hoboken, NJ: John Wiley & Sons; 2012.

24. Fioratou E, Flin R, Glavin R, Patey R. Beyond monitoring: distributed situation awareness in anaesthesia. *Br J Anaesth.* 2010;**105**(1):83–90.

25. Stanton NA, Stewart R, Harris D, Houghton RJ, Baber C, McMaster R, et al. Distributed situation awareness in dynamic systems: theoretical development and application of an ergonomics methodology. *Ergonomics.* 2006;**49**(12–13):1288–1311.

26. Lehto MR, Nah FFH, Yi JS. Decision-making models, decision support, and problem solving. In: Salvendy G (ed) *Handbook of Human Factors and Ergonomics*, pp. 192–242. Hoboken, NJ: John Wiley & Sons; 2012.

27. Stiegler MP, Tung A. Cognitive processes in anesthesiology decision making. *Anesthesiology.* 2014;**120**(1):204–217.

28. Stiegler MP, Ruskin KJ. Decision-making and safety in anesthesiology. *Curr Opin Anaesthesiol.* 2012;**25**(6):724–729.

29. Rhee AJ, Valentin-Salgado Y, Eshak D, Feldman D, Kischak P, Reich DL, et al. Team training in the perioperative arena: a methodology for implementation and auditing behavior. *Am J Med Qual.* 2017;**32**(4):369–375.

30. Baker DP, Salas E, King H, Battles J, Barach P. The role of teamwork in the professional education of physicians: current status and assessment recommendations. *Jt Comm J Qual Patient Saf.* 2005;**31**(4):185–202.

31. Chute RD, Wiener EL. Cockpit-cabin communication: II. Shall we tell the pilots? *Int J Aviat Psychol.* 1996;**6**(3):211–231.

32. American College of Surgeons (ACS) Committee on Perioperative Care. Statement on distractions in the operating room. *Bull Am Coll Surg.* 2016;**101**(10):42–44.

33. Widmer LW, Cumin D, Lombard B, Torrie J, Civil N, Weller J. More than talking about the weekend: content of case-irrelevant communication within the OR team. *World J Surg.* 2018;**42**(7):2011–2017.

34. Boyd M, Torrie J, Boyd M, Frengley R, Garden A, Ng WL, et al. Read-back improves information transfer in simulated clinical crises. *BMJ Qual Saf.* 2014;**23**(12):989–993.

35. Weller JM, Torrie J, Boyd M, Frengley R, Garden A, Ng WL, et al. Improving team information sharing with a structured call-out in anaesthetic emergencies: a randomized controlled trial. *Br J Anaesth.* 2014;**112**(6):1042–1049.

36. Bodor R, Nguyen BJ, Broder K. We are going to name names and call you out! Improving the team in the academic operating room environment. *Ann Plast Surg.* 2017;**78**(5 Suppl 4):S222–S224.

37. Green B, Oeppen RS, Smith DW, Brennan PA. Challenging hierarchy in healthcare teams—ways to flatten gradients to improve teamwork and patient care. *Br J Oral Maxillofac Surg.* 2017;**55**(5):449–453.

38. Brindley PG, Reynolds SF. Improving verbal communication in critical care medicine. *J Crit Care.* 2011;**26**(2):155–1559.

39. Krage R, Zwaan L, Tjon Soei Len L, Kolenbrander MW, van Groeningen D, Loer SA, et al. Relationship between non-technical skills and technical performance during cardiopulmonary resuscitation: does stress have an influence? *Emerg Med J.* 2017;**34**(11):728–733.

40. Morris GP, Morris RW. Anaesthesia and fatigue: an analysis of the first 10 years of the Australian Incident Monitoring Study 1987–1997. *Anaesth Intensive Care.* 2000;**28**(3):300–304.

41. McClelland L, Holland J, Lomas JP, Redfern N, Plunkett E. A national survey of the effects of fatigue on trainees in anaesthesia in the UK. *Anaesthesia.* 2017;**72**(9):1069–1077.

42. Rall M, Gaba D, Howard SK, Dieckmann P. Human performance and patient safety. In: Miller RD, Cohen NH, Eriksson LI, Fleisher LA, Wiener-Kronish JP, Young WL (eds) *Miller's Anesthesia*, 8th ed, pp. 106–166. Philadelphia, PA: Elsevier/Saunders; 2015.

43. Small SD. Simulation applications for human factors and systems evaluation. *Anesthesiol Clin.* 2007;**25**(2):237–259.

44. Lipman SS, Daniels KI, Carvalho B, Arafeh J, Harney K, Puck A, et al. Deficits in the provision of cardiopulmonary resuscitation during simulated obstetric crises. *Am J Obstet Gynecol.* 2010;**203**(2):179.e1–5.

45. Frengley RW, Weller JM, Torrie J, Dzendrowskyj P, Yee B, Paul AM, et al. The effect of a simulation-based training intervention on the performance of established critical care unit teams. *Crit Care Med.* 2011;**39**(12):2605–2611.

46. Williams AL, Lasky RE, Dannemiller JL, Andrei AM, Thomas EJ. Teamwork behaviours and errors during neonatal resuscitation. *Qual Saf Health Care.* 2010;**19**(1):60–64.

47. Hughes KM, Benenson RS, Krichten AE, Clancy KD, Ryan JP, Hammond C. A crew resource management program tailored to trauma resuscitation improves team behavior and communication. *J Am Coll Surg.* 2014;**219**(3):545–551.

48. Gardner AK, Ahmed RA, George RL, Frey JA. In situ simulation to assess workplace attitudes and effectiveness in a new facility. *Simul Healthc.* 2013;**8**(6):351–358.

49. Murray AW, Beaman ST, Kampik CW, Quinlan JJ. Simulation in the operating room. *Best Pract Res Clin Anaesthesiol.* 2015;**29**(1):41–50.

50. Wayne DB, Didwania A, Feinglass J, Fudala MJ, Barsuk JH, McGaghie WC. Simulation-based education improves quality of care during cardiac arrest team responses at an academic teaching hospital: a case-control study. *Chest.* 2008;**133**(1):56–61.

51. Draycott T, Sibanda T, Owen L, Akande V, Winter C, Reading S, et al. Does training in obstetric emergencies improve neonatal outcome? *BJOG.* 2006;**113**(2):177–182.

52. Andreatta P, Saxton E, Thompson M, Annich G. Simulation-based mock codes significantly correlate with improved pediatric patient cardiopulmonary arrest survival rates. *Pediatr Crit Care Med.* 2011;**12**(1):33–38.

53. Hardy JB, Gouin A, Damm C, Compère V, Veber B, Dureuil B. The use of a checklist improves anaesthesiologists' technical and non-technical performance for simulated malignant hyperthermia management. *Anaesth Crit Care Pain Med.* 2018;**37**(1):17–23.

54. Tan GM. A medical crisis management simulation activity for pediatric dental residents and assistants. *J Dent Educ.* 2011;**75**(6):782–790.

55. Breuer G, Knipfer C, Huber T, Huettl S, Shams N, Knipfer K, et al. Competency in managing cardiac arrest: a scenario-based evaluation of dental students. *Acta Odontol Scand.* 2016;**74**(4):241–249.

56. Marshall S. The use of cognitive aids during emergencies in anesthesia: a review of the literature. *Anesth Analg.* 2013;**117**(5):1162–1171.

57. Soar J, Deakin CD, Lockey A, Nolan J, Perkins G. *Adult Advanced Life Support Guidelines.* London: Resuscitation Council UK; 2015.

58. Neal JM, Mulroy MF, Weinberg GL, American Society of Regional Anesthesia and Pain Medicine. American Society of Regional Anesthesia and Pain Medicine checklist for managing local anesthetic systemic toxicity: 2012 version. *Reg Anesth Pain Med.* 2012;**37**(1):16–18.

59. Frerk C, Mitchell VS, McNarry AF, Mendonca C, Bhagrath R, Patel A, et al. Difficult Airway Society 2015 guidelines for management of unanticipated difficult intubation in adults. *Br J Anaesth.* 2015;**115**(6):827–848.

60. Müller M, Jürgens J, Redaèlli M, Klingberg K, Hautz WE, Stock S. Impact of the communication and patient hand-off tool SBAR on patient safety: a systematic review. *BMJ Open.* 2018;**23**;8(8):e022202.

61. Marshall SD, Sanderson P, McIntosh CA, Kolawole H. The effect of two cognitive aid designs on team functioning during intra-operative anaphylaxis emergencies: a multi-centre simulation study. *Anaesthesia.* 2016;**71**(4):389–404.

62. Marshall SD. Helping experts and expert teams perform under duress: an agenda for cognitive aid research. *Anaesthesia.* 2017;**72**(3):289–295.

63. Haynes AB, Weiser TG, Berry WR, Lipsitz SR, Breizat AH, Dellinger EP, et al. A surgical safety checklist to reduce morbidity and mortality in a global population. *N Engl J Med.* 2009;**360**(5):491–499.

64. Gillespie BM, Chaboyer W, Thalib L, John M, Fairweather N, Slater K. Effect of using a safety checklist on patient complications after surgery: a systematic review and meta-analysis. *Anesthesiology.* 2014;**120**(6):1380–1389.

65. Bergs J, Hellings J, Cleemput I, Zurel Ö, De Troyer V, Van Hiel M, et al. Systematic review and meta-analysis of the effect of the World Health Organization surgical safety checklist on postoperative complications. *Br J Surg.* 2014;**101**(3):150–158.

66. Neuhaus C, Spies A, Wilk H, Weigand MA, Lichtenstern C. 'Attention everyone, time out!': safety attitudes and checklist practices in anesthesiology in Germany. A cross-sectional study. *J Patient Saf.* 2021;**17**(6):467–471.

67. Russ S, Rout S, Caris J, Mansell J, Davies R, Mayer E, et al. Measuring variation in use of the WHO surgical safety checklist in the operating room: a multicenter prospective cross-sectional study. *J Am Coll Surg.* 2015;**220**(1):1–11.e4.

68. Dharampal N, Cameron C, Dixon E, Ghali W, Quan ML. Attitudes and beliefs about the surgical safety checklist: just another tick box? *Can J Surg.* 2016;**59**(4):268–275.

69. Pemberton MN. Surgical safety checklists and understanding of never events, in UK and Irish dental hospitals. *Br Dent J.* 2016;**220**(11):585–589.

70. Leape LL. The checklist conundrum. *N Engl J Med.* 2014;**370**(11):1063–1064.

71. Chang HH, Lee JJ, Cheng SJ, Yang PJ, Hahn LJ, Kuo YS, et al. Effectiveness of an educational program in reducing the incidence of wrong-site tooth extraction. *Oral Surg Oral Med Oral Pathol Oral Radiol Endod.* 2004;**98**(3):288–294.

72. Hill MR, Roberts MJ, Alderson ML, Gale TC. Safety culture and the 5 steps to safer surgery: an intervention study. *Br J Anaesth.* 2015;**114**(6):958–962.

19

Orofacial pain

Stanley Sau Ching Wong and Chi Wai Cheung

Introduction

Orofacial pain disorders are a common clinical problem experienced by a quarter of the general population, and about 10% is chronic.[1,2] In the latest International Association for the Study of Pain (IASP) classification of chronic pain, chronic headache or orofacial pain is defined as headache or orofacial pain that occurs on at least 50% of the days during at least 3 months, and lasting at least 2 hours per day.[3] Persistent facial pain has an incidence ratio of 38.7 per 100,000 person years.[4] It is more common in women and the incidence increases with age.[4] Both acute and chronic facial pain results in significant impairment in quality of life.[1] Patients with facial pain may experience serious challenges in everyday activities such as eating, brushing teeth, talking, and cleaning of the face. These pain-related problems can negatively impact patients' psychosocial function for long periods of time.

Pain in the face is generally separated from headache. This is because transmission from the second (maxillary) and third (mandibular) trigeminal branches is responsible for pain in the facial region, whereas headaches are due to pain transmission via the first trigeminal (ophthalmic) branch. The trigeminal nerves innervate numerous anatomical structures including the lips, teeth, upper pharynx, uvula, soft palate, anterior two-thirds of the tongue, face, muscles of mastication and facial expression, nasal and oral mucosa, cornea, temporomandibular joints, dura mater, intracranial vessels, tooth pulp, and ears. The sensory innervation of the face, head, and neck is complex. The three branches of the trigeminal nerve and the upper cervical nerves (C2–C4) that innervate the posterior head and neck together form the trigeminocervical network[5,6] (**Fig. 19.1**). This results in complex pain referral patterns, and orofacial pain, headache, and neck pain are often closely related. In addition, there are many anatomical structures in the head, face, and neck that can be the source of pain. These include the eyes, nose, teeth, tongue, sinuses, muscles, and temporomandibular joints. Anatomical complexity has often led to difficulties in forming accurate diagnoses in patients with orofacial pain. Effective treatment of chronic orofacial pain depends on a precise diagnosis. Since chronic orofacial pain conditions are often complex and associated with psychosocial dysfunction, optimal management requires a multidisciplinary biopsychosocial approach.

Assessment for orofacial pain

History

Comprehensive assessment requires history, physical examination, and investigations. The history needs to follow the principles of a biopsychosocial approach and address the biological, psychological, social, and functional aspects of the patient. Diagnosis of the underlying pain condition is important but can be challenging due to the complex innervation of related structures and numerous potential causes. It is important to also be aware of conditions affecting the head, neck, shoulders, and upper back when searching for the cause of orofacial pain. The mouth and the face are important for many social activities, and an assessment of the functional impact on these activities is essential.

The patient should be given the opportunity to describe the presenting pain problem. Issues in the chief complaint include the date of onset, location, duration, pain intensity, quality of pain, changes over time, aggravating and relieving factors, and any other associated symptoms. Intensity of pain can be rated using a 0–10

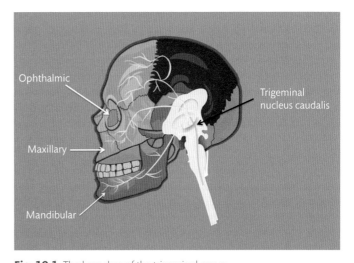

Fig. 19.1 The branches of the trigeminal nerve.
Reproduced with permission from Bartsch T, Goadsby PJ. The trigeminocervical complex and migraine: current concepts and synthesis. *Current pain and headache reports.* 2003;7(5):371–6.

numerical rating scale, with 10 representing the worse possible pain. It can also be described as mild, moderate, or severe. How the pain interferes with activities such as sleep, work, talking, and eating is an important indicator of the impact and severity of the pain condition. It is important to work out the anatomical distribution of the pain. In trigeminal neuralgia, for example, the location of pain is within the dermatomal distribution of the affected trigeminal branch. The quality and pattern of pain can also be used to aid diagnosis. For example, neuropathic pain is more likely to be described as sharp, burning, pins and needles, and lancinating. It is useful to determine whether the pain is episodic or continuous, to determine the duration of each pain attack, and any periods of remission. Patients with trigeminal neuralgia typically experience short episodes of severe pain, versus patients with persistent idiopathic facial pain (PIFP) who experience a persistent throbbing and aching pain. It is important to know what worsens or improves the pain. For example, is it worsened by light touch such as brushing the face, or other activities such as chewing or talking? The presence of associated symptoms should be sought. These may include symptoms such as facial numbness, itchiness, or crepitation. As patients with orofacial pain may have sought medical care from many practitioners before, a detailed account of past treatment and its efficacy should be obtained. In addition, the past medical history including details such as any history of trauma or dental procedures should be recorded. A psychosocial history is important. This should include questions about the presence of depression, anxiety, and social stressors. Patients should also be evaluated on how they adapt to chronic pain and whether they have barriers such as pain catastrophizing, fear avoidance, and passive coping. Any pending or planned disability claims or litigation should also be noted.

Physical examination

The physical examination should be conducted systematically in order to aid the diagnosis. It should be guided by the history. Red flag conditions such as underlying tumours that require definitive treatment need to be excluded. A complete examination of the face, head and neck, oral cavity, and neurological system should be performed. The teeth should be examined since dental problems are a common cause of orofacial pain. The ears and nose should be inspected, including otoscopic examination. Any swellings, lesions, signs of previous trauma, and discolouration should be looked for. Lymphadenopathy over the anterior and lateral neck and the submandibular region needs to be excluded. The carotid arteries and superficial temporal arteries should be examined, and tenderness on palpation may indicate a vascular pathology such as temporal arteritis. A neurological examination needs to include the cranial nerves. In particular, the fifth cranial nerve is important, as it innervates the majority of the face, head, and oral cavity. This includes sensory testing of the skin distributions of all three trigeminal branches (ophthalmic, maxillary, and mandibular). Sensory modalities that should be tested include light touch, pinprick, temperature, and the presence of dynamic allodynia. Prominent neurological deficit may suggest significant underlying pathology. The masticatory muscles should be inspected for change in size and palpated for any familiar pain. The temporomandibular joint should be assessed for obvious swelling, tenderness, range of motion, and crepitation. The cervical spine, neck muscles, shoulders, and upper back should also be examined, since they may be associated with orofacial pain.

Investigations

Investigations are ordered according to information gathered from the history and physical examination. Investigations include laboratory tests, imaging studies, and diagnostic blocks.

Laboratory tests are not routinely needed. Blood tests may be required to look for metabolic, haematological, and autoimmune disorders. Blood taking for human leukocyte antigen (HLA)-B*15:02 is needed prior to commencing carbamazepine and oxcarbazepine to avoid the occurrence of severe cutaneous reactions.

Imaging studies may sometimes be indicated to look for structural pathologies in the head and neck region. Dental radiographs are inexpensive and provide information about the teeth and jaws. Computed tomography is good for providing images of bony structures in the maxillofacial skeleton such as the nose and sinuses, temporomandibular joints, and the skull base. Magnetic resonance imaging (MRI) is the investigation of choice for assessing soft tissues. It can be used to assess the oropharyngeal and nasopharyngeal structures, as well as the anatomy of the temporomandibular joints. It can also be used to look for intracranial pathologies. Patients with symptoms suggestive of trigeminal neuralgia should have an MRI performed to look for vascular compression of the trigeminal nerve root or other secondary causes such as tumours or multiple sclerosis (Fig. 19.2).

When diagnosis is uncertain, diagnostic blocks may be considered using injection of local anaesthetic. A significant positive response in pain reduction after a diagnostic block would suggest that the targeted structure is a significant pain generator, while a negative response would suggest the presence of a different source of pain. This may be useful in differentiating from referred pain conditions. Nerves, muscles, or joints can all be targets of diagnostic local anaesthetic blocks.

Classification

There have been different classifications for orofacial pain disorders. These include the International Classification of Headache Disorders (ICHD), the American Academy of Orofacial Pain, and

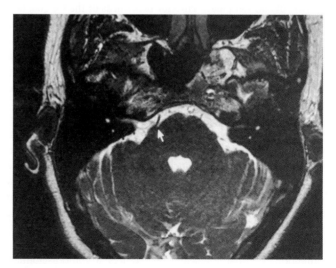

Fig. 19.2 MRI showing vascular compression of the trigeminal nerve root in a patient with trigeminal neuralgia (white arrow).

the Diagnostic Criteria for Temporomandibular Disorders (DC/TMD).[7-9] Classification of headache disorders is mostly based on the ICHD, which is now in its third edition and also includes orofacial pain disorders.[7] However, the ICHD classification is not comprehensive with respect to orofacial pain disorders, especially dental pain disorders and temporomandibular disorders (TMDs). A comprehensive and complete classification system for orofacial pain disorders is lacking. This limitation may have contributed to a relatively slower progress in the field of orofacial pain research. In order to fill this gap, the IASP created a task force that worked closely with the World Health Organization, the International Headache Society, the IASP special interest group on orofacial and head pain (OFHA-SIG), the American Academy of Orofacial Pain, and the International Network for Orofacial Pain and Related Disorders Methodology to come up with a standardized classification system for chronic headache and orofacial pain disorders. The classification only describes chronic pain conditions, defined as persistent or recurrent pain lasting >3 months. Chronic headache or orofacial pain is separated into chronic primary headache or orofacial pain and chronic secondary headache or orofacial pain. The criteria for chronic primary pain are as follows: (1) persist or recurs >3 months, (2) is associated with significant emotional distress and/or functional disability, and (3) symptoms are not better accounted for by another diagnosis.[10] Examples include chronic migraine and PIFP. Pain is defined as secondary when it is clearly associated with an identifiable disease, trauma, or other factors.[3] The majority of the secondary headache disorders are classified according to the ICHD-3.

One advantage of the new IASP classification is a more detailed systematic categorization of orofacial pain disorders, which has not been done previously. This classification has been accepted by the International Headache Society and IASP. Close cooperation between these two major societies will increase the likelihood that this classification is widely adopted in the future. The list of primary and secondary headache and orofacial pain disorders, as classified under the new IASP classification, are shown in **Box 19.1**.

Specific chronic orofacial pain disorders

Trigeminal neuralgia

Trigeminal neuralgia is an uncommon neuropathic facial pain condition involving one or more divisions of the trigeminal nerve. It is usually characterized by short episodes of severe unilateral facial pain and can result in significant disruption of psychosocial function due to its detrimental effects on many normal daily activities such as eating and talking. Trigeminal neuralgia can be classified as classical, secondary, or idiopathic according to the new IASP classification.[11] Classical trigeminal neuralgia is when there is vascular compression resulting in morphological changes of the trigeminal nerve root. It is classified as secondary trigeminal neuralgia when an underlying structural lesion or disease affects the trigeminal nerve. Idiopathic trigeminal neuralgia is when there is no identifiable cause in a patient with clinically diagnosed trigeminal neuralgia.

Clinical features

Patients with trigeminal neuralgia suffer severe facial pain in the distribution of the branches of the trigeminal nerve. The second

---

Box 19.1 List of primary and secondary headache and orofacial pain disorders with their ICD-10 code if applicable

Chronic primary headache or orofacial pain
Chronic migraine without or with aura (G43.3)
Chronic tension-type headache (G44.22)
Chronic trigeminal autonomic cephalalgias (TACs):
    Chronic cluster headache (G44.02)
    Chronic paroxysmal hemicranias (G44.04)
    Short-lasting unilateral neuralgiform headache with conjunctival injection and tearing (SUNCT) (G44.05)
    Hemicrania continua (G44.51)
Chronic primary temporomandibular disorder pains
    Myalgia (M79.1)
    Myofascial pain with referral
    Arthralgia (M26.62)
Chronic burning mouth
    Glossodynia (K14.6)
Chronic primary orofacial pain
    Orofacial pain as a presentation of primary headache
    Presentation idiopathic dentoalveolar pain
    Atypical facial pain (persistent idiopathic facial pain) (G50.1)

Chronic secondary headache or orofacial pain
Chronic headache/orofacial pain attributed to trauma or injury to the head and/or neck
Chronic headache/orofacial pain attributed to cranial or cervical vascular disorder
Chronic headache/orofacial pain attributed to nonvascular intracranial disorder
Chronic headache attributed to substance or its withdrawal
Chronic headache/orofacial pain attributed to infection
Chronic headache/orofacial pain attributed to disorder of homeostasis or their nonpharmacological treatment
Chronic headache/orofacial pain attributed to disorder of the cranium, neck, eyes, ears, sinuses, salivary glands, and oral mucosa
Chronic dental pain
    Diseases of pulp and periapical tissue (K04)
    Other diseases of hard tissue of teeth (K03)
Chronic neuropathic orofacial pain
    Pain attributed to a lesion or disease of the trigeminal nerve including trigeminal neuralgia (primary parent: chronic peripheral neuropathic pain)
    Other cranial and regional neuralgias and neuropathies
Chronic secondary temporomandibular disorder pain
    Chronic secondary orofacial muscle pain
        Systemic disorder or trauma
    Chronic secondary temporomandibular joint pain
        Systemic disorder, trauma or infection

IASP Classification, Benoliel et al, Pain. 2019 Jan;160(1):60–68.

---

and third trigeminal branches are most frequently affected.[12] Bilateral involvement is rare in classical trigeminal neuralgia, and its presence is suggestive of secondary trigeminal neuralgia.[13] The pain is intense, occurs suddenly, and is transient in nature. The duration of each pain attack is usually a few seconds to 2 minutes; however, there may be numerous recurring pain attacks each day. The nature of the pain is stabbing, electric shock-like, burning, sharp, and shooting. The patient is typically pain free in between attacks. However, a subgroup of patients also have a continuous dull, burning, or aching background pain of a lower intensity, and this appears to affect women more frequently.[14] The distribution of background pain is the same as that of the intense pain attacks.

Very often pain is triggered by non-painful stimuli to the affected face. Therefore, patients with trigeminal neuralgia may encounter extreme pain and difficulty when engaging in normal daily activities such as chewing, talking, brushing their teeth, or touching their face.[12]

Epidemiology

The incidence of trigeminal neuralgia ranges from 4.3 to 27 per 100,000 people each year.[15–17] It affects women more commonly than men, and in those aged between 50 and 69 years.[15] For classical trigeminal neuralgia, the average age of onset is 53 years, and for secondary trigeminal neuralgia the average age of onset is younger, at 43 years.[12,18]

Aetiology

The underlying pathophysiology is focal demyelination of the primary trigeminal afferents close to where the trigeminal root enters into the pons.[19–21] In classical trigeminal neuralgia, this is due to compression of the trigeminal nerve root by a blood vessel, usually an artery in the cerebellopontine cistern. In secondary trigeminal neuralgia, an identifiable structural lesion is present. The most common causes are multiple sclerosis with a plaque affecting the trigeminal nerve root or a space-occupying lesion in the cerebellopontine cistern (e.g. meningioma, arteriovenous malformation, or epidermoid tumours).[22,23] It has been hypothesized that focal demyelination results in hyperexcitable nerve fibres, which can lead to ectopic excitation and high-frequency discharges.[24,25] Hyperactivity of the primary afferent neurons may also result in central sensitization of neurons in the spinal trigeminal nucleus.[21,26]

Treatment

Pharmacotherapy

Carbamazepine (400–1200 mg/day) and oxcarbazepine (900–1800 mg/day) should be given as first-line treatment.[27,28] They work by blocking voltage-gated sodium channels, which stabilizes hyperexcited neural membranes and reduces repetitive firing. They have excellent analgesic efficacy and carbamazepine has a number needed to treat of 1.7.[29] They are highly effective for paroxysmal pain, but are generally less effective for concomitant continuous pain.[28] Carbamazepine has a number needed to harm of 3.4 for minor adverse events and 24 for severe adverse events.[27] Common adverse effects include nausea, drowsiness, dizziness, diplopia, and increased levels of transaminases. Hyponatraemia may also occur. Uncommon but serious adverse effects include allergic rash, hepatoxicity, systemic lupus erythematous, Stevens–Johnson syndrome, and aplastic anaemia. An electrocardiogram is necessary before prescription because atrioventricular block is a contraindication. In Chinese, Thai, and Malaysian populations, HLA-B*15:02 polymorphism is associated with carbamazepine- and oxcarbazepine-induced severe cutaneous reactions (Stevens–Johnson syndrome and toxic epidermal necrolysis).[30–33] Screening for HLA-B*15:02 is recommended prior to starting these drugs. Oxcarbazepine has similar efficacy to carbamazepine, but is more tolerable and has less potential for drug interaction, and therefore may be preferred.[34] Treatment failure is often due to intolerable side effects instead of a lack of drug efficacy. Interruption or dose reduction has been shown to occur in 27% of patients on carbamazepine and 18% of patients on oxcarbazepine.[35]

Other pharmacological agents for trigeminal neuralgia include lamotrigine, baclofen, pregabalin, gabapentin, botulinum toxin A, and phenytoin. These can be used as monotherapy or as adjuncts with carbamazepine or oxcarbazepine.[36] Recommendations for these drugs are weak and based on low quality of evidence.[36] For patients suffering from severe acute exacerbations, infusion of lidocaine or fosphenytoin may be effective.[28,36] Hospital admission may be required for rehydration and adjustment of analgesic medication.

Surgical and neuroablative procedures

Medical management should be used first. Surgical management may be offered when medical treatment is ineffective or the patient is unable to tolerate the side effects.[36] Surgical procedures available include microvascular decompression, and other percutaneous neuroablative procedures: radiofrequency thermocoagulation, gamma knife surgery, balloon compression, and glycerol rhizolysis (**Fig. 19.3**). Microvascular decompression is recommended as the first-line surgical option in patients with classical trigeminal neuralgia where neurovascular contact of the trigeminal nerve root with morphological changes is demonstrated.[36] The chance of success after microvascular decompression is significantly higher in patients with classical trigeminal neuralgia than those with idiopathic trigeminal neuralgia. However, a significant proportion of patients with idiopathic trigeminal neuralgia also benefit from microvascular decompression. Compared to other percutaneous neuroablative procedures, microvascular decompression is associated with the longest duration of pain relief.[37–41] It has been reported that between 61% and 80% of patients were pain free at 4–5 years after microvascular decompression.[38,39,42] However, this is a major operation requiring craniotomy and posterior fossa exploration. Minor complications include aching or burning pain, sensory loss, or transient cranial nerve dysfunction. Major complications are rare. The incidence of stroke is around 0.3%, major cranial nerve dysfunction is 2%, and death is 0.2%.[43] Patients unwilling to be exposed to these risks can be offered other neuroablative procedures. All these alternative interventional procedures have also been shown to be effective. The trigeminal ganglion is targeted chemically in glycerol rhizolysis, thermally in radiofrequency thermocoagulation, and mechanically in balloon compression (**Fig. 19.3**). Beams of radiation are used to target the trigeminal nerve root in gamma knife surgery. These procedures are less invasive and associated with less major adverse effects compared to microvascular decompression. Minor complications such as sensory loss, masticatory problems, and new burning pain can occur.[27] There is currently no evidence to show any superiority in efficacy of one neuroablative procedure over another. Furthermore, it is also unclear whether microvascular decompression or any of the other neuroablative procedures are more effective for idiopathic trigeminal neuralgia where neurovascular contact with morphological changes is not present.[36] For patients with idiopathic trigeminal neuralgia, neuroablative procedures may be more appropriate than microvascular decompression.

(a)

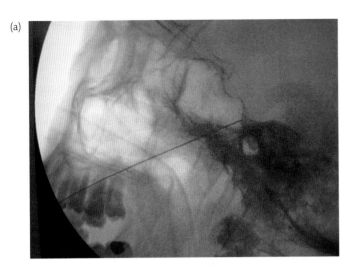

(b)

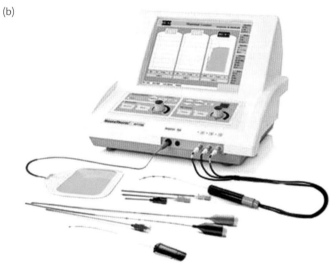

Fig. 19.3 Radiofrequency thermocoagulation of the trigeminal ganglion. (a) Fluoroscopic image demonstrating needle position for targeting the trigeminal ganglion. (b) Radiofrequency machine and cannulas for delivering thermocoagulation.
Reproduced with permission from Neurotherm.

Glossopharyngeal neuralgia

Glossopharyngeal neuralgia is a rare neuropathic pain condition affecting the distribution of the glossopharyngeal nerve. Similar to trigeminal neuralgia, glossopharyngeal neuralgia can be caused by neurovascular compression of the glossopharyngeal nerve. In secondary (symptomatic) glossopharyngeal neuralgia, it can be due to neck trauma, multiple sclerosis, tumours, and Chiari I malformation.[44] In most secondary causes, there is damage to the nerve or nucleus, and the term glossopharyngeal neuropathy is more appropriate.

Clinical features

Patients suffer from short attacks of sharp, stabbing pain located in the ear, posterior part of the tongue, tonsillar fossa, or angle of the mandible. Pain is triggered by activities such as swallowing, talking, yawning, sneezing, and coughing. Pain intensity is usually severe, and can prevent patients from eating. Patients commonly

experience remissions and recurrences. According to the predominant location of the pain, glossopharyngeal neuralgia can be further subdivided into oropharyngeal and otalgic forms. Vagal symptoms such as bradycardia, syncope, or even cardiac arrest can accompany pain attacks 10% of the time.[45] Mild sensory deficits may also occur. When an underlying pathology is identifiable, continuous pain is usually present in addition to paroxysmal pain attacks. There may also be prominent sensory deficits or missing gag reflex.

Epidemiology and aetiology

Glossopharyngeal neuralgia is a very rare pain disorder and has an incidence of around 0.8 per 100,000.[46]

Similar to trigeminal neuralgia, neurovascular conflict from vascular compression of the nerve root entry zone of the glossopharyngeal nerve is thought to be the cause of pain in most patients.[47] There have also been reports of rare familial cases, which may be due to mutations of the voltage-gated sodium channel genes.[48] Associated bradycardia and syncope may be a result of involvement of vagal afferents and afferents from the carotid sinus.[44]

Treatment

The treatment options are similar to that of trigeminal neuralgia. As the disorder is very rare, there is a paucity of available evidence. Carbamazepine and oxcarbazepine are usually effective. Gabapentin and pregabalin may also be useful. Microvascular decompression can be considered when pharmacological treatment is ineffective, and is associated with a high success rate.[49] A study reported that it resulted in long-term pain relief in 84.7% of patients.[50] Percutaneous radiofrequency thermocoagulation, surgical rhizotomy, and stereotactic radiosurgery are other therapeutic options.[51–53]

Temporomandibular disorders

The most common orofacial pain conditions are TMDs—used to describe pain and dysfunction of the temporomandibular joints, masticatory muscles, and associated tissues.[54,55] Chronic pain from TMDs can negatively impair quality of life and is associated with both psychosocial and functional impairment. TMDs are associated with other comorbidities such as bruxism, depression, irritable bowel syndrome, and chronic fatigue.[56] The DC/TMD is a valid and reliable method that can be used for the diagnosis and classification of TMDs.[8] It consists of two components: a physical domain called axis 1 and a psychosocial domain called axis 2. TMD pain can be divided into three main subgroups: (1) myalgia, (2) arthralgia, and (3) headache attributed to TMDs. Myalgia describes pain originating from the muscles and is the most common TMD condition.[57] Arthralgia, which refers to pain from the joint, most often occurs together with myalgia.[58] Headache attributed to a TMD is pain over the temple region as a result of pain-related TMD, and is aggravated by jaw movement and function. The importance of this diagnosis is that TMD treatment would be indicated for these patients. For TMDs, early diagnosis, explanation, and management is important for better outcomes.

Clinical features

Patients with TMDs can experience pain from the temporomandibular joint or masticatory muscles. The pain can be located in the cheek, temporal regions, or preauricular area and can radiate to other areas. Pain is usually moderate in intensity, and can be both intermittent and persistent. Aggravating factors include activities such as chewing, talking, and yawning. Audible clicking, popping, or grating sounds and limitation of range of motion of the temporomandibular joints are also prominent symptoms. Other clinical features include crepitus, locking, and an inability to open the mouth wide. The most common clinical sign is tenderness on palpation of the pericranial muscles and temporomandibular joint. Patients with TMDs may also have other symptoms such as tension-type headache, neck and back pain, depression, and anxiety.[54] There is a poor correlation between patient-reported severity of pain and pathological changes.[59]

Epidemiology

The prevalence of TMDs in the general population is around 10–15% for adults and 4–7% for adolescents.[60,61] The incidence of first-onset painful TMD has been reported to be between 3% and 4% per year.[62] Women are more frequently affected than men, occurring most commonly during child-bearing age (20–40 years old). There are no sex differences during childhood. TMD pain occurred as a single episode in 12%, recurrent episodes in 65%, and persistent pain in 19% of patients according to the large OPPERA study.[63] TMD pain most commonly occurred together in both muscle and joint (73% of incident cases), followed by muscle pain alone (23%).[62]

Aetiology

The aetiology of TMD pain is thought to be multifactorial and biopsychosocial, including genetic factors, hormonal factors, trauma, endogenous opioid function, central sensitization, and psychosocial factors. Genetic variation can influence the development of TMD pain, and there is an association with the two genes *HTR2A* and *COMT*.[64] However, the degree of association with TMD pain may be limited.[65] As TMDs affect women more commonly, oestrogen has been postulated to play a role. Oestrogen may affect temporomandibular joint inflammation and nociceptive responses.[54] However, there is contradictory evidence regarding the association between oestrogen levels and TMD pain, with some studies showing association with low oestrogen levels while others show association with high oestrogen levels.[66] Therefore, the overall evidence is weak and inconclusive. Trauma may also contribute to the development of TMD, whether it is macrotrauma or microtrauma. Macrotrauma may occur after injuries following procedures such as intubation or dental treatment. Microtrauma may be caused by habits such as bruxism, tongue thrusting, bracing of the jaw, and pen chewing.[54] Peripheral sensitization of myofascial sensory afferent neurons and central sensitization in the spinal dorsal horn, trigeminal nucleus, and supraspinal neurons may also contribute to the development and persistence of TMD pain.[54] Psychosocial factors can predispose, precipitate, and prolong TMD pain.[67] Patients with TMD pain have higher levels of stress, anxiety, depression, pain catastrophizing, and somatic awareness.[68] In the OPPERA study, the factors most strongly associated with onset of TMD pain were perceived stress, past stressful life events and negative affect.[69]

Treatment

Management of TMD pain includes reversible and irreversible approaches. Reversible options are typically conservative methods and should be considered first. Between 75% and 90% of patients respond positively to simpler, less invasive treatment.[70]

Reversible and conservative treatment

Patients with TMD pain should be educated and reassured about the benign nature of the condition. Behavioural therapies are important and effective for self-management of TMD pain.[71] It includes education, biofeedback, cognitive behavioural therapy, habit reversal, and relaxation techniques. Cognitive behavioural therapy aims to train patients to actively cope with their pain. It covers techniques to manage pain-related anxieties, pain flare-ups, sleep hygiene, and communication strategies with family. Cognitive behavioural therapy has been shown to improve pain control, mood, and activity in TMD pain sufferers.[72] Therapeutic jaw exercises appear to have low to moderate effects for TMD pain, and are usually part of patient self-care programmes.[71] Jaw exercises can help with coordination, relaxation, and strengthening of muscles. Passive stretching can improve range of motion of the temporomandibular joint. Occlusal appliance therapy is commonly used for TMD pain (Fig. 19.4). They allow coverage and protection of both the upper and lower teeth, and can be used at night for individuals who grind or clench their teeth. Occlusal appliances can also relax the jaw muscles and reduce the load on the temporomandibular joint.[54] They have also been shown to reduce headache attributed to TMDs.[73]

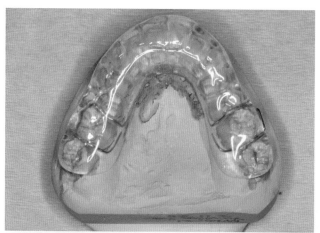

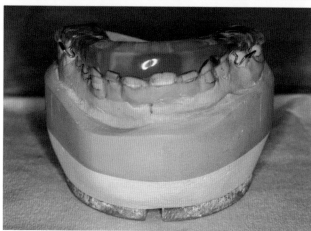

Fig. 19.4 Occlusal appliance for patients with temporomandibular disorder.

Pharmacological treatment can be used for pain management. These include non-steroidal anti-inflammatory drugs, paracetamol, diazepam, tricyclic antidepressants, glucocorticoids, propranolol, and antiepileptic drugs. However, there is insufficient evidence to enable strong conclusions about the effectiveness of these drugs for TMD pain.[74] The use of preventive analgesic drugs such as tricyclic antidepressants and antiepileptic drugs may be preferable because the adverse effect profile of acute analgesic drugs may not be as suitable for a chronic pain condition.

Irreversible approaches

According to the American Association for Dental Research, irreversible approaches should not be used as the primary management for TMD.[75] There is a lack of evidence to support the use of orthodontics and occlusal equilibration. Arthroscopic surgery and arthrocentesis have been shown to reduce pain intensity and improve function.[72,76] However, evidence regarding long-term outcomes is lacking. Many patients respond positively to conservative management; therefore, surgical management is only indicated in a small number of patients who have severe disability and are unresponsive to conservative treatment for at least 6 months.[54] These patients should have an intra-articular disorder, degenerative joint disease, or disease clearly affecting the temporomandibular joint.[72]

Auriculotemporal neuralgia

This is a rare neuropathic pain disorder where patients experience pain over the temple, ear, preauricular area, temporomandibular joint, and the parotid area. The pain is unilateral and of moderate to severe intensity. The pain characteristic is stabbing, aching, or throbbing. It may be associated with paraesthesia and tenderness over the preauricular and temporal areas. Pain attacks can last from a few seconds to 30 minutes, and patients may also have background pain.[44] Auriculotemporal neuralgia is a rare disorder with an estimated prevalence of 0.2–0.4%,[77,78] affecting middle-aged females more commonly. The auriculotemporal nerve may be affected and entrapped as it runs through the lateral pterygoid muscle. It may also be compressed by synovial cysts, malformation or aneurysm of the middle meningeal artery, fracture of the mandibular condyle, or perineural spread of tumour.[44] Local anaesthetic block of the auriculotemporal nerve with or without steroids has been shown to provide positive analgesic effect. Pharmacological drug options include carbamazepine, oxcarbazepine, and gabapentin.[77,78]

Geniculate neuralgia

Geniculate neuralgia is characterized by the occurrence of short episodes of pain located in the auditory canal, and can radiate to the parieto-occipital area. The pain is always unilateral, stabbing, electric shock-like in nature, and located deep in the ear. Problems with lacrimation, salivation, or taste may also be present. This pain condition is very rare, and a systematic review that searched from 1935 to 2012 found <150 cases.[79] Patients are usually elderly. Similar to trigeminal neuralgia, it is thought to be due to microvascular compression. Pharmacological treatment of geniculate neuralgia includes the use of carbamazepine, oxcarbazepine, lamotrigine, and gabapentin. Microvascular decompression and transection of the geniculate nerve and ganglion are possible surgical options.[79]

Persistent idiopathic facial pain

Previously known as atypical facial pain, PIFP is a distressful, chronic orofacial pain disorder. It is defined by the ICHD-3 as persistent facial pain and/or oral pain, with varying presentations, but recurring daily for >2 hours per day over >3 months, in the absence of a clinical neurological deficit.[7] It is often diagnosed when other possible causes have been excluded. The pathophysiology is not well understood, and it is difficult to treat effectively.

Clinical features

Patients with PIFP typically suffer from persistent, unilateral facial pain that is deep and poorly localized. The pain persists over a long duration of time, is present daily, is there for most of the day, and is not associated with periods of remission.[80] The characteristic of the pain is usually aching, burning, throbbing, and stabbing.[80–82] The distribution of pain may not be dermatomal and can spread to the upper or lower jaws, and even to the face and neck. In addition, the location, characteristics, and associated features of the pain can change over time. The severity of the pain ranges from mild to severe. Onset of pain is often associated with minor surgical procedures including invasive dental procedures.[83] There should be no clinically detectable neurosensory impairment in PIFP. This is in contrast to painful traumatic trigeminal neuropathy, where neurosensory changes should be present on clinical examination.[84] Patients with PIFP may also have other chronic orofacial pain or headache syndromes.[80] PIFP is associated with psychiatric conditions, with anxiety and depression being the most common symptoms. Pain may be worsened with emotional stress.

Epidemiology

The estimated incidence rate of PIFP is 4.4 per 100,000 years, and lifetime prevalence is around 0.03%.[4,16] Females are more likely to have PIFP, and the mean age of onset is in the mid-40s.[80]

Aetiology

The pathophysiology of PIFP is not well known, and may be due to a combination of biological and psychological factors. Many patients with PIFP have a history of minor trauma and subclinical sensory changes detected with quantitative sensory testing.[81,82] Patients with PIFP have been shown to have increased brainstem neuronal excitability, impaired inhibitory function at the prefrontal cortex, and hypofunction of the dopaminergic pathway.[85–88] These findings suggest that PIFP may be a neuropathic pain syndrome. However, there are also patients with PIFP who have no significant changes in the trigeminal somatosensory pathways, which suggests that it may not always be a neuropathic pain syndrome.[85] Therefore, there may be different subtypes of PIFP, with some patients having a greater neuropathic component. The association between PIFP and psychiatric disorders such as depression suggests that psychological factors may also play a prominent role.

Treatment

There is no curative treatment for PIFP. Since patients often suffer from biological and psychological comorbidities, a multidisciplinary approach is required. Pharmacological options includes antidepressants (e.g. tricyclic antidepressants and serotonin–noradrenaline reuptake inhibitors) and anticonvulsants (e.g. pregabalin and gabapentin).[89] First-line drug treatment is usually oral amitriptyline 25–100 mg daily.[90] Second-line drug treatment includes other antidepressants such as venlafaxine, duloxetine, and fluoxetine, and anticonvulsants such as pregabalin and gabapentin.[89–92] While these drugs have been shown to provide analgesic benefit, the level of evidence is low. The addition of cognitive behavioural therapy together with antidepressant therapy has been shown to improve outcomes.[89,93] Stress coping strategies and treatment of unresolved psychological problems are important as part of the overall management of PIFP.[94] Hypnosis may be a useful option for pain reduction.[95] Complementary and alternative medicine can also be tried, although the overall level of evidence is limited.[96]

Interventional pain procedures should be considered when conservative management is ineffective, although the level of supporting evidence is weak. The intervention associated with the most success is pulsed radiofrequency of the sphenopalatine ganglion, which has been shown to reduce pain and opioid consumption[97,98] (**Fig. 19.5**). Pulsed radiofrequency of the sphenopalatine ganglion is therefore the recommended interventional treatment for PIFP.[90,98] Other potential interventional procedures that require further evaluation include peripheral nerve field stimulation and botulinum toxin injection.[99,100]

Acute herpes zoster

Acute herpes zoster results from the reactivation of dormant varicella virus from the sensory ganglia. It is characterized by the development of a painful maculopapular or vesicular rash over the affected dermatome. It is usually defined as acute when the duration of pain is <3 months. Apart from the face, acute herpes zoster can affect other regions of the body. The thoracic region is most commonly affected, followed by trigeminal (usually the ophthalmic nerve), cervical, and then the lumbar regions.[101] Acute herpes zoster can result in severe pain. It usually resolves over a few weeks, but some patients go on to develop chronic post-herpetic neuralgia (PHN).

Clinical features

The most prominent clinical feature of acute herpes zoster is the acute onset of maculopapular or vesicular rash. Herpes zoster affecting one of the three branches of the trigeminal nerve is responsible for pain and rash over the face.[102] The ophthalmic branch is most commonly affected. Rash and pain over the tympanic membrane, auditory canal, auricle, and skin over the mastoid process occurs when the geniculate ganglion of the facial nerve is affected. Sometimes, vesicles may be present in the anterior third of the tongue or on the hard palate. The motor branches of the facial nerve may also be affected, which results in facial palsy. This is called Ramsay Hunt syndrome.

Ninety to ninety-five per cent of patients will experience pain and other symptoms such as tingling, itchiness, and numbness.[103] Pain usually occurs prior to onset of the rash. Patients typically suffer from continuous pain of a burning, throbbing, and aching quality. They may also have stabbing and shooting pain. Mechanical allodynia is prominent over the affected dermatome.

Acute herpes zoster may also result in other non-pain complications, which are important for the clinician to recognize. Around 10–15% of herpes zoster infections involve the ophthalmic division of the trigeminal nerve.[104] Serious eye complications can occur in 25–50% of patients with ophthalmic herpes zoster. These include keratitis, iritis, and glaucoma.[105] More rarely, patients may have necrotizing retinitis and optic neuritis. In trigeminal herpes zoster, ophthalmoplegia may occur as a result of involvement of cranial nerves III, IV, and XI. Patients may experience tinnitus, hearing loss, vertigo, nausea, hoarseness, and dysphagia as a result of involvement of the cranial nerves VIII, IX, X, and XI. A rare complication of acute herpes zoster is stroke due to the virus travelling from the trigeminal ganglion to the cerebral arteries. In addition, herpes zoster may also be complicated by bacterial superinfection and pneumonia.[106]

Diagnosis is usually straightforward due to the presence of skin rash and vesicles. When symptoms are not obvious, laboratory tests can be used to aid diagnosis. These include direct immunofluorescence assay for varicella zoster virus antigen or polymerase chain reaction assay for varicella zoster virus DNA from the base of the lesions or cerebrospinal fluid samples.[107]

Epidemiology

The estimated global annual incidence of herpes zoster is between 3 and 5 per 1000 person years.[108] The incidence increases with increased age. Individuals who are immunocompromised, have chronic pulmonary disease, kidney disease, autoimmune disease, or depression have a higher risk of developing herpes zoster infection.[109] As varicella zoster virus vaccination becomes more common for both children and the elderly, the incidence in the future may change.

Aetiology

Acute herpes zoster is due to reactivation of the varicella zoster virus that has been dormant in the sensory ganglia after primary infection. Reactivation of the virus causes inflammatory changes in the skin, nerve, ganglion, and spinal cord. Virus activation results in damage to the cell bodies and axons of nerve fibres. Inflammatory changes induce sensitization of peripheral nociceptors, which exacerbates pain transmission.

Treatment

Acute herpes zoster is usually self-limiting. The goal of treatment is to reduce pain, limit the duration of disease, and prevent complications. Systemic antivirals such as aciclovir, valaciclovir, and famciclovir can reduce pain intensity and reduce the duration of acute disease.[110] They are recommended for all immunocompetent patients with acute herpes zoster who have one or more of the following: age 50 years or older, moderate to severe pain, moderate or severe rash, and non-truncal involvement.[111] They should ideally be started within 72 hours after appearance of rash.[110] Antivirals should be given intravenously for immunocompromised patients, and those with complicated herpes zoster.[110]

Mild to moderate pain can be treated with paracetamol, nonsteroidal anti-inflammatory drugs, and weak opioids such as tramadol. When pain is severe, strong opioids may be required. Oxycodone has been shown to be more effective than gabapentin for severe herpes-related pain.[110] Corticosteroids in combination with antiviral agents can reduce pain, but due to their adverse effect profile, they should only be considered in patients with severe pain and in the absence of any contraindications to steroid use. Antineuropathic pain medications such as gabapentinoids and tricyclic antidepressants may also be effective. Most pharmacological drugs, including antivirals and corticosteroids, do not reduce the

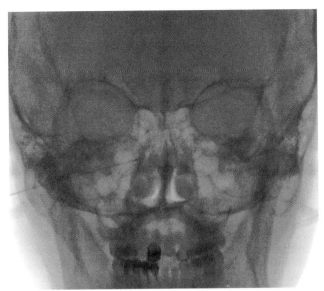

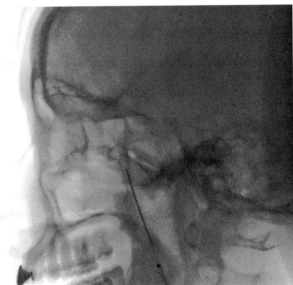

Fig. 19.5 Fluoroscopic images of the needle position for pulsed radiofrequency of the sphenopalatine ganglion.

Reproduced with permission from Bayer E, Racz GB, Miles D, Heavner J. Sphenopalatine ganglion pulsed radiofrequency treatment in 30 patients suffering from chronic face and head pain. *Pain practice: the official journal of World Institute of Pain.* 2005;5(3):223-7.

risk of developing PHN. Administration of low-dose amitriptyline (25 mg once daily for 90 days) has been shown to reduce the prevalence of PHN.[112] Stellate ganglion nerve blocks, when performed early, may reduce acute pain intensity and the incidence of PHN in patients with trigeminal herpes zoster.[113]

Post-herpetic neuralgia

PHN can be defined as pain that persists for >3 months after acute herpes zoster. It causes chronic neuropathic pain, and results in impairment of general activity, sleep, mood, and quality of life. Patients with PHN are more likely to have symptoms of anxiety and depression.[114] Risk factors for PHN include the presence of severe acute pain, prodromal pain, severe rash, and old age.[109] In addition, patients with ophthalmic herpes zoster are twice as likely to develop PHN compared to those with other types of herpes zoster.

Clinical features

Patients with PHN can experience one or more of the following three types of pain: spontaneous continuous pain, paroxysmal pain, and evoked pain. Continuous pain is described as burning, throbbing, and gnawing over the affected dermatome. Paroxysmal pain usually occurs spontaneously without provocation, and typically has a lancinating quality. Evoked pain occurs in response to normally innocuous stimuli. The most common form of evoked pain is dynamic mechanical allodynia, which occurs in around half of the patients.[115] This is a hallmark feature of PHN and is often the most distressing and debilitating clinical feature. It can adversely affect everyday activities such as cleaning the face. Patients may also have pinprick hyperalgesia and heat or cold allodynia. Numbness and paraesthesia are also common. One out of six patients experience itchiness.[103] The pain eventually disappears in >95% of patients with PHN, and rarely recurs after spontaneous remission.[116]

Epidemiology

The incidence and prevalence of PHN may differ depending on the duration used to define persistent pain. The incidence rate has been suggested to be 3.9 per 100,000 person years.[4] The incidence increases steeply with increased age. The incidence rate increases from 2 in people aged between 40 and 49 to 11.9 in people between 70 and 79 years old, and up to 44.2 per 100,000 person years in those >80 years old.

Aetiology

PHN is caused by neuronal injury affecting both the peripheral and central nervous system. The injury results in spontaneous discharges and lowering of activation threshold in both the peripheral and central neurons. In the 'irritable nociceptor' model, cutaneous C-fibres become sensitized, which lowers their threshold for activation and increases the rate and magnitude of nerve discharge.[117] This results in spontaneous pain and allodynia, as well as minimal sensory loss. In the 'deafferentation model', there is peripheral deafferentation that causes reorganization in the spinal dorsal horn. There is loss of sensitized peripheral C-fibres, and this leads to sprouting of A-β fibres that are responsible for mechanical stimuli. This sprouting results in connection of the A-β fibres with pain transmitting neurons in the spinal cord. Such reorganization causes sensory loss and allodynia in response to light moving mechanical stimuli. The above mechanisms may exist together in the same patient. Constant barrage of nerve signals from the peripheral nervous system to the spinal cord can lead to central sensitization with chronic excitability of second-order neurons.[118]

Treatment

Pharmacological management of PHN generally follows guidelines for neuropathic pain treatment.[119] Antivirals and corticosteroids are not useful. First-line treatment includes tricyclic antidepressants, and gabapentinoids.[120] Serotonin–noradrenaline reuptake inhibitors are first-line drugs for neuropathic pain, but no published randomized controlled trials have looked at these drugs specifically for PHN. Tramadol, an opioid agonist and serotonin–noradrenaline reuptake inhibitor, and topical lidocaine are recommended as second-line therapy,[120] and 5% lidocaine patches can be beneficial, especially in elderly patients who may not tolerate the side effects of systemic drugs. Strong opioids and botulinum toxin are recommended as third-line therapy. Botulinum toxin has been shown to be effective in reducing PHN pain, but the follow-up duration of the studies were only up to 3 months.[121,122] Strong opioids, such as oxycodone, should only be used in patients with severe pain refractory to other treatments, as they are only mildly effective, and are not associated with long-term analgesic benefit.[119] Furthermore, there is increasing concern about opioid-related overdose, death, diversion, misuse, and morbidity.[123] Capsaicin 8% patch is effective for managing cervical, thoracic, and lumbar PHN, and is recommended as a second-line therapy for PHN.[101] However, it is not licensed for PHN affecting the trigeminal and geniculate nerves. Peripheral nerve stimulation has the potential to be a useful therapeutic option for facial PHN, but there is currently a paucity of studies in this area.[124,125]

The most evidence-based method for preventing acute herpes zoster and PHN is vaccination. Live attenuated varicella zoster vaccine is available. Vaccination of people aged >60 years has been shown to reduce the incidence of herpes zoster by 51%, and the incidence of PHN by 66%.[126] It should be recommended in immunocompetent patients aged ≥60 years.[127]

Conclusion

Orofacial pain disorders are an important clinical problem that can adversely impact psychosocial health, quality of life, and function. Innervation of the face, head, and neck is complex and closely interlinked. This results in complex referral patterns that make diagnosis particularly challenging. Previous classification systems did not comprehensively cover all headache and orofacial pain conditions. The new IASP classification for headache and orofacial pain disorders provides a more comprehensive and standardized classification system that also adequately covers orofacial pain disorders. Orofacial pain is difficult to manage. Therefore, a biopsychosocial approach is needed in the assessment and management. Red flag pathologies that require definitive treatment should be identified if present. Many patients with orofacial pain also have comorbid psychological conditions, and these need to be adequately managed in order to achieve optimal outcomes. Both pharmacological and non-pharmacological therapies should be used. In patients who are refractory to conservative treatment, more invasive interventional pain procedures should be considered.

REFERENCES

1. Shueb SS, Nixdorf DR, John MT, Alonso BF, Durham J. What is the impact of acute and chronic orofacial pain on quality of life? *J Dent*. 2015;**43**(10):1203–1210.
2. McMillan AS, Wong MC, Zheng J, Lam CL. Prevalence of orofacial pain and treatment seeking in Hong Kong Chinese. *J Orofac Pain*. 2006;**20**(3):218–225.
3. Benoliel R, Svensson P, Evers S, Wang SJ, Barke A, Korwisi B, et al. The IASP classification of chronic pain for ICD-11: chronic secondary headache or orofacial pain. *Pain*. 2019;**160**(1):60–68.
4. Koopman JS, Dieleman JP, Huygen FJ, de Mos M, Martin CG, Sturkenboom MC. Incidence of facial pain in the general population. *Pain*. 2009;**147**(1–3):122–127.
5. Le Doare K, Akerman S, Holland PR, Lasalandra MP, Bergerot A, Classey JD, et al. Occipital afferent activation of second order neurons in the trigeminocervical complex in rat. *Neurosci Lett*. 2006;**403**(1–2):73–77.
6. Bartsch T, Goadsby PJ. The trigeminocervical complex and migraine: current concepts and synthesis. *Curr Pain Headache Rep*. 2003;**7**(5):371–376.
7. Headache Classification Committee of the International Headache Society (IHS). The International Classification of Headache Disorders, 3rd edition. *Cephalalgia*. 2018;**38**(1):1–211.
8. Schiffman E, Ohrbach R, Truelove E, Look J, Anderson G, Goulet JP, et al. Diagnostic criteria for temporomandibular disorders (DC/TMD) for clinical and research applications: recommendations of the International RDC/TMD Consortium Network and Orofacial Pain Special Interest Group. *J Oral Facial Pain Headache*. 2014;**28**(1):6–27.
9. De Leeuw R, Klasser G. *Orofacial Pain: Guidelines for Assessment, Diagnosis, and Management*, 5th ed. Chicago, IL: Quintessence Publishing Company; 2013.
10. Nicholas M, Vlaeyen JWS, Rief W, Barke A, Aziz Q, Benoliel R, et al. The IASP classification of chronic pain for ICD-11: chronic primary pain. *Pain*. 2019;**160**(1):28–37.
11. Cruccu G, Finnerup NB, Jensen TS, Scholz J, Sindou M, Svensson P, et al. Trigeminal neuralgia: new classification and diagnostic grading for practice and research. *Neurology*. 2016;**87**(2):220–228.
12. Maarbjerg S, Gozalov A, Olesen J, Bendtsen L. Trigeminal neuralgia—a prospective systematic study of clinical characteristics in 158 patients. *Headache*. 2014;**54**(10):1574–1582.
13. Maarbjerg S, Di Stefano G, Bendtsen L, Cruccu G. Trigeminal neuralgia—diagnosis and treatment. *Cephalalgia*. 2017;**37**(7):648–657.
14. Maarbjerg S, Gozalov A, Olesen J, Bendtsen L. Concomitant persistent pain in classical trigeminal neuralgia—evidence for different subtypes. *Headache*. 2014;**54**(7):1173–1183.
15. Katusic S, Beard CM, Bergstralh E, Kurland LT. Incidence and clinical features of trigeminal neuralgia, Rochester, Minnesota, 1945–1984. *Ann Neurol*. 1990;**27**(1):89–95.
16. Mueller D, Obermann M, Yoon MS, Poitz F, Hansen N, Slomke MA, et al. Prevalence of trigeminal neuralgia and persistent idiopathic facial pain: a population-based study. *Cephalalgia*. 2011;**31**(15):1542–1548.
17. MacDonald BK, Cockerell OC, Sander JW, Shorvon SD. The incidence and lifetime prevalence of neurological disorders in a prospective community-based study in the UK. *Brain*. 2000;**123** (Pt 4):665–676.
18. De Simone R, Marano E, Brescia Morra V, Ranieri A, Ripa P, Esposito M, et al. A clinical comparison of trigeminal neuralgic pain in patients with and without underlying multiple sclerosis. *Neurol Sci*. 2005;**26** Suppl 2:S150–S151.
19. Rappaport ZH, Govrin-Lippmann R, Devor M. An electron-microscopic analysis of biopsy samples of the trigeminal root taken during microvascular decompressive surgery. *Stereotact Funct Neurosurg*. 1997;**68**(1–4 Pt 1):182–186.
20. Lutz J, Thon N, Stahl R, Lummel N, Tonn JC, Linn J, et al. Microstructural alterations in trigeminal neuralgia determined by diffusion tensor imaging are independent of symptom duration, severity, and type of neurovascular conflict. *J Neurosurg*. 2016;**124**(3):823–830.
21. Obermann M, Yoon MS, Ese D, Maschke M, Kaube H, Diener HC, et al. Impaired trigeminal nociceptive processing in patients with trigeminal neuralgia. *Neurology*. 2007;**69**(9):835–841.

22. Nomura T, Ikezaki K, Matsushima T, Fukui M. Trigeminal neuralgia: differentiation between intracranial mass lesions and ordinary vascular compression as causative lesions. *Neurosurg Rev.* 1994;**17**(1):51–57.

23. Jensen TS, Rasmussen P, Reske-Nielsen E. Association of trigeminal neuralgia with multiple sclerosis: clinical and pathological features. *Acta Neurol Scand.* 1982;**65**(3):182–189.

24. Devor M, Amir R, Rappaport ZH. Pathophysiology of trigeminal neuralgia: the ignition hypothesis. *Clin J Pain.* 2002;**18**(1):4–13.

25. Calvin WH, Devor M, Howe JF. Can neuralgias arise from minor demyelination? Spontaneous firing, mechanosensitivity, and afterdischarge from conducting axons. *Exp Neurol.* 1982;**75**(3):755–763.

26. Dubner R, Sharav Y, Gracely RH, Price DD. Idiopathic trigeminal neuralgia: sensory features and pain mechanisms. *Pain.* 1987;**31**(1):23–33.

27. Cruccu G, Gronseth G, Alksne J, Argoff C, Brainin M, Burchiel K, et al. AAN-EFNS guidelines on trigeminal neuralgia management. *Eur J Neurol.* 2008;**15**(10):1013–1028.

28. Di Stefano G, Truini A, Cruccu G. Current and innovative pharmacological options to treat typical and atypical trigeminal neuralgia. *Drugs.* 2018;**78**(14):1433–1442.

29. Wiffen PJ, Derry S, Moore RA, McQuay HJ. Carbamazepine for acute and chronic pain in adults. *Cochrane Database Syst Rev.* 2011;**1**:CD005451.

30. Chen CB, Hsiao YH, Wu T, Hsih MS, Tassaneeyakul W, Jorns TP, et al. Risk and association of HLA with oxcarbazepine-induced cutaneous adverse reactions in Asians. *Neurology.* 2017;**88**(1):78–86.

31. Tassaneeyakul W, Tiamkao S, Jantararoungtong T, Chen P, Lin SY, Chen WH, et al. Association between HLA-B*1502 and carbamazepine-induced severe cutaneous adverse drug reactions in a Thai population. *Epilepsia.* 2010;**51**(5):926–930.

32. Chouchi M, Kaabachi W, Tizaoui K, Daghfous R, Aidli SE, Hila L. The HLA-B*15:02 polymorphism and Tegretol((R))-induced serious cutaneous reactions in epilepsy: an updated systematic review and meta-analysis. *Revue Neurol.* 2018;**174**(5):278–291.

33. Tangamornsuksan W, Chaiyakunapruk N, Somkrua R, Lohitnavy M, Tassaneeyakul W. Relationship between the HLA-B*1502 allele and carbamazepine-induced Stevens-Johnson syndrome and toxic epidermal necrolysis: a systematic review and meta-analysis. *JAMA Dermatol.* 2013;**149**(9):1025–1032.

34. Beydoun A. Safety and efficacy of oxcarbazepine: results of randomized, double-blind trials. *Pharmacotherapy.* 2000;**20**(8 Pt 2):152s–158s.

35. Di Stefano G, La Cesa S, Truini A, Cruccu G. Natural history and outcome of 200 outpatients with classical trigeminal neuralgia treated with carbamazepine or oxcarbazepine in a tertiary centre for neuropathic pain. *J Headache Pain.* 2014;**15**:34.

36. Bendtsen L, Zakrzewska JM, Abbott J, Braschinsky M, Di Stefano G, Donnet A, et al. European Academy of Neurology guideline on trigeminal neuralgia. *Eur J Neurol.* 2019;**26**(6):831–849.

37. Brisman R. Microvascular decompression vs. gamma knife radiosurgery for typical trigeminal neuralgia: preliminary findings. *Stereotact Funct Neurosurg.* 2007;**85**(2–3):94–98.

38. Linskey ME, Ratanatharathorn V, Penagaricano J. A prospective cohort study of microvascular decompression and Gamma Knife surgery in patients with trigeminal neuralgia. *J Neurosurg.* 2008;**109** Suppl:160–172.

39. Pollock BE, Schoeberl KA. Prospective comparison of posterior fossa exploration and stereotactic radiosurgery dorsal root entry zone target as primary surgery for patients with idiopathic trigeminal neuralgia. *Neurosurgery.* 2010;**67**(3):633–638.

40. Haridas A, Mathewson C, Eljamel S. Long-term results of 405 refractory trigeminal neuralgia surgeries in 256 patients. *Zentralbl Neurochir.* 2008;**69**(4):170–174.

41. Jellish WS, Benedict W, Owen K, Anderson D, Fluder E, Shea JF. Perioperative and long-term operative outcomes after surgery for trigeminal neuralgia: microvascular decompression vs percutaneous balloon ablation. *Head Face Med.* 2008;**4**:11.

42. Wang DD, Raygor KP, Cage TA, Ward MM, Westcott S, Barbaro NM, et al. Prospective comparison of long-term pain relief rates after first-time microvascular decompression and stereotactic radiosurgery for trigeminal neuralgia. *J Neurosurg.* 2018;**128**(1):68–77.

43. Barker FG, 2nd, Jannetta PJ, Bissonette DJ, Larkins MV, Jho HD. The long-term outcome of microvascular decompression for trigeminal neuralgia. *N Engl J Med.* 1996;**334**(17):1077–1083.

44. O'Neill F, Nurmikko T, Sommer C. Other facial neuralgias. *Cephalalgia.* 2017;**37**(7):658–669.

45. Blumenfeld A, Nikolskaya G. Glossopharyngeal neuralgia. *Curr Pain Headache Rep.* 2013;**17**(7):343.

46. Pearce JM. Glossopharyngeal neuralgia. *Eur Neurol.* 2006;**55**(1):49–52.

47. Tanrikulu L, Hastreiter P, Dorfler A, Buchfelder M, Naraghi R. Classification of neurovascular compression in glossopharyngeal neuralgia: three-dimensional visualization of the glossopharyngeal nerve. *Surg Neurol Int.* 2015;**6**:189.

48. Wang Y, Yu CY, Huang L, Riederer F, Ettlin D. Familial neuralgia of occipital and intermedius nerves in a Chinese family. *J Headache Pain.* 2011;**12**(4):497–500.

49. Patel A, Kassam A, Horowitz M, Chang YF. Microvascular decompression in the management of glossopharyngeal neuralgia: analysis of 217 cases. *Neurosurgery.* 2002;**50**(4):705–710.

50. Rey-Dios R, Cohen-Gadol AA. Current neurosurgical management of glossopharyngeal neuralgia and technical nuances for microvascular decompression surgery. *Neurosurg Focus.* 2013;**34**(3):E8.

51. Isamat F, Ferran E, Acebes JJ. Selective percutaneous thermocoagulation rhizotomy in essential glossopharyngeal neuralgia. *J Neurosurg.* 1981;**55**(4):575–580.

52. Ma Y, Li YF, Wang QC, Wang B, Huang HT. Neurosurgical treatment of glossopharyngeal neuralgia: analysis of 103 cases. *J Neurosurg.* 2016;**124**(4):1088–1092.

53. O'Connor JK, Bidiwala S. Effectiveness and safety of Gamma Knife radiosurgery for glossopharyngeal neuralgia. *Proc (Bayl Univ Med Cent).* 2013;**26**(3):262–264.

54. List T, Jensen RH. Temporomandibular disorders: old ideas and new concepts. *Cephalalgia.* 2017;**37**(7):692–704.

55. Durham J, Newton-John TR, Zakrzewska JM. Temporomandibular disorders. *BMJ.* 2015;**350**:h1154.

56. Hoffmann RG, Kotchen JM, Kotchen TA, Cowley T, Dasgupta M, Cowley AW, Jr. Temporomandibular disorders and associated clinical comorbidities. *Clin Pain.* 2011;**27**(3):268–274.

57. List T, Dworkin SF. Comparing TMD diagnoses and clinical findings at Swedish and US TMD centers using research diagnostic criteria for temporomandibular disorders. *J Orofac Pain.* 1996;**10**(3):240–253.

58. Schiffman EL, Truelove EL, Ohrbach R, Anderson GC, John MT, List T, et al. The research diagnostic criteria for temporomandibular disorders. I: overview and methodology for assessment of validity. *J Orofac Pain.* 2010;**24**(1):7–24.

59. Cairns B, List T, Michelotti A, Ohrbach R, Svensson P. JOR-CORE recommendations on rehabilitation of temporomandibular disorders. *J Oral Rehabil.* 2010;**37**(6):481–489.

60. Nilsson IM, List T, Drangsholt M. Prevalence of temporomandibular pain and subsequent dental treatment in Swedish adolescents. *J Orofac Pain.* 2005;**19**(2):144–150.

61. Macfarlane TV, Glenny AM, Worthington HV. Systematic review of population-based epidemiological studies of oro-facial pain. *J Dent.* 2001;**29**(7):451–467.

62. Slade GD, Bair E, Greenspan JD, Dubner R, Fillingim RB, Diatchenko L, et al. Signs and symptoms of first-onset TMD and sociodemographic predictors of its development: the OPPERA prospective cohort study. *J Pain.* 2013;**14**(12 Suppl):T20–T32. e1–3.

63. Dworkin SF. The OPPERA study: act one. *J Pain.* 2011;**12**(11 Suppl):T1–T3.

64. Smith SB, Maixner DW, Greenspan JD, Dubner R, Fillingim RB, Ohrbach R, et al. Potential genetic risk factors for chronic TMD: genetic associations from the OPPERA case control study. *J Pain.* 2011;**12**(11 Suppl):T92–T101.

65. Visscher CM, Lobbezoo F. TMD pain is partly heritable. A systematic review of family studies and genetic association studies. *J Oral Rehabil.* 2015;**42**(5):386–399.

66. Berger M, Szalewski L, Bakalczuk M, Bakalczuk G, Bakalczuk S, Szkutnik J. Association between estrogen levels and temporomandibular disorders: a systematic literature review. *Prz Menopauzalny.* 2015;**14**(4):260–270.

67. LeResche L, Mancl LA, Drangsholt MT, Huang G, Von Korff M. Predictors of onset of facial pain and temporomandibular disorders in early adolescence. *Pain.* 2007;**129**(3):269–278.

68. Macfarlane TV, Kenealy P, Kingdon HA, Mohlin B, Pilley JR, Mwangi CW, et al. Orofacial pain in young adults and associated childhood and adulthood factors: results of the population study, Wales, United Kingdom. *Community Dent Oral Epidemiol.* 2009;**37**(5):438–450.

69. Fillingim RB, Ohrbach R, Greenspan JD, Knott C, Diatchenko L, Dubner R, et al. Psychological factors associated with development of TMD: the OPPERA prospective cohort study. *J Pain.* 2013;**14**(12 Suppl):T75–T90.

70. Greene CS. The etiology of temporomandibular disorders: implications for treatment. *J Orofac Pain.* 2001;**15**(2):93–105.

71. Story WP, Durham J, Al-Baghdadi M, Steele J, Araujo-Soares V. Self-management in temporomandibular disorders: a systematic review of behavioural components. *J Oral Rehabil.* 2016;**43**(10):759–770.

72. List T, Axelsson S. Management of TMD: evidence from systematic reviews and meta-analyses. *J Oral Rehabil.* 2010;**37**(6):430–451.

73. Ekberg EC, Nilner M. Treatment outcome of short- and long-term appliance therapy in patients with TMD of myogenous origin and tension-type headache. *J Oral Rehabil.* 2006;**33**(10):713–721.

74. Mujakperuo HR, Watson M, Morrison R, Macfarlane TV. Pharmacological interventions for pain in patients with temporomandibular disorders. *Cochrane Database Syst Rev.* 2010;**10**:CD004715.

75. Greene CS. Managing patients with temporomandibular disorders: a new 'standard of care'. *Am J Orthod Dentofacial Orthop.* 2010;**138**(1):3–4.

76. Al-Baghdadi M, Durham J, Araujo-Soares V, Robalino S, Errington L, Steele J. TMJ disc displacement without reduction management: a systematic review. *J Dent Res.* 2014;**93**(7 Suppl):37s–51s.

77. Ruiz M, Porta-Etessam J, Garcia-Ptacek S, de la Cruz C, Cuadrado ML, Guerrero AL. Auriculotemporal neuralgia: eight new cases report. *Pain Med.* 2016;**17**(9):1744–1748.

78. Speciali JG, Goncalves DA. Auriculotemporal neuralgia. *Curr Pain Headache Rep.* 2005;**9**(4):277–280.

79. Tang IP, Freeman SR, Kontorinis G, Tang MY, Rutherford SA, King AT, et al. Geniculate neuralgia: a systematic review. *J Laryngol Otol.* 2014;**128**(5):394–399.

80. Maarbjerg S, Wolfram F, Heinskou TB, Rochat P, Gozalov A, Brennum J, et al. Persistent idiopathic facial pain—a prospective systematic study of clinical characteristics and neuroanatomical findings at 3.0 Tesla MRI. *Cephalalgia.* 2017;**37**(13):1231–1240.

81. Siqueira SR, Siviero M, Alvarez FK, Teixeira MJ, Siqueira JT. Quantitative sensory testing in trigeminal traumatic neuropathic pain and persistent idiopathic facial pain. *Arq Neuropsiquiatr.* 2013;**71**(3):174–179.

82. Baad-Hansen L, Abrahamsen R, Zachariae R, List T, Svensson P. Somatosensory sensitivity in patients with persistent idiopathic orofacial pain is associated with pain relief from hypnosis and relaxation. *Clin J Pain.* 2013;**29**(6):518–526.

83. Nobrega JC, Siqueira SR, Siqueira JT, Teixeira MJ. Differential diagnosis in atypical facial pain: a clinical study. *Arq Neuropsiquiatr.* 2007;**65**(2A):256–261.

84. Benoliel R, Zadik Y, Eliav E, Sharav Y. Peripheral painful traumatic trigeminal neuropathy: clinical features in 91 cases and proposal of novel diagnostic criteria. *J Orofac Pain.* 2012;**26**(1):49–58.

85. Lang E, Kaltenhauser M, Seidler S, Mattenklodt P, Neundorfer B. Persistent idiopathic facial pain exists independent of somatosensory input from the painful region: findings from quantitative sensory functions and somatotopy of the primary somatosensory cortex. *Pain.* 2005;**118**(1–2):80–91.

86. Jaaskelainen SK, Forssell H, Tenovuo O. Electrophysiological testing of the trigeminofacial system: aid in the diagnosis of atypical facial pain. *Pain.* 1999;**80**(1–2):191–200.

87. Derbyshire SW, Jones AK, Devani P, Friston KJ, Feinmann C, Harris M, et al. Cerebral responses to pain in patients with atypical facial pain measured by positron emission tomography. *J Neurol Neurosurg Psychiatry.* 1994;**57**(10):1166–1172.

88. Hagelberg N, Forssell H, Aalto S, Rinne JO, Scheinin H, Taiminen T, et al. Altered dopamine D2 receptor binding in atypical facial pain. *Pain.* 2003;**106**(1–2):43–48.

89. Weiss AL, Ehrhardt KP, Tolba R. Atypical facial pain: a comprehensive, evidence-based review. *Curr Pain Headache Rep.* 2017;**21**(2):8.

90. Cornelissen P, van Kleef M, Mekhail N, Day M, van Zundert J. Evidence-based interventional pain medicine according to clinical diagnoses. 3. Persistent idiopathic facial pain. *Pain Pract.* 2009;**9**(6):443–448.

91. Forssell H, Tasmuth T, Tenovuo O, Hampf G, Kalso E. Venlafaxine in the treatment of atypical facial pain: a randomized controlled trial. *J Orofac Pain.* 2004;**18**(2):131–137.

92. Nagashima W, Kimura H, Ito M, Tokura T, Arao M, Aleksic B, et al. Effectiveness of duloxetine for the treatment of chronic nonorganic orofacial pain. *Clin Neuropharmacol.* 2012;**35**(6):273–277.

93. Zakrzewska JM. Multi-dimensionality of chronic pain of the oral cavity and face. *J Headache Pain.* 2013;**14**:37.

94. Zakrzewska JM. Chronic/persistent idiopathic facial pain. *Neurosurg Clin N Am.* 2016;**27**(3):345–351.

95. Abrahamsen R, Baad-Hansen L, Svensson P. Hypnosis in the management of persistent idiopathic orofacial pain—clinical and psychosocial findings. *Pain*. 2008;**136**(1–2):44–52.

96. Nguyen CT, Wang MB. Complementary and integrative treatments: atypical facial pain. *Otolaryngol Clin N Am*. 2013;**46**(3):367–382.

97. Bayer E, Racz GB, Miles D, Heavner J. Sphenopalatine ganglion pulsed radiofrequency treatment in 30 patients suffering from chronic face and head pain. *Pain Pract*. 2005;**5**(3):223–227.

98. Akbas M, Gunduz E, Sanli S, Yegin A. Sphenopalatine ganglion pulsed radiofrequency treatment in patients suffering from chronic face and head pain. *Braz J Anesthesiol*. 2016;**66**(1):50–54.

99. Klein J, Sandi-Gahun S, Schackert G, Juratli TA. Peripheral nerve field stimulation for trigeminal neuralgia, trigeminal neuropathic pain, and persistent idiopathic facial pain. *Cephalalgia*. 2016;**36**(5):445–453.

100. Cuadrado ML, Garcia-Moreno H, Arias JA, Pareja JA. Botulinum neurotoxin type-A for the treatment of atypical odontalgia. *Pain Med*. 2016;**17**(9):1717–1721.

101. Haanpää M, Rice A, Rowbotham M. Treating herpes zoster and postherpetic neuralgia. *Pain Clin Updates*. 2015;**23**(4):1–8.

102. Haanpaa M, Laippala P, Nurmikko T. Allodynia and pinprick hypesthesia in acute herpes zoster, and the development of postherpetic neuralgia. *J Pain Symptom Manage*. 2000;**20**(1):50–58.

103. van Wijck AJM, Aerssens YR. Pain, itch, quality of life, and costs after herpes zoster. *Pain Pract*. 2017;**17**(6):738–746.

104. Liesegang TJ. Herpes zoster ophthalmicus natural history, risk factors, clinical presentation, and morbidity. *Ophthalmology*. 2008;**115**(2 Suppl):S3–S12.

105. Nagel MA, Gilden D. Complications of varicella zoster virus reactivation. *Curr Treat Options Neurol*. 2013;**15**(4):439–453.

106. Johnson RW, Bouhassira D, Kassianos G, Leplege A, Schmader KE, Weinke T. The impact of herpes zoster and post-herpetic neuralgia on quality-of-life. *BMC Med*. 2010;**8**:37.

107. Cohen JI. Clinical practice: herpes zoster. *N Engl J Med*. 2013;**369**(3):255–263.

108. Kawai K, Gebremeskel BG, Acosta CJ. Systematic review of incidence and complications of herpes zoster: towards a global perspective. *BMJ Open*. 2014;**4**(6):e004833.

109. Forbes HJ, Bhaskaran K, Thomas SL, Smeeth L, Clayton T, Langan SM. Quantification of risk factors for herpes zoster: population based case-control study. *BMJ*. 2014;**348**:g2911.

110. Werner RN, Nikkels AF, Marinovic B, Schafer M, Czarnecka-Operacz M, Agius AM, et al. European consensus-based (S2k) guideline on the management of herpes zoster—guided by the European Dermatology Forum (EDF) in cooperation with the European Academy of Dermatology and Venereology (EADV). Part 2: treatment. *J Eur Acad Dermatol Venereol*. 2017;**31**(1):20–29.

111. Dworkin RH, Johnson RW, Breuer J, Gnann JW, Levin MJ, Backonja M, et al. Recommendations for the management of herpes zoster. *Clin Infect Dis*. 2007;**44** Suppl 1:S1–S26.

112. Bowsher D. The effects of pre-emptive treatment of postherpetic neuralgia with amitriptyline: a randomized, double-blind, placebo-controlled trial. *J Pain Symptom Manage*. 1997;**13**(6):327–331.

113. Makharita MY, Amr YM, El-Bayoumy Y. Effect of early stellate ganglion blockade for facial pain from acute herpes zoster and incidence of postherpetic neuralgia. *Pain Physician*. 2012;**15**(6):467–474.

114. Bouhassira D, Chassany O, Gaillat J, Hanslik T, Launay O, Mann C, et al. Patient perspective on herpes zoster and its complications: an observational prospective study in patients aged over 50 years in general practice. *Pain*. 2012;**153**(2):342–349.

115. Truini A, Galeotti F, Haanpaa M, Zucchi R, Albanesi A, Biasiotta A, et al. Pathophysiology of pain in postherpetic neuralgia: a clinical and neurophysiological study. *Pain*. 2008;**140**(3):405–410.

116. Reda H, Greene K, Rice FL, Rowbotham MC, Petersen KL. Natural history of herpes zoster: late follow-up of 3.9 years (n= 43) and 7.7 years (n=10). *Pain*. 2013;**154**(10):2227–2233.

117. Fields HL, Rowbotham M, Baron R. Postherpetic neuralgia: irritable nociceptors and deafferentation. *Neurobiol Dis*. 1998;**5**(4):209–227.

118. Dworkin RH, Gnann JW Jr, Oaklander AL, Raja SN, Schmader KE, Whitley RJ. Diagnosis and assessment of pain associated with herpes zoster and postherpetic neuralgia. *J Pain*. 2008;**9**(1 Suppl 1):S37–S44.

119. Finnerup NB, Attal N, Haroutounian S, McNicol E, Baron R, Dworkin RH, et al. Pharmacotherapy for neuropathic pain in adults: a systematic review and meta-analysis. *Lancet Neurol*. 2015;**14**(2):162–173.

120. Colloca L, Ludman T, Bouhassira D, Baron R, Dickenson AH, Yarnitsky D, et al. Neuropathic pain. *Nat Rev Dis Primers*. 2017;**3**:17002.

121. Apalla Z, Sotiriou E, Lallas A, Lazaridou E, Ioannides D. Botulinum toxin A in postherpetic neuralgia: a parallel, randomized, double-blind, single-dose, placebo-controlled trial. *Clin J Pain*. 2013;**29**(10):857–864.

122. Xiao L, Mackey S, Hui H, Xong D, Zhang Q, Zhang D. Subcutaneous injection of botulinum toxin a is beneficial in postherpetic neuralgia. *Pain Med*. 2010;**11**(12):1827–1833.

123. Ray WA, Chung CP, Murray KT, Hall K, Stein CM. Prescription of long-acting opioids and mortality in patients with chronic noncancer pain. *JAMA*. 2016;**315**(22):2415–2423.

124. Kurklinsky S, Palmer SC, Arroliga MJ, Ghazi SM. Neuromodulation in postherpetic neuralgia: case reports and review of the literature. *Pain Med*. 2018;**19**(6):1237–1244.

125. Lerman IR, Chen JL, Hiller D, Souzdalnitski D, Sheean G, Wallace M, et al. Novel high-frequency peripheral nerve stimulator treatment of refractory postherpetic neuralgia: a brief technical note. *Neuromodulation*. 2015;**18**(6):487–493.

126. Oxman MN, Levin MJ, Johnson GR, Schmader KE, Straus SE, Gelb LD, et al. A vaccine to prevent herpes zoster and postherpetic neuralgia in older adults. *N Engl J Med*. 2005;**352**(22):2271–2284.

127. Le P, Sabella C, Rothberg MB. Preventing herpes zoster through vaccination: new developments. *Cleve Clin J Med*. 2017;**84**(5):359–366.

Index